HYPERACTIVE CHILDREN GROWN UP
SECOND EDITION

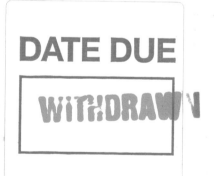

DATE DUE

WITHDRAWN

HYPERACTIVE CHILDREN GROWN UP
Second Edition
ADHD IN CHILDREN, ADOLESCENTS, AND ADULTS

GABRIELLE WEISS
LILY TROKENBERG HECHTMAN
Montreal Children's Hospital

Foreword by Russell A. Barkley

THE GUILFORD PRESS
New York   *London*

© 1986, 1993 The Guilford Press
A Division of Guilford Publications, Inc.
72 Spring Street, New York, NY 10012

Printed in the United States of America

This book is printed on acid-free paper.

Last digit is print number: 9 8 7 6 5 4 3 2

Library of Congress Cataloging-in-Publication Data

Hyperactive children grown up: ADHD in children, adolescents, and
    adults / Gabrielle Weiss, Lily Trokenberg Hechtman; foreword by
    Russell A. Barkley.—2nd ed.
        p.   cm.
    ISBN 0-89862-039-2 (hard).—ISBN 0-89862-596-3 (pbk.)
    1. Attention-deficit hyperactivity disorder—Longitudinal studies.
    2. Attention-deficit hyperactivity disorder—Treatment—Longitudinal
    studies.   I. Hechtman, Lily Trokenberg.
    [DNLM: 1. Attention Deficit Disorder with Hyperactivity.
    2. Longitudinal Studies.   WL 348 W429h 1993]
    RJ506.H9W44   1993
    616.85'89—dc20
    DNLM/DLC
    for Library of Congress   ·   93-6950
                                                                              CIP

In the interest of protecting the privacy of individuals, most
names and identifying details have been altered.

When the adults who had been hyperactive were asked what had helped them most to overcome their childhood difficulties, their most common reply was that someone (usually a parent or teacher) had believed in them. . . .

This book is dedicated to all children who have to struggle hard to overcome difficulties while growing up to become adults. And to people in their lives who believed in them.

To the memory of my mother and father, Drs. Margarethe and Erwin H. Loewenfeld, for the gift of their example. To my husband, Michael, for all he has done for me during our 37 years together. To my daughters, Margaret and Jacqueline, and their husbands, Larry Schibuk and Bill Steinberg, with love and respect. Finally, to my grandchildren, Ben, 11 years, David, 10, Rebecca, 7, Elizabeth, 6, Heidi, 3, and Douggie, 2, who have brought magic into the present, and the past into the future.—GABRIELLE WEISS

To my parents, Sam and Rose Trokenberg, for their devotion and unselfishness. To my husband, Peter, for his encouragement and generosity of spirit. To my children, Kenneth and Jeremy, for meeting the many challenges of my absences with such competence, good humor, and understanding. And to the memory of Mrs. Downing who for 15 years mothered us all.—LILY TROKENBERG HECHTMAN

FOREWORD

One of the earliest follow-up studies of hyperactive children and certainly one of the best of those conducted prospectively was the series of studies published by Gabrielle Weiss and Lily Hechtman and their colleagues at the Montreal Children's Hospital during the 1970s and 1980s. Since then, others—including Rachel Gittelman and her colleagues at the New York State Psychiatric Institute, Jan Loney and associates at the University of Iowa, and James Satterfield of the National Center for Hyperactive Children (California)—have initiated such prospective longitudinal studies of children with hyperactivity, now called Attention-Deficit Hyperactivity Disorder (ADHD). Later, I initiated my own follow-up investigations of a large sample of ADHD and normal children at the Medical College of Wisconsin in Milwaukee, studies that continue to this day. Most of these studies began at a time when ADHD was known as "hyperactivity," "the hyperactive child syndrome," or "minimal brain dysfunction." Unlike now, there were no consensus criteria then to guide the clinician or clinical scientist in the selection of children for such research. What criteria were available were often vague (as in the DSM-II), idiosyncratic among clinicians, and loosely applied, if at all, in practice. Much to their credit, Drs. Weiss and Hechtman were among the first to begin developing research criteria for the definition and study of such children. They were also among the first investigators to realize the scientific richness of following such a group of children prospectively with clinical and laboratory psychological measures. Such measures could more rigorously evaluate the nature of problems experienced by these children, which had only been descriptively noted in prior, less rigorous research.

Over the last 27 years, Drs. Weiss and Hechtman have continued to monitor and track their hyperactive and control subjects, inviting them to return periodically to the clinic for re-evaluations and to share their personal life stories with the project staff. This is no small task: Follow-up research of this sort is time-consuming, frustrating, and very demanding on the skills of the investigators to pursue every lead in relocating subjects as they move about the country and play out the developmental trajectories of their earlier years. It demands extreme patience and persistence as well as grace in gently and humanely contacting subjects and repeatedly imposing upon their lives to share their development with clinical science for the betterment of others afflicted with ADHD. We must be thankful beyond measure that Drs. Weiss and Hechtman did so, and that all the subjects and their families cooperated so generously with the demands of the study. Their work has provided major revelations for the rest of us who toil in the clinical and scientific trenches to help children with ADHD and their families, and, more recently, those adults who continue to have the disorder. The results of this almost 30-year effort to follow these individuals have yielded substantial insights into the course, outcome, causes, and treatment of ADHD, and have been of great import in appreciating the underlying nature of the disorder. Even more fascinating to me has been the rich vein of information the more recent adult outcome studies from this project have yielded on just how ADHD expresses itself in adulthood.

For years the clinical field struggled against the entrenched clinical lore that hyperactive or ADHD children outgrow their disorder, although there was never the slightest bit of scientific data that supported such a claim. Drs. Weiss and Hechtman provided the field with some of the first objectively obtained and undeniable evidence that the disorder continues in many, though not all, children clinically diagnosed with the condition. Even among those who no longer met full criteria for the disorder, evidence accumulated to show that residual symptoms still affected the lives of many. Here was some of the earliest truly prospectively obtained data to show that as it develops, ADHD comes to predominantly affect the very fabric of daily existence.

Unlike other flagrant psychiatric disorders whose symptoms are so extreme, atypical, bizarre, or grotesque that they may fascinate or horrify and are highly obvious, ADHD expresses itself by its subtle, pernicious impact upon the individual's ability to meet life's daily, often petty, responsibilities—one's relationship to friends, family, and offspring; one's capacity to pursue productive and successful work; the ability to engage in the process of education for self-improvement; and even the ability to demonstrate love, fidelity, and trust in close relationships with loved ones. Thus, ADHD is not a "glitzy" disorder or one that is culturally *de rigueur* for the moment. It is less obvious, more silent, but more pervasive in its influence on the capacity to successfully meet life's daily demands and challenges. Its effects over development may be glacially slow but ever-persistent in eroding one's self-esteem, relations with others, and success in school, often leading to a life of dramatic underachievement relative to one's actual creative, intellectual, and academic abilities. No other source so thoroughly, accurately, and scholarly demonstrated these points than the first edition of *Hyperactive Children Grown Up* in 1986. That book became the best single source on the course and outcome of hyperactive or ADHD children. It not only brought together all of the findings from Drs. Weiss and Hechtman's earlier publications but placed them in the context of the most comprehensive review of the follow-up literature yet published on the disorder. There simply was no other such volume to guide both clinician and scientist on these matters. If I may speak for the field of ADHD, we are forever grateful to them for that endeavor.

So it is easy to understand my delight in seeing the second edition of this unique book. To their existing chapters Drs. Weiss and Hechtman have added others on new developments in the field, such as those concerning genetic and biological evidence that accumulated in the literature since the publication of the first edition, and on the evaluation and management of ADHD in adults. In doing so, the authors have ensured that this will continue to be the best single source on the course and outcomes of hyperactive children.

Most touching and poignant in their first edition were the reminiscences of Ian Murray, one of the hyperactive subjects who had been followed in Drs. Weiss and Hechtman's research. I have shared this brief autobiography with many adults with ADHD as part of their counseling about the disorder. Their reaction has been uniformly positive in finding within it much insight about themselves and much relief in realizing that others such as Mr. Murray had struggled with the disorder as they had been doing. I have also directed thousands of clinicians to it to use in counseling their own clients. Ian Murray's courage in sharing his personal life, warts and all, has helped more people in their journey of discovery about the disorder and themselves than he will ever know. One of the treasured features of this second edition is his updating of this sketch with a postscript about his life since 1986. Despite his apparently mixed feelings in preparing these reminiscences for our edification, he should take great comfort from knowing how many others he is likely to continue to help through his own insights about his ADHD. I personally wish to thank him here for his contributions to both editions.

Only a very small group of scientists devote their entire careers to the singular study of ADHD; it is a small club indeed, and Drs. Weiss and Hechtman are among them. From such scientists we often gain not just the benefits of their scientific findings, but the wisdom that arises from their constant immersion into the lives of their ADHD subjects. If they are perceptive and open to all of the information that comes their way in the process, and not just to the quantitative scores from their interviews, scales, and tests, they truly enlighten us with a considerably deeper understanding of and appreciation for the essence of the disorder and its management. More than most, Drs. Weiss and Hechtman have been so perceptive, and have shared this wisdom with us, both in their first edition and again here. For it is the unwritten obligation of every clinical scientist to not simply take information from subjects or merely add to the accumulated knowledge in the literature, but to improve the lot of the lives of those we have studied and other similarly afflicted. Drs. Weiss and Hechtman have done so and continue fulfilling that obligation here. One unquestionable measure of the significance of any literature is how well it withstands the "tooth of time." This second edition will undoubtedly do so, giving us lasting value for years to come.

RUSSELL A. BARKLEY, PhD
Worcester, Massachusetts

ACKNOWLEDGMENTS

We wish to express gratitude particularly to our two collaborators in the follow-up research: Terrye Perlman and Daphne Tuck. As became apparent, doing a long-term follow-up study is a very unique task fraught with special pleasures and serious frustrations.

We are grateful to Terrye Perlman, MS, for her assistance with the data collection and general organization of the data for analysis. She developed a very special and caring relationship with the subjects, who often turned to her after their evaluation if they were in difficulties. She counseled several of them (normals and hyperactives) after completion of the study.

Daphne Tuck with tenacity traced the subjects and dealt heroically every now and again with rejection and rudeness on the telephone, followed by frequent "failures to show up" for appointments resulting in more recalls, etc. Hyperactives, unlike controls, were very difficult to reach by telephone: they were always "out," doing something, and usually did not reply to letters. At intervals we dealt with our frustration by calling in the evenings, all four of us together for mutual support, offering interviews to subjects "anywhere"—at home, at a restaurant, or wherever the subject wished it. Similarly, we attempted to reduce the number of "refusals" in every way we could think of. As one of us remarked in a "down period" regarding some subjects who had refused to be seen, "I feel like a third-rate salesman selling a fourth-rate product." Nevertheless, the joys of doing this study more than balanced the frustrations. The pleasure of seeing the gradual maturation and change over the many years of children growing into adults was a unique experience which taught all of us a great deal about human nature and human development.

Dr. Tom Milroy, a psychiatrist who worked with us and who assessed the subjects "blind," was most helpful in freeing up evening hours for this purpose. We are grateful for his assistance.

We wish to thank Rhonda Amsel, PhD, statistician in the Department of Psychology, McGill University, for her expertise and advice on statistics for the study and for her responsibility in its analysis. Her patience with our team was truly beyond understanding. Our thanks are due also to Miriam Edelson for her help in putting an unbelievably massive amount of data onto cards for computer analysis.

We also wish to thank our colleagues across the United States, some of them doing similar work: Drs. Rachel Gittelman-Klein, Jan Loney, Keith Conners, Judith Rapoport, Carol Whalen, Barbara Henker, Jim Satterfield, and many others. They were always generous in their sharing of data and good counsel. Dr. Ron Lipman had a major role in shepherding us through the ups and downs of long-term research and was always encouraging and enthusiastic, which we appreciated enormously.

Certain key people have had a major role at various periods in this research. Dr. J. S. Werry helped initiate the study and injected his enthusiasm and skills; even after he left the project he remained interested and helpful. Dr. Klaus Minde (Professor of Psychiatry, University of Toronto) was an integral part of the research particularly during the 5-year follow-up study, and has helped us subsequently with constructive criticism and ideas. Finally, Dr. Virginia Douglas at McGill University, well known for her own studies (which have contributed greatly to the field), was our friend and teacher of research methodology from the beginning.

For the major source of funding for the research described in the book we are grateful to Health and Welfare Canada and to the Psychopharmacology Branch of the National Institute of Mental Health. Ms. Natalie Reatig of NIMH was consistently supportive and helpful.

Thanks also to the American Academy of Child Psychiatry for permission to reprint material from two of our earlier publications (Hyperactives as Young Adults: Initial Predictors of Adult Outcome, by L. Hechtman, G. Weiss, T. Perlman, & R. Amsel, *Journal of the American Academy of Child Psychiatry*, 23:250–261, 1984; Psychiatric Status of Hyperactives as Adults: A Controlled Prospective 15-Year Follow-Up of 63 Hyperactive Children, by G. Weiss, L. Hechtman, T. Milroy, & T. Perlman, *Journal of the American Academy of Child Psychiatry*, 24:211–221, 1985).

Finally, we are most grateful to Mrs. Daphne Tuck, Ms. Gwynneth Whittingham, Mrs. Margaret Campeau, and Miss Maria Ponte who have typed the manuscript, and to the MCH Research Institute who gave financial support to see us through at times of difficulty.

We thank all those young people who participated in the series of follow-up studies over 15 or more years. We are grateful to them for their willingness to share the stories of their lives with us and for the many insights they have given us. They became very much a part of us and we will not forget them.

PREFACE

The prospective follow-up of hyperactive children, the results of which are described in this book, began in 1960 when Dr. John S. Werry (now Professor of Psychiatry, University of Auckland, N.Z.) and Dr. Gabrielle Weiss were young and boisterous first-year Residents in Child Psychiatry at the Montreal Children's Hospital. Dr. Taylor Statten, the then Director of the Department of Psychiatry, encouraged and supported them to initiate a research project in the field of child psychiatry as early as possible in their training.

The choice of hyperactive children for subject matter of study was motivated by the inherent interest in a condition which seemed to have both biological and psychosocial antecedents. Moreover, this childhood problem manifested itself by symptoms likely to be responsive to psychoactive agents, and both J. S. W. and G. W. were particularly interested in the area of pediatric psychopharmacology, a field which Dr. Leon Eisenberg and Dr. Keith Conners were beginning to pioneer with studies using adequate methodology. Another motivating factor was that our outpatient department had many children (mainly boys) who exhibited the symptoms of this syndrome.

Our experience in recruiting hyperactive children suitable for the study was perhaps more complex than is suggested by our clear inclusion and exclusion criteria described in Chapter 5. Our adherence to the inclusion and exclusion criteria was always strictly maintained. However, within those bounds, during periods when many children were referred to us for the study, we included the more severely hyperactive. During lean periods, when referrals were more sparse, we probably also included some of the milder cases. No child was ever included who was not hyperactive both at home and at school. Since the Conners Parent and Teacher Rating Scales were not yet constructed, we used a modified version of what was later known as the Werry–Weiss–Peters Hyperactivity Scale.

Writing this book has been a great pleasure. During the course of this long-term study we have learned many things about hyperactive children, adolescents, and adults which are not revealed by "statistically significant group differences" alone. While some of our clinical observations have been reported in various publications, many others have been able to be discussed only in this book. These psychiatric "impressions" fill the interstitial spaces between empirical findings of many investigators and of our own studies. It is very much hoped that the children whom we saw develop into adolescence and then adulthood, and whose joys and struggles we witnessed, will come to life for the readers of this book and that this will enhance the understanding of them for those who live with them or who teach or treat them.

Empirical findings, clinical impressions, and theoretical considerations have all been included. We have taken great care not to confuse these three different aspects.

With respect to terminology, we have decided to stick with "the hyperactive child" or "the hyperactive child syndrome" because these were the terms we applied to these children in our publications. Of course, we recognize that there is not "one hyperactive child" but several subgroups among them, and also we regard the DSM-III terminology Attention Deficit Disorder with Hyperactivity as an advance. Our theoretical approach to the condition is to view the constellation of symptoms as the final common pathway of a variety of biopsychosocial interacting antecedents. Whether or not this symptom complex fulfills the criteria of a syndrome is discussed in Chapter 1. The authors take the point of view that it would be a mistake at this stage of our knowledge to throw out the notion of a syndrome.

The book starts with a brief overview of classic and recent findings related to the hyperactive syndrome. This is followed by a section on the main characteristics of the condition seen at different ages, with a selected literature review pertinent to the developmental period discussed. The major aim of the book is to summarize for the reader the growing body of retrospective and prospective outcome studies of hyperactive children as adolescents and adults, including details of our own 10- and 15-year controlled prospective follow-up studies of hyperactive children. We have attempted to give readers a wide-ranging and detailed review of a large number of areas related to the adult hyperactive.

Each chapter is written in such a way as to provide the reader with a review of the particular area, its controversial issues, available data relating to these diverse views, possible conclusions, and, where appropriate, directions for future interventions and research. Thus, each chapter stands on its own as a discussion of a particular area. To accomplish this, different aspects of the same studies are referred to in different chapters rather than summarizing an entire study in one place only. Specifically, chapters deal with psychiatric status, antisocial behavior, drug and alcohol use and abuse, and work record, as well as physiological issues and family factors. On a more philosophical and clinically descriptive note are the chapters dealing with beliefs and values, self-esteem and social skills, and life-styles. Wherever appropriate actual case histories are presented to illustrate points discussed.

A separate section of the book deals with possible predictors of outcome. Treatment issues are dealt with briefly throughout the book with regard to particular stages of development, and a separate section is devoted to the treatment of the adult hyperactive.

Another section of the book discusses how hyperactive adults viewed the treatment they received when they were children, and what factors they found helpful or harmful as they were growing up. This section ends appropriately with a chapter written by Ian Murray, who describes in candid and vivid terms his subjective experience in growing up hyperactive and in being a "subject" in a long-term follow-up study.

The book is intended to be of interest to researchers and clinicians (psychologists, social workers, pediatricians, general practitioners, and psychiatrists). It is also intended to be informative and useful for teachers, parents of hyperactive children, and those who were hyperactive themselves. Some chapters will be of more interest to researchers, others to clinicians, others to teachers, parents, or hyperactive adults.

Our main purpose was to collect the body of information now available on the outcome of this condition and its predictive aspects and to make it meaningful to the reader. In doing this we sincerely hope that we have generated interest in these children and in the type of personal involvement and interventions, at various ages, which may potentially result in better long-term outcomes.

SECOND EDITION: 1993

This edition has a postscript to Chapter 21 and four new chapters. In Ian Murray's postscript, he shares his adult experiences and how he has handled the various challenges posed by Attention-Deficit Hyperactivity Disorder (ADHD). The first of the new chapters, Chapter 22, describes recent research on genetic transmission, neurobiological aspects, and the importance of comorbidity in ADHD. Chapter 23 summarizes recent findings on the use of medication for this condition. Chapter 24 describes various forms of psychosocial treatment for ADHD, including behavior modification, parent training, social skills interventions, academic skills training and remediation, and individual psychotherapy, and ends with a description of a multimodal (multiple-treatment) approach to the treatment of children with ADHD. Chapter 25 discusses the assessment, diagnosis, and treatment of ADHD in adulthood.

CONTENTS

I. OVERVIEW

CHAPTER 1. OVERVIEW OF CHILDHOOD SYNDROME   3

Historical Background and Terminology, 3; Current Research Interest in the Syndrome, 7; Does the Hyperactive Syndrome Exist?, 9; Clinical Aspects of Diagnosis and Assessment, 15

II. THE SYNDROME SEEN DEVELOPMENTALLY

CHAPTER 2. INFANCY, TODDLER, PRESCHOOLER   21

Crying, 23; Sleep Difficulties, 23; Vocalization, 24; Feeding Difficulties, 24; Appearance, 24; Smiling, 25; Cuddling, 25; Effect of the "Difficult" Infant and Toddler on the Mother–Child Relationship, 25; The Preschooler, 27; Treatment of Hyperactive Preschoolers, 31

CHAPTER 3. THE HYPERACTIVE CHILD IN
ELEMENTARY SCHOOL   35

Problems Related to Activity, 36; Attentional Difficulties, 37; Impulsivity, 40; Reinforcement Issues in the Learning of Hyperactive Children, 41; Poor School Achievement, 42; Poor Self-Esteem and Depression, 43; Difficulties in Social Interactions at Home and at School, 44; Peer and Teacher Relationships, 44; Treatment, 45

CHAPTER 4. HYPERACTIVES AS ADOLESCENTS   50

Retrospective Studies, 53; Prospective Studies, 55

III. ADULTHOOD

CHAPTER 5. THE ADULT HYPERACTIVE:
PSYCHIATRIC STATUS   61

Retrospective Studies, 62; Follow-Back Studies, 64; Ten-Year Prospective Controlled Follow-Up Study from the Montreal Children's Hospital, 66; Fifteen-Year Prospective Follow-Up Study from the Montreal Children's Hospital, 70; Similarities and Differences of the Various Studies of Adult Outcome, 81

CHAPTER 6. ANTISOCIAL BEHAVIOR   84

Adolescent Outcome Studies: Prospective and Retrospective, 84; Studies of Families of Hyperactives, 87; Adult Psychiatric Disorders in Patients with Histories Suggesting Childhood Hyperactivity, 88; Adult Outcome Studies of Hyperactive Children: Prospective and Retrospective, 90; Ten-Year Prospective Controlled Follow-Up Study, 93; Fifteen-Year Controlled Prospective Follow-Up Study, 97; Limitations of Specific Diagnostic Criteria Scales, 103; Similar and Divergent Findings, 104; Summary, 105

CHAPTER 7. VALUES AND BELIEFS   107

Results, 107; Discussion, 113

CHAPTER 8. DRUG AND ALCOHOL USE AND ABUSE   118

Follow-Up Studies of Adolescent Hyperactives: Prospective and Retrospective, 119; Studies of Adult Psychiatric Patients (Including Alcoholics) with Possible Histories of Childhood Hyperactivity, 122; Studies of Families of Hyperactive Children, 124; Follow-Up Studies of Adult Hyperactives: Prospective and Retrospective, 125; Drug and Alcohol Use and Abuse at Ten-Year Follow-Up, 129; Drug and Alcohol Use and Abuse at Fifteen-Year Follow-Up, 136

CHAPTER 9. WORK RECORD   142

Fifteen-Year Follow-Up: Work Status, 144

CHAPTER 10. SELF-ESTEEM AND SOCIAL SKILLS   150

Adolescent Follow-Up Studies, 150; Adult Follow-Up Studies, 153; Ten-Year Follow-Up Study, 154; Fifteen-Year Prospective Follow-Up, 158

CHAPTER 11. PHYSIOLOGICAL MEASURES   162

Physiological Differences in Hyperactive Children, 163; Physiological Measures in Adulthood, 169

CHAPTER 12. FAMILIES OF HYPERACTIVES   180

Sibling Studies, 180; Parental Studies: Interactional Aspects, 183; Parental Studies: Genetic Aspects, 186; Long-Term Follow-Up of Families of Hyperactive Children, 189; Summary, 204

CHAPTER 13. LIFE-STYLES AND ILLUSTRATIVE CASE HISTORIES   205

Fairly Normal Outcome Group, 205; Group with Continuing Symptoms of the Hyperactive Syndrome and/or Social, Emotional, and Interpersonal Problems, 209; Group with More Serious Psychiatric or Antisocial Disturbance, 214; Conclusions, 218

IV. PREDICTIVE FACTORS

CHAPTER 14. PREDICTIVE FACTORS PERTAINING
TO THE CHILD   221

Introduction, 221; Child's Age at Referral, 222; Degree of Central Nervous System
Abnormality, 222; IQ or Intelligence, 224; Symptoms at Referral, 226

CHAPTER 15. PREDICTIVE FACTORS PERTAINING
TO THE FAMILY   230

Mental Health of Family Members, 230; Parent–Child Relationship: Child-Rearing
Practices, 232; Socioeconomic Status, 234; Overall Family Functioning, 236

CHAPTER 16. PREDICTIVE FACTORS PERTAINING
TO TREATMENT   238

Psychotherapy, Counseling, Remedial Education, 238; Drug Treatment, 240; Young-
Adult Outcome of Hyperactives Who Received Long-Term Stimulant Treatment in
Childhood, 242

CHAPTER 17. INTERRELATIONSHIP OF VARIOUS
PREDICTIVE FACTORS   257

Results, 259; Discussion and Summary, 268

V. TREATMENT ISSUES

CHAPTER 18. CLINICAL VIGNETTES OF PSYCHOTHERAPY
AT DIFFERENT AGES   275

Case Example: Derrick, 276; Case Example: David, 277; Case Example: Randy, 277;
Case Example: Henry, 278; Case Example: Jimmy, 278

CHAPTER 19. THE EFFICACY OF MEDICATION ON
HYPERACTIVE ADOLESCENTS AND ADULTS   281

Stimulant Therapy of Hyperactive Adolescents, 281; Stimulant Therapy of Hyperactive
Adults, 284

VI. THE HYPERACTIVE ADULT LOOKS BACK

CHAPTER 20. ADULT HYPERACTIVE SUBJECTS' VIEW
OF THEIR TREATMENT IN CHILDHOOD
AND ADOLESCENCE   293

Types of Comments Made Regarding Parents, 295; Types of Comments Made Regarding
Teachers, 295; Types of Comments Made about Maturation, 296; Types of Responses
Regarding the Effect of Medication, 296; Impressions from the Subjects' Responses, 299;
Summary, 300

CHAPTER 21. LOOKING BACK: REMINISCENCES FROM
CHILDHOOD AND ADOLESCENCE   301

   Ian Murray

VII.   NEW DEVELOPMENTS IN ATTENTION-DEFICIT
HYPERACTIVITY DISORDER

CHAPTER 22. RECENT BIOLOGICAL AND
DIAGNOSTIC ISSUES   329

   Genetic Studies of Children with ADHD, 329; Neurobiological Developments,
   336; Comorbidity and Subgroups of Children, 345

CHAPTER 23. MEDICATION TREATMENT OF ADHD   348

   Prevalence of Stimulant Use, 348; History of Stimulant Use, 348; Effectiveness of
   Stimulants, 349; Adverse Effects (Side Effects) of Stimulants, 353; Long-Acting
   Stimulants, 358; Mechanism of Stimulant Action, 359; Stimulant Absorption
   and Metabolism, 359; Drug Interactions, 360; Nonstimulant Drugs in the
   Treatment of ADHD, 361; Conclusion, 365

CHAPTER 24. PSYCHOSOCIAL TREATMENT OF ADHD   366

   Behavior Modification, 366; Parent Training, 369; Social Skills Interventions,
   374; Academic Skills Training and Remediation, 376; Individual Psychotherapy,
   377; Multimodal Treatment, 381

CHAPTER 25. ASSESSMENT, DIAGNOSIS, AND
TREATMENT OF ADULT ADHD   384

   Introduction: The Existence of Adult ADHD, 384; Diagnostic Assessment, 387;
   Clinical Assessment of Individual Symptoms, 391; Two Case Vignettes, 393;
   Differential Diagnosis, 398; Treatment of Adult ADHD, 400

CHAPTER 26. CONCLUSIONS   407

REFERENCES   413

AUTHOR INDEX   457

SUBJECT INDEX   469

HYPERACTIVE CHILDREN GROWN UP
SECOND EDITION

OVERVIEW

CHAPTER ONE

OVERVIEW OF CHILDHOOD SYNDROME

The gods did not reveal, from the beginning,
All things to us; but in the course of time
Through seeking we may learn, and know things better.

But as for certain truth, no man has known it,
Nor will he know it; neither of the gods,
Nor yet of all the things of which I speak.
And even if by chance he were to utter
The final truth, he would himself not know it;
For all is but a woven web of guesses.
—Xenophanes, ca. 500 B.C

In that several excellent books[1-3] are now available on the various
aspects of this syndrome in childhood; it would be absurd to attempt
here a review of the field. Instead, this chapter is intended as a general
introduction to various interesting areas which are of value to the
reader in understanding historical and current thinking related to
hyperactivity in childhood. The following areas will be discussed:

1. Historical background and terminology
2. Current research interest in the syndrome
3. Does the hyperactive syndrome exist?
4. Clinical aspects of diagnosis and assessment

HISTORICAL BACKGROUND AND TERMINOLOGY

The many diagnostic labels given to children who show clusters of
symptoms such as poor sustained attention, hyperactivity, impulsivity,
and sometimes learning disabilities and/or conduct problems generally
reflect various historical concepts related either to the etiology of the
disorder (Minimal Brain Damage Syndrome, Minimal Brain Dysfunction, Developmental Hyperactivity) or to what were considered its

3

cardinal manifestations (Hyperactive Impulse Disorder, Hyperactive Child Syndrome, and more recently Attention Deficit Disorder with Hyperactivity).

Still[4] in 1902 was the first to describe children who had a cluster of behavioral problems which he termed "defects in moral control," and he recognized that the condition occurred more commonly in boys. He described the children as having hyperactivity, learning difficulties, conduct disorders, and poor attention, and felt that the etiology was probably organic (e.g., inborn differences of temperament), but that environmental factors might also play a role.

As far back as the early Greeks, connections have been made between organic factors (body humors) and personality and behavior. Prior to Still's description of the syndrome, the 19th-century medical literature contained many detailed case histories of personality and behavioral changes following accidents which resulted in brain damage. After the First World War, an epidemic of encephalitis lethargica was noted to result in postencephalitic behavior disorders in some of its child victims.[5,6] The children were described in much the same way as Still had earlier described them, namely as having hyperactivity, impulsivity, antisocial behavior, and emotional lability. They were referred to by Kahn and Cohen[7] in 1934 as being "organically driven," and these clinicians felt the problem was due to damage in the brain stem. At that time, special residential treatment centers were established to treat these children who had behavioral sequelae following encephalitis lethargica, and it was noted that the behavioral problems could be improved by residential treatment but that relapse occurred if the children were returned to maladjusted parents.[8] It was implicitly recognized even then that "etiology" may be multiple, namely organic and environmental.

The discovery of the "paradoxical quietening effect" and marked behavioral and school improvement of hyperactive children treated with Benzedrine (a racemic mixture of dextro- and levoamphetamine) by Bradley[9] in 1937 was another landmark. This finding may have influenced the selection of the term "Minimal Brain Dysfunction" (MBD) which came into use to describe these children in the 1960s, even though the concept of a unique paradoxical effect on hyperactive children was later shown not the exist.[10] For example, Wender in 1973 suggested that one of the common properties of this heterogeneous group of children diagnosed as MBD is the dramatic response of many of them to treatment with stimulants and antidepressant drugs.[11] Bradley's original finding in 1937 that children with diverse psychopathology responded favorably to stimulants has remained largely forgotten.

Historically, the designation "Minimal Brain Damage Syndrome," which preceded the terminology "MBD," originated from the work of Strauss and Werner which began in the 1930s. These workers differentiated a group of brain-damaged from non-brain-damaged retarded children and described the former as having difficulties in perception, concept formation, language, emotion, and behavior. The brain-damaged retarded children were described as hyperactive ("motor disinhibition"), distractible ("driven hither and yon by outside stimulation"), impulsive ("cannot master planful action"), perseverative ("perseveration . . . which obstructs the child's understanding of purposeful action"), and as having cognitive deficits (e.g, foreground–background difficulties). Strauss and Kephart suggested in Volumes 1 and 2 of *Psychopathology and Education of the Brain-Injured Child*[12] that if children with known brain damage (as detected in their studies by a neurological examination and/or history suggestive of brain damage) showed specific behavioral and cognitive problems, then children exhibiting these same difficulties but without any evidence of brain damage probably suffered from brain damage. However, the latter could not be diagnosed because the neurological examination is known to be fallible. The authors were aware of the circularity of their reasoning but felt justified in their assumption.

The popularity of the terminology Minimal Brain Damage Syndrome in the 1940s and 50s probably resulted from Strauss's optimistic emphasis on the importance of early recognition of the syndrome so that affected children could be identified as young as possible and treated by placing them into special educational settings where their learning would be enhanced. Cruikshank, Kephart, Getman (an optometrist), and Barsch all shared Strauss's concept and urged that the "special educational" classes should utilize special cubicles to reduce external distractions.[13] As late as 1972, Clemmens and Kenny[14] reported that in some school systems it was still the practice to require a neurological examination and an electroencephalogram (EEG) before children were accepted. This was so in spite of the knowledge at the time that children with learning disabilities and/or hyperactivity may have a normal neurological examination and EEG.

The concept of a Minimal Brain Damage Syndrome was further reinforced in 1959 by Knobloch and Pasamanick,[15] who compared birth histories of 500 children referred for behavior problems with a matched control group of 350 children from the same socioeconomic statuses,[16] and found that the behavior-disordered children had significantly more complications of pregnancy and that the most common behavioral syndrome was hyperactivity. They postulated "a continuum of reproductive casualty" ranging from severe abnormalities (cerebral palsy, mental retardation) to minimal sequelae (e.g., learning disorders and hyperactivity).

Clements and Peters[17] in the 1960s suggested broadening the term Minimal Brain Damage to include also constitutional factors and temperament and coined the term MBD. These workers were aware of the two opposing views: (1) Birch's admonition[18] that if we postulate brain damage we should demonstrate it given the fact that many children with this syndrome do not have signs of frank brain damage; (2) the attitude in child guidance clinics (influenced by the psychoanalytic movement), where good parents were sometimes unnecessarily blamed for their children's problems and it was suggested to the parents that "there was some magical subtle aberration in their attitudes and behavior" (p. 195).[17] In coining the terminology MBD Clements and Peters wrote, "It is necessary to take into account the full spectrum of causality from the unique genetic combination that each individual is to his gestation and birth experiences, to his interaction with significant persons, and finally to the stresses and emotional traumata of later life, after his basic reaction patterns have been laid down" (p. 195).[17]

At the Oxford Conference in 1962, Ronald MacKeith,[19] in the article "Minimal Brain Damage—A Concept Discarded," gave the historical warning that the children included under the new diagnosis MBD were heterogeneous and that future effort should be diverted toward subclassifying them. Unfortunately, this overinclusive terminology is hard to eliminate from clinical use.

The concept of a "maturational lag,"[20] which was postulated by Lauretta Bender to explain various behavior disorders including schizophrenia, was implied in the term "Developmental Hyperactivity." The concept of a maturational or developmental lag for this condition has recently been challenged in that it implies that children will outgrow the symptoms of the hyeractive syndrome. While this view was initially held by pediatricians,[21] it is contradicted by the controlled follow-up studies (see subsequent chapters), all of which indicate that many children do not outgrow the disorder.

As early as 1957 Laufer and Denhoff[22] gave an excellent description of this syndrome, which they termed "Hyperkinetic Impulse Disorder." Their terminology was based on core symptoms of restlessness and impulsivity and did not imply any etiology, although from their own research these workers felt that the damage lay in the diencephlon. Roscoe Dykman and associates[23] and Virginia Douglas,[24] prominent psychologists who have spent much of their professional lives researching and conceptualizing this syndrome, have indicated that faulty attention and disorders of inhibitory control are cardinal features of the syndrome. Their thinking influenced a change of terminology in 1980 from DSM-II's "Hyperkinetic Reaction of Childhood" to DSM-III's "Attention Deficit Disorder with or without Hyperactivity" (ADD[H] or ADD).[25] The DSM-III terminolgy, which attempted to define the syndrome operationally, has now achieved widespread use as well as serving the function of stimulating further research. It will be discussed in more detail in Chapter 3. In this book the decision was made to use the older terminology because most of the research described in subsequent chapters was carried out before the new terminology came into use.

This brief historical account highlights some interesting aspects of the hyperactive syndrome.

1. The description of the syndrome is not new in the medical literature and appeared as early as 1902.

2. The interaction between organic factors and the environment in the perpetuation of the behavioral syndrome was recognized already in the 1930s with respect to children whose behavior problems followed encephalitis lethargica.

3. The terminology of the syndrome has changed over time since it was first described, and the changes generally reflected current views of either etiology (e.g., MBD) or a cardinal symptom considered to be the most fundamental aspect of the syndrome (e.g., Attention Deficit Disorder).

4. The terminology Minimal Brain Damage Syndrome, which was popular from the 1940s to the 1960s reflected circular reasoning concepts of etiology. Nevertheless, it led to social changes such as setting up isolated cubicles in classrooms intended to cut out extraneous stimuli for these children, solutions which were based on clinical impressions poorly documented by evidence.

CURRENT RESEARCH INTEREST IN THE SYNDROME

It has been estimated that between 1957 and 1960 31 articles were published in the scientific literature on the hyperactive child syndrome. Between 1960 and 1975 there were 2000 articles, and from 1977 to 1980 (a period of only 3 years) 700 articles were published.[3]

Within the past 20 years, this condition has clearly become the most-researched and best-known of the childhood behavior disorders. In speculating on the reasons for this, several possibilities come to mind:

1. It is the most common single condition (or constellation of symptoms) referred to child psychiatry clinics.[1]

2. The condition is severe enough to be very distressing to teachers and parents, and in a more subtle way to the children themselves.

3. Unlike more serious and rarer conditions like autism, the syndrome offers possibilities for useful intervention.

4. The nature of the deficits seen in the hyperactive child syndrome lend themselves to research and intervention by practitioners in many disciplines, notably child psychiatrists, neurologists, pediatricians, epidemiologists, psychologists, educators, and biochemists.

5. The rediscovery in the 1960's (through the use of more refined research methodology, namely double-blind, placebo-controlled drug studies) of the efficacy of the stimulant drugs on both behavioral and cognitive aspects of the syndrome. Most of these studies indicated that 70–80% of any group of hyperactive children were considerably benefited on a short-term basis. Great optimism was thus generated, which resulted in widespread use of stimulants in the United States for children whose diagnosis was not always clearly established. As Maslow once said: "If the only tool you have is a hammer, then it is very tempting to treat everything as though it were a nail" (quoted by Milman[26] in Ross and Ross[3]). Subsequently, much research focused on establishing specific target symptoms responsive to stimulants as well as dose-response-curve issues. Finally, studies appeared attempting to assess long-term efficacy of stimulants.[27-31]

6. The discovery in the 1970s by the use of controlled prospective[32,33] and retrospective[34] studies that the hyperactive child syndrome was not limited to childhood, and that children do not necessarily outgrow this condition. The fact of psychiatric, social, and cognitive impairment continuing into adolescence and adulthood was established. This paved the way for further research to try to determine what factors could predict both poor and good outcome.[35] It is this aspect, as well as the various manifestations of the childhood syndrome in adult life, which is the subject of the present book.

If the above helped generate widespread research interest in the hyperactive syndrome (and in the past 5 years the number of publications is still increasing), we have to ask ourselves whether all the effort has been worthwhile. Robert Sprague, a key researcher in the field, wrote, ". . . such a mass of contradictory and misleading literature confounds. . . ."[36] Ross and Ross[3] in their newly revised textbook comment that intervention research in hyperactivity has too often been uncontrolled and short term, without assessing either long-term effect or generalization into natural settings. They also emphasized the difficulties of comparing results across studies which have used different methodologies and inclusion criteria and finally researchers demonstrating the same findings over and over again.

While these points are well made, the reader should bear in mind that research on the hyperactive child led the field of research in child psychopathology. We see the painstaking slowness in generating a solid body of empirical data as the growing pains of beginning research in a complex area. For example, much current research is focusing on "childhood depression." The researcher interested in this equally complex condition can learn both from the mistakes and from the resultant better grasp of crucial methodological issues which arose from research on hyperactivity.

Certainly in the past 5 years new research findings concerning the hyperactive syndrome have led to some interesting questions, not the least of which is the controversy over the existence of a syndrome of hyperactivity apart from that of conduct disorder.

DOES THE HYPERACTIVE SYNDROME EXIST?

The clinical picture has wide agreement among investigators and clinicians. Hyperactive children have a short attention span, high distractibility, and an inability to cut out extraneous stimuli when trying to attend to a task. They are impulsive in behavior and on cognitive tasks, they do not "stop, look, and listen,"[37] and they jump in where angels fear to tread. They speak out of turn and impulsively interrupt adults. They have a hard time regulating their activity to conform with expected social norms, and may be actually overactive or inappropriately active. They tend to have poor frustration tolerance and are often poor at losing games, waiting in line, obeying rules of a game, etc. The main presenting symptoms vary according to the age of the child referred, and for this reason subsequent chapters are devoted to discussions of the syndrome at different ages. All these attributes are well summarized in DSM-III under the diagnosis ADD(H). The clinical picture is so well known that one is almost embarrassed to describe it once again. What is less well known are the conceptual difficulties in calling these symptoms one syndrome and giving them the status of a diagnosis.

In a thought-provoking review article, David Shaffer and Lawrence Greenhill[38] questioned the value of the concept of the hyperactive child syndrome. They felt that on the grounds of postdictive, concurrent, and predictive validity there was insufficient evidence for the presence of a syndrome. Postdictive validity required that there be a common etiology, which would direct the clinician to the underlying psychopathology or neurophysiology. Concurrent validity required that the children who are diagnosed as hyperactive differ from other deviant children on grounds other than the presence of the defining symptoms. This does not mean that all hyperactive children must have identical symptoms, but rather that some generalizations should be able to be made about the clinical state by virtue of belonging to the diagnosis. Predictive validity would be present if in spite of diverse etiology, prediction could be made about the natural history, final outcome, and response to treatment.

In their perusal of the literature, Shaffer and Greenhill conclude that a diagnosis of the hyperactive child syndrome tells little about etiology and does not allow generalizations to be made about clinical state. Finally, after reviewing the available follow-up studies, they found that these indicated widely different outcomes, so that in their view the syndrome lacks also predictive validity. They concluded that there is little validity or clinical usefulness for the diagnostic concept of the hyperactive child syndrome.

With respect to postdictive validity, no one etiology has been demonstrated for the hyperactive syndrome. Various possible biological etiologies or at least correlates exist, which were summarized in an excellent review article by Rapoport et al.[39] They discuss the following:

1. Prenatal and perinatal risk, referring to Knobloch and Pasamanick's findings[15] (see p. 5) and the results of the Kauai study,[40] which indicated that there was a group of children whose environment was not good enough to compensate for perinatal trauma to the brain. In these children conditions like the hyperactive syndrome were present. The collaborative project of the National Institute of Neurological Diseases and Strokes (NINDS) followed 50,000 pregnancies until the children were 7 years old. Hyperactivity was one of four factors at age 7 which could be predicted from prenatal variables.[41]

2. Some studies have shown that hyperactive children compared to normals have a greater number of soft neurological signs.[42] However, both the specificity of this finding for hyperactive children compared to other disturbed children and its significance are obscure.

3. Rapoport and Quinn[43] and Waldrop and Halverson[44] reported the association of minor physical anomalies with children who were hyperactive.

4. Review articles[45,46] are now available which summarize the data related to underarousal of some hyperactive children.

5. Toxic substances appear to be causal in some hyperactive children. For example, high levels of lead in the blood of some hyperactive children are improved by chelation therapy.[47] In addition, Fetal Alcohol Syndrome has been demonstrated by Shaywitz et al. to result sometimes in hyperactivity.[48]

6. Genetic factors may be causal, [49-51] and the evidence for this is discussed in Chapter 12.

7. Biochemical abnormalitites have been postulated to lead to the syndrome of hyperactivity. Much work is currently proceeding to

clarify the issue. Various investigators have postulated from their findings that hyperactive children have deficiencies in dopamine transmission.[52,53]

In addition to the above, a recent study from Sweden[54] of 141 hyperactive children (selected from 4000 kindergarten children) who were evaluated 2 years later at age 7 and compared to 59 normal controls indicated a remarkably strong correlation of hyperactivity with signs of cerebral dysfunction (87% of the children who had pervasive hyperactivity also had signs of brain dysfunction).

One may conclude that biological correlates clearly exist, some of which are causal. However, as Rapoport *et al.*[39] pointed out, some of the correlates sometimes lack specificity for the hyperactive syndrome and may also be present in other disturbed children. Furthermore, as shown in the Kauai study,[40] organic antecedents interact with psychosocial factors which may be stronger predictors. Many investigators now take an interactional view of causality and consider the hyperactive syndrome to be the final common path of various antecedent variables, which include both biological and psychosocial factors.

There is an interesting parallel in medicine which makes one realize that other well-known diagnoses do not have postdictive validity. Let us take hypertension as an example. The etiology of this condition may be renal pathology, an adrenal tumor, or most commonly "essential," that is, "unknown etiology." In the latter (essential hypertension) antecedent variables are both organic (e.g., family history of hypertension—i.e., a genetic factor) and psychosocial (environmental stress, personality structure, etc.). In other words, there are a variety of interacting antecedent variables or etiologies. Nevertheless, the condition has concurrent validity; that is, you can predict clinical state by symptoms other than those which constitute the diagnosis, for example headaches and, in time, symptoms related to secondary renal and cardiac or brain pathology. The condition has predictive validity (made use of by every insurance company), and there is improvement of outcome if the condition is treated.

With respect to the hyperactive child syndrome, there are some analogies. Only a small percentage of hyperactive children have a single known organic pathology. The majority have varying degrees of biological (brain damage or dysfunction) and psychosocial antecedent variables.

Recent findings indicate that the syndrome has concurrent validity. If a child is diagnosed to be pervasively hyperactive, he or she is more likely to have concomitant:

1. Cognitive deficits (including lower IQ)[55,56]
2. Reading retardation[56]

3. More severe other psychiatric problems[55]

4. Neurodevelopmental difficulties (i.e., signs and symptoms of MBD)[54]

5. Symptoms of the syndrome which are likely to endure (see Chapter 5)

As has been mentioned, the main purpose of this book is to review findings and discuss theoretical implications of the various follow-up studies of the manifestation of the syndrome in adult life. While agreeing with Shaffer that there are some discrepancies in the findings of outcome, we are more impressed by the similarity of the results from very widely different kinds of studies, all of which agree on some fundamental outcome issues, suggesting that there exists a fairly high predictive validity.

Michael Rutter[57] has recently summarized in a masterful review article the various difficulties in making a diagnosis of the hyperactive syndrome in spite of the widely accepted behavioral symptoms. He concluded that the notion of a hyperactive syndrome begins to look rather illusionary.

We will discuss briefly some of the difficulties he referred to regarding the concept of hyperactivity as a distinct syndrome.

1. Studies by Kenny et al. in 1971[58] and Lambert et al. in 1978[59] showed that there was relatively low agreement among parents, teachers, and clinicians as to which children were reported as hyperactive. This low level of agreement may have two quite different reasons. One possibility is that interobserver reliability is indeed poor—that is, two people looking at the same time at the same child do not agree on whether the behavior is hyperactive. (This has not been demonstrated in the literature.) A second reason for the poor correlation of different defining systems is that a given child may be situationally hyperactive, that is, hyperactive either at home or at school or in the physician's office. When a child is hyperactive in all these situations, he or she is said to be "pervasively" hyperactive, as opposed to "situationally" hyperactive. The confusion between pervasive and situational hyperactivity has plagued the literature, and even the current nomenclature of DSM-III. The latter suggests that when parents' reports do not agree with teachers' reports of hyperactivity, the latter should be given preference. Barkley[60] has suggested that the disorder should be diagnosed only when it is "pervasive" and has drawn attention to the lack of clarity regarding this issue in the DSM-III diagnosis of ADD(H). In all the studies described subsequently in this book, which were carried out at the Montreal Children's Hospital, the children to be included in the follow-up had to be hyperactive both at home and at school. It was felt

when the studies were initiated in the early 1960s that when hyperactive symptoms were specific to one situation there was a stronger possibility that the child was reacting to that situation, be it in the home or in the classroom.

2. A second problem regarding the hyperactive syndrome mentioned by Rutter is the difference in prevalence of the hyperactive child syndrome between the United States and Britain. Figures in Britain used to be given as 1 in 1000[61] and as 5% in the United States.[62] There are important new data on this apparent discrepancy, which previously most of us felt was due only to diagnostic criteria differences between United States and Britain—namely that the British workers excluded hyperactive–aggressive children from the hyperactive child syndrome diagnosis and included them in the conduct disorder category. Now we know that this discrepancy was also confounded by confusing pervasively and situationally hyperactive children. Lambert *et al.*[59] found that 1.2% of 5000 children living in the East Bay area near San Francisco were hyperactive when diagnosed by the parents *and* the teacher *and* the physician. In an attempt to confirm this finding from the United States, Schachar and coworkers[55] returned to the Isle of Wight in 1975–1976, 5 years after their initial studies, and once again sent questionnaires to teachers and parents of all 14- and 15-year-old adolescents on the island. Of approximately 2000 children, 500 were excluded, mostly because parents failed to return the questionnaire. The 25% who could not be followed represented a more deviant subgroup (lower socioeconomic status, more likely to be rated by teacher as disturbed, initially more hyperactive, and having lower scores on cognitive tests). Hence, the finding that 2% of the children who were contacted were pervasively hyperactive represents, if anything, an understatement. We can conclude that when the issue of pervasive versus situational hyperactivity is addressed, prevalence figures are remarkably constant for the hyperactive syndrome in the United States and in Britain.

3. Rutter also suggested that the poor agreement between different measures of hyperactivity—for example, the many mechanical devices available (actometer, watch, ballistographic cushion, photoelectric systems, etc.), direct observational methods in natural settings, and questionnaires—muddies the definition of the syndrome. A mechanical device measures quantity of activity. Teachers' or parents' ratings on a questionnaire may measure quantity, but are more likely to measure mainly the type of non-task-oriented and annoying activity characteristic of hyperactive children. Our feeling is that good correlation between these two types of measurement would be highly unlikely, for they obviously measure different things.

4. Until recently, few investigators could demonstrate by statistical techniques (e.g., factor analysis) a factor for hyperactivity.[63] More recently, Shachar et al.[55] found that combining both parent and teacher scales of the Rutter questionnaire at ages 10 and 15, resulted in a restricted factor of these items. These were "very restless," "squirmy," and "cannot settle to anything," which represented one dimension in the ratings of both sexes in pervasively hyperactive children. They called this factor the "hyperactivity factor." In addition, the empirically derived syndromes of Achenbach[64] include a narrow-band Hyperactivity Disorder (including attention deficit). Loney and coworkers have demonstrated that a factor of hyperactivity could be obtained if the ratings of a child were derived from one source, for example, the teacher or the parent.[65]

While Loney has cautioned against a tendency to rely solely on factor-analytic studies in the issue of syndrome status for hyperactivity,[66] the most recent study on this issue gave clear evidence of the existence of an independent factor of hyperactivity. Trites and Laprade[67] carried out factor-analytic studies on Conners teacher ratings of 9000 elementary-school children. They found a factor of hyperactivity which accounted for the greatest proportion of the variance. When these investigators looked at the overlap between their factors of conduct disorder and hyperactivity, they found a group of children who were hyperactive and not conduct disordered. These authors suggest that their findings provide evidence for an independent syndrome of hyperactivity in a sample of Canadian children.

5. Finally, there is the as yet unsolved problem of the overlap with conduct disorders. Schachar et al.'s findings[55] indicated that pervasively hyperactive children had a higher likelihood of conduct disorders, which were present in two-thirds of the pervasively hyperactive children and in one-half of the situationally hyperactive group ($p < .01$). This finding of the large overlap between hyperactive and aggressive (or conduct-problem) children has been found by virtually all workers, including systematic studies by Stewart and coworkers[68] in Iowa and by McGee and associates in Dunedan, New Zealand.[69] Whether or not there is anything to be gained by separating diagnostically conduct disorders without hyperactivity and hyperactivity with or without conduct disorders is not only a semantic issue. The issue rests on whether these conditions are distinct with respect to treatment and outcome.

The concerns of Shaffer, Greenhill, Rutter, and others regarding the existence of a distinct syndrome have been dealt with in detail. Empirical findings described as well as alternate explanations for the difficulties they have raised clearly lead, in the opinion of the authors, to the conclusion that a syndrome of hyperactivity exists. It is also clear that clinically most (but not all) children diagnosed as hyperactive have some degree of concurrent conduct disorder, at least at some stage of their development.

With respect to future research, the following considerations are worth taking into account:

1. It is important to study situationally and pervasively hyperactive children separately. They may well differ on the grounds of etiology, phenomenology, response to treatment, and outcome, or they may differ from one another in degree of severity only.

2. It is equally important in future studies to try to separate out children who are hyperactive without conduct disorders (this constitutes only a small minority of the referred children), children who are hyperactive and have conduct disorders (the majority), and those who only have conduct disorders. While this separation is important, it is easier to make "on paper" than when actually evaluating a child. Conduct problems may be mild, or present in only some situations, or present during certain years of development and not during other years.

3. Too much of the research has focused on comparing "hyperactive" children with *normal* controls. As Rutter has frequently pointed out, this is interesting, but tells us nothing about the specificity of the syndrome. Further research on any aspect of hyperactivity would do well to concentrate also on comparing groups of "hyperactive" children (with and without conduct disorder) who are pervasive in their hyperactivity with mixed and pure groups of other disturbed children as well as with normal controls.

4. Much research on stimulant medication has focused on its effect in improving concentration and increasing reflectivity and task-oriented behavior. Much too little work exists on the effect of stimulants on sociability, conduct problems, aggression, and learning, and on the long-term benefit of stimulant treatment. Also, more studies are required on the effects of various treatments (other than stimulants) on hyperactive children from the preschool age to adulthood.

CLINICAL ASPECTS OF DIAGNOSIS AND ASSESSMENT

Since this chapter has focused so far on theoretical aspects, we will conclude with some key clinical issues regarding diagnosis and assessment. The diagnosis of hyperactivity is never made on the basis of a single symptom. Clinically, a number of symptoms (behavioral and sometimes cognitive difficulties) clustered together in one child form the syndrome. This syndrome is present usually in some form from early childhood, although it may not be diagnosed until the child enters school. Hyperactivity and related symptoms may also occur as concomitants of other diagnoses such as childhood psychosis, autism, cerebral palsy, and mental retardation. Most studies of hyperactive children exclude children with the above primary diagnoses.

The following operational criteria are listed in DSM-III for ADD(H):

A. Inattention (at least three of the following)
   1. Often fails to finish things he or she starts
   2. Often does not seem to listen
   3. Easily distracted
   4. Has difficulty concentrating on schoolwork or other tasks requiring sustained attention
   5. Has difficulty sticking to a play activity
B. Hyperactivity (at least two of the following)
   1. Runs about or climbs on things excessively
   2. Has difficulty sitting still or fidgets excessively
   3. Has difficulty staying seated
   4. Moves about excessively during sleep
   5. Is always on the go or acts as if "driven by a motor"
C. Impulsivity (at least three of the following)
   1. Often acts before thinking
   2. Shifts excessively from one activity to another
   3. Has difficulty organizing work (this not due to cognitive impairment)
   4. Needs a lot of supervision
   5. Frequently calls out in class
   6. Has difficulty awaiting turn in games or group situations
D. Onset before the age of 7
E. Duration of at least 6 months
F. Not due to schizophrenia, affective disorder, or severe or profound mental retardation

Barkley[60] has expressed the view held by many clinicians and researchers that the above DSM-III criteria represent an improvement over other classifications. However, he noted the lack of norms at different ages for determining abnormality of symptoms and the failure to clarify whether the condition is pervasive or situational. Others have commented on the degree of overlap between symptoms even across categories.

Since the main problems complained about by parents depend on the age of the child, the subsequent chapters are devoted to the syndrome as it manifests most typically during different development periods, including adolescence.

A comprehensive multidisciplinary assessment is required for diagnosis in order to formulate the optimal treatment plan, which must be directed to whatever deficits exist in the child, family, and school. The following types of evaluation are usually carried out.

1. A history of the pregnancy, delivery, and the child's developmental milestones from infancy on. A parental history of hyperactivity, alcoholism, sociopathy, hysteria, may be looked for.

2. Assessment of the child's behavioral aberrations; the specific symptoms present, their severity and frequency, the degree to which individual symptoms are situational; the duration of the problem.

3. An educational assessment to determine if a specific learning disability is present and if so, its nature. This is a great importance for remedial educational measures.

4. Assessment of the intrapsychic processes in the child, how he or she views himself or herself, family, peers, school; what personality strengths the child possesses.

5. Assessment of the interactions of the child and family. Cause and effect are irrelevant at the point of diagnosis after years of interaction. Parents frequently require help to interact constructively, and their guilt and blaming of one another needs to be addressed.

6. Assessment of the child's classroom. Is the educational environment conducive to learning? Sometimes specific remedial programs can be incorporated into the regular school curriculum. In our experience, it was rare that a "special education class" was required. The relationship between the child and teacher may require help, and the teacher can benefit from being brought into the treatment team as an important member, for assessment, diagnosis, and management.

7. Assessment of the child's neurological status if there is any suspicion of a neurological lesion. Routine neurological examinations of hyperactive children are usually negative except for the presence of soft signs whose significance is not kown. EEG's often show diffuse dysrhythmias which tend to disappear in adolescence. Again, the significance is not known.

In conclusion, hyperactivity in childhood, now termed ADD(H), has a long history of terminologies reflecting different theories of etiology or current thinking on key symptoms of the syndrome. The syndrome for various reasons has attracted a great deal of research, some of which has thrown doubt on the existence of a specific syndrome. In the authors' opinion, there is substantial evidence for the existence of a syndrome of hyperactivity. Various biological measures can be shown to correlate with the hyperactive syndrome, but these correlations are nonspecific and are overshadowed by psychosocial parameters. To make a diagnosis, a careful assessment of biological and psychosocial factors is requried and is carried out usually by professionals of different disciplines.

THE SYNDROME
SEEN DEVELOPMENTALLY

CHAPTER TWO

INFANCY, TODDLER, PRESCHOOLER

The Childhood shows the man,
As morning shows the day.
—from *Paradise Regained*, by John Milton, 1608–1674

Few systematic, controlled prospective studies exist of infants who are later diagnosed as having the hyperactive child syndrome. What information we have is usually obtained from mother's retrospective accounts of their memory of the infancy of the child whom they have brought for assessment and treatment of the various behavioral and cognitive difficulties of the syndrome. There is some evidence that mothers' memories of their children's infancy are selective, and it is quite likely that this would apply in the situation where a problem child is brought for help. One may speculate that mothers are more likely to remember difficulties in the infancy of children who later have "problems" than of those who become "normal" children.

Another reason why we have relatively little information is that in spite of the wide public interest in the hyperactive child syndrome, the condition is relatively rare if pervasiveness (that is, presence of the syndrome in all situations) is required for the diagnosis. Thus prevalence figures of between 1% and 2% are given by British and American surveys.[1,2] This requires that for every infant who later becomes pervasively hyperactive, 99 other infants would have to be systematically observed in order to study precursors of the syndrome. This would be an expensive project, and to overcome this problem investigators have attempted to select what may be a "vulnerable" infant population for the development of the syndrome: for example, those who at birth have neurological abnormalities, perinatal distress, low birth weight, congenital anomalies, and so on. Even this strategy is not always helpful, since we know relatively little about the various possibly interacting etiologies of the syndrome. Several studies exist which have followed a large number of normal infants from birth till they are in elementary or high school. For example, the Kauai study[3] followed over 1000 pregnancies for almost 20 years. In this study it was concluded that perinatal distress by itself predicted only mental retardation and cerebral palsy, but that perinatal distress and low socioeconomic status or inadequate homes predicted various behavioral abnormalities. This finding indicated the interaction of more than one antecedent variable to produce behavioral abnormalities, and the necessity of using multivariate statistical techniques for determining interacting prognostic indicators. With respect to the hyperactive child syndrome, in the present state of our knowledge we have to view it as the final common path of various interacting etiologies.

We know from the systematic follow-up studies available that once a diagnosis is made different clusters of symptoms are prominent at different developmental periods,[4] and that symptoms may continue into adult life.[5] Knowing this, it is probable that different clusters of symptoms might indeed be present from infancy on, as precursors or manifestations of the syndrome before the diagnosis is made. Final conclusions must await further systematic studies rather than relying on mother's retrospective accounts or clinical case reports of experienced clinicians.[6]

Perhaps some hyperactive children manifest precursors of the syndrome from the beginning of life, while others manifest the syndrome when they begin to walk; mothers frequently observe, "He never walked, he always ran." Yet other children do not manifest the syndrome until the preschool or early school years. Probably "manifesting" the syndrome and diagnosis of the syndrome are two different things. Actual diagnosis is often not made until the expectation on the part of society of what is required of the child exceeds the child's ability to conform to the expected norm. For example, at about age 3 there is an increased expectation regarding the abilities of the child. If development is proceeding according to established norms of the society, the child is now expected to play cooperatively, listen to adult instructions, and use symbolic language. The hyperactive 3-year-old will have difficulties in some or all of these areas and may "manifest" the syndrome at this time. Diagnosis may not be made until society can no longer tolerate these manifestations, for example, in a nursery or day care center.

An early study carried out by Werry and associates at the Montreal Children's Hospital[7] suggested that one-third of a group of mothers of hyperactive children reported difficulties in the first year of life of their children. The problems were similar to those described by Campbell et al.[8] and related to excessive crying or drowsiness, colic, feeding problems, and sleep disturbances. The nonspecific and variable nature of the disturbances suggested early difficulties in the mother-child relationship.

Each of the common complaints made by mothers about the infancy of hyperactive children will be discussed briefly. This information was obtained from various accounts of the retrospective memories of mothers and from the careful observations of clinicians like Nichamin,[6] who has had experience with infants who were diagnosed as having cerebral dysfunction. It should be remembered that the following difficulties apply to only a minority (30%) of "hyperactive infants," a term which is used purely for convenience in spite of the fact that it is misleading.

CRYING

In an early study it was reported that colic is more common in the infancy of hyperactive children compared to normal control children.[7] In this study the investigators probably did not clarify for the mothers the difference between true colic and frequent crying periods unrelated to colic. The latter commence earlier than colic (often in the first days of life), last longer, and are less paroxysmal and less piercing. The crying may be of normal pitch or shrill and high pitched, as described by Wolff and coworkers.[10] These infants were described as being difficult or impossible to soothe by the usual efforts made by mothers, such as rocking, holding, cuddling, carrying, changing, feeding, and so on. Mothers usually try different ways of soothing in vain. Their very efforts as well as the crying itself result in longer periods of high arousal and shorter periods of positive, quiet mother–infant interaction. This in itself is likely to affect emotional development, which is dependent on the quality and security of the attachment to the mother. Cognitive development may also become impaired because the infant is less free to "take in" the external environment. For example, an infant who cries much of the time will "babble" less, and there will be less time for what is called "mirroring," something mothers do naturally to help their infants smile responsively, imitate them in various ways, and generally interact positively with them.

SLEEP DIFFICULTIES

Mothers remember some "hyperactive infants" as excessively sleepy and unresponsive in the first months of life and others as having difficulties sleeping and being overreactive. The former are often underactive as infants and the latter overactive. In those with poor sleep, mothers frequently describe sleep, once achieved, as being restless, which suggests that the ratio of deep sleep to rapid-eye-movement (REM) sleep is disturbed. If this is shown to be true, it would be interesting, in that the same area of the brain is involved in both attention and deep sleep.[11] It must be remembered that sleep architecture has not been found to be disturbed in hyperactive school-age children (see Chapter 11). It has not as yet been studied in hyperactive infants or preschoolers. The "hyperactive infant" may awake with a startle reaction, followed by screaming. Once again the mother's efforts to soothe generally fail.

VOCALIZATION

During the course of the first year of life normal infants commence a variety of vocalization (babbling). These vocalizations are precursors of speech, and some "hyperactive infants" do not babble till over a year old; speech (first words, phrases, and short sentences) may be delayed. Fiedler *et al.*[12] found much atypical behavior during the first year of life in those who failed a speech screening examination at age 3. Later, in a 7-year follow-up evaluation, both behavioral disturbances and neurological dysfunctions were found.

FEEDING DIFFICULTIES

Some mothers of hyperactive children report feeding difficulties in the infancy of their children. These may be related to poor sucking or crying during feeding, or in later months hyperactive infants may become picky eaters. Some infants are described as irregular in their wish for food. As was suggested with other difficulties in infancy, the significance of these problems relates to what a "difficult" infant may do to generate problems in the mother–infant relationship rather than to poor nutrition.

APPEARANCE

Minor physical anomalies have been described by Waldrop *et al.*[13] to predict later poor attention span, peer aggression, and impulsivity. Some of these anomalies are related to the head and face and thus may affect to varying degrees the appearance of the child. Others affect hands or feet and are less obvious to others. Head and facial irregularities include abnormalities in the head circumference, fine, electric hair, widely spaced eyes, skin folds at the corners of their eyes (epicanthal folds), low-seated ears, adherent earlobes, malformed or asymmetrical ears, high palate, and so on. These irregularities were labeled by Wender as FLK (funny-looking kid), and whatever the cause, the effect is certainly that the mother is less likely to get approval and admiration of her infant by others. Later, the child with minor anomalies may "feel" different from others and suffer loss of self-esteem, even if the defect is very minimal.

SMILING

The infant who cries more often and who is generally irritable (as has been described for the infancy of some hyperactive children) also smiles less often. Smiling is well known to elicit a warm maternal response, and mothers create all kinds of games to elicit their infant's smiling response. An infant who rarely smiles will be less rewarding to the mother.

CUDDLING

It has been our clinical impression that some "hyperactive" infants and toddlers are described by their mothers as not being cuddly. Instead, they are hypertonic and may not enjoy being held. This leads to a lack of mutuality with the mother since cuddling and being held are interactive behaviors particularly enjoyable to most mothers and infants.

EFFECT OF THE "DIFFICULT" INFANT AND TODDLER ON THE MOTHER-CHILD RELATIONSHIP

Winnicott's[14] concept of the "good-enough mother" is relevant to the difficult infant. Many mothers are good enough for normal infants, but when they have an infant difficult to soothe, who cries frequently, sleeps poorly, and does not reward them but makes them feel incompetent, then anger, helplessness, lowered self-esteem, anxiety, and guilt are initiated in the mothers, and these negative feelings interact with the baby's temperament, producing vicious cycles and insecure attachment in the infant. This in itself, apart from the other problems the infant has, will have an effect on future development and personality formation. Winnicott's "good-enough mother" will in contrast recognize that "this baby is more difficult," but will not feel that this is her failing. Rather, she does what she can and continues to feel that she is a good mother. She is able to become attached to this difficult infant, while recognizing that she will more often feel tired and frustrated. This kind of self-confidence in the mother probably comes from having been "well mothered" herself and from having a stable personality. However, it helps if the "hyperactive" infant is not her firstborn baby and if previous babies were easier. Even those researchers who hold a purely biological view of the etiology of the hyperactive syndrome will not disagree with the concept that the infant and mother interact from the moment of birth and that much will depend on the relative success or failure of this interaction. The quality of the attachment to the mother (or primary caretaker) is likely to affect future personality formation and play its part in the final outcome.

Battle and Lacey,[15] looking at correlates of maternal and child motor activity from infants and mothers in the Fels longitudinal study, reported a lack of harmony in the early mother–child relationship of children who later developed behavior problems which would probably now be diagnosed as "hyperactive." Their data were collected from 1939 to 1957, and the term "hyperkinetic child" was just beginning to be recognized toward the end of this period. The mothers of the "hyperactive" boys felt negative about their babies, interacted less, and were less affectionate. In turn, hyperactive infants were less compliant to their mothers and other adults. Cause and effect would be difficult to separate, so that all we can conclude is that some mothers are good enough even for difficult infants, while other mothers are made to feel irritable, inadequate, and guilty and will react negatively to or withdraw from difficult infants.

Mash and Johnston,[16] studying 16 families with hyperactive children (mean age 5 years) and 24 families with older hyperactive children (mean age 8 years), found that particularly the mothers of the younger hyperactive children reported a markedly higher level of stress than mothers of normal children. The lower the maternal self-esteem, the worse was the mother's perception of the child's problem. The authors suggest that "low self esteem and maternal stress are likely to be, in part, a reaction to having a child who is perceived as difficult. However, such feelings are equally likely to influence the parent–child relationship in ways which may exacerbate the child's difficulties and the parents' subsequent perception of these difficulties" (p. 97).

Pediatricians in primary-care practice can be very helpful in diagnosing difficulties early in the mother–infant, parent–child interaction and fostering parenting skills and self-esteem in those parents who require it.

THE PRESCHOOLER

At 3 and 4 years of age the number of referrals for "hyperactivity" rises. The reasons for this increase are probably multiple. It was previously mentioned in this chapter that as a result of normally expected maturational changes by age 3, society's expectations of children rise markedly and now include specific types of abilities which the hyperactive may find difficult. A second reason for increased referral is probably the widespread publicity the syndrome has received in the lay press and the general belief that the earlier any condition is referred the more effective the treatment. Thirdly, at this age the mother of a "hyperactive" youngster encounters the community's rejection of her child, which may take the form of other mothers not wanting the youngster in their home (even accompanied by his or her mother), or, as mentioned, a nursery teacher who wishes the child to be withdrawn and may suggest referral.

Pelham and Bender,[17] studying an older group of hyperactive children, found that they were highly rejected by peers even after a period of familiarity as short as 2 hours. In a preschool peer-nomination study Milich and coworkers[18] established that 154 preschoolers, rating 86 preschool male peers, rejected those whom teachers had designated as "aggressive." Those whom teachers described as "hyperactive" (on the 39-item Conners Teacher Rating Scale and Swanson, Nolan, and Pelham [SNAP] checklist) were nominated either as more rejected or as more popular. The latter rating might have been an artificial one arising from the inclusion of one of four items rated by the preschoolers, namely: "who runs around the room a lot." This item may pick out the very active normal children, who are generally liked by others.

It was in response to a sharp increase of referrals from pediatricians of 3- and 4-year olds whose mothers wanted to know if their children were "hyperactive" to our psychiatry outpatient department at the Montreal Children's Hospital that Schleifer and coworkers[19] decided to carry out a systematic study of 28 children, all referred for symptoms of "hyperactivity, difficulty paying attention, not listening, and not responding to normal praise and punishment." We solicited 26 normal children from the nurseries in the community who were matched with the hyperactive preschoolers on IQ (Stanford–Binet), socioeconomic status (Hollingshead), and age. The purpose of the study was to compare the two groups via structured laboratory tests, in an observation nursery specially set up for this purpose, and through observation in the child's home. We also wished to do a controlled study of the efficacy of methylphenidate in this age group. Nursery observations were made during periods of free play (when the teachers kept their interaction with the children to a minimum) by the method used by Morgenstern,[20] and during half-hour periods of "structured play" (when the children were required to sit around a table and carry out a variety of tasks) by the methods of Emerich.[21] Each experimental nursery contained three hyperactive and three control children, together with two nursery teachers. Each nursery group met once weekly for 9 weeks. All the children were initially screened to exclude cerebral palsied, epileptic, retarded, and psychotic children, or children with autistic features. Those included in the study were then given tests designed to measure dimensions of reflectivity–impulsivity (Early Childhood Matching Familiar Figures Test, ECMFFT), field independence (Embedded Figures Test, EFT), and motor impulsivity (Draw a Line Slowly Test, DALST).

Great variability was found in the group of hyperactive preschoolers when observations were made of their behavior in the nursery and of their results on cognitive tasks, even though their mothers' presenting complaints were all fairly similar. Typical of these were, "He is on the go all the time," "cannot stick to anything," "cannot play alone," "is into everything," and, most annoying of all, "does not listen" or "Nothing helps, neither praise nor punishment: we can spank him, and he will cry for a minute, but then go on to do the very same thing again."

Although all the mothers had fairly similar complaints and most of them had begun to feel very negative about their youngsters, finding the problems they presented unbearable, in the nursery only 11 of 28 hyperactive children were observed to have behavior problems. The two nursery teachers could not distinguish the remaining 17 hyperactive children from the normal children. We therefore divided the group of hyperactive children into two subgroups, one of which we called "true hyperactives" and the other "situational hyperactives," in that their behavioral difficulties were present only in some situations, for example, at home.

Direct observations of the children in the nursery indicated the following:

In the *free-play period* there were no significant differences between the interactions of the hyperactives as a group and those of the control children, nor were any significant differences observed between "true" and "situational" hyperactive children. This probably indicates that normal preschool children become very active in free-play situations that their behavior and interactions resemble those of hyperactive children.

In contrast to the above findings, observations made on "up" and "away" dimensions of activity and on "aggression" during the *structured nursery period* were significantly different for the whole group of hyperactives compared with the control group and were also significantly different for the "true" compared with the "situational" hyperactives. "Up" was the number of times the child got up but did not leave his or her chair; "away" referred to the number of times the child left the table completely. Aggression was measured by the following: attacking others by teasing, throwing things, kicking, hitting, or biting. This indicates that observations made during "structured" play more sensitively distinguish the two groups; in other words, sitting still during "structured" activity was best accomplished by the normal children and least well by the "true" hyperactives; the "situational" hyperactives "scored" in between.

We hypothesized that the etiology might differ for the two groups of hyperactive children, with the "true" hyperactives being more likely to have an "organic" etiology and the "situational" hyperactives being more likely to come from more disturbed families. Two psychiatrists together visited each home and scored the degree of parental frustration versus satisfaction, time spent with the child, and extent of use of physical punishment. Contrary to our hypothesis, the parents of "true" hyperactives scored worse on the home observation scale, showing more frustration and more use of physical punishment. This may indicate that the more severe and pervasively hyperactive a child is, the more he or she contributes to the family's difficulties. On a family rating scale with mother as informant compiled in the hospital, both hyperactive groups had more disturbed families than did normal controls.

Tests of reflectivity–impulsivity (ECMFFT) significantly distinguished the whole group of hyperactive children from the normal children, whereas tests of field independence (EFT) and motor impulsivity (DALST) failed to distinguish the whole group of hyperactives from the normal children but significantly distinguished the "true" hyperactives from the normal children. The auditory Continuous Performance Test (CPT) did not distinguish between the groups. We felt the version which we used was too hard for our sample of children.

A 3-year follow-up of the children in this study was carried out by Susan Campbell and coworkers.[22] Of the original group, 15 of 28 hyperactive children and 16 of 26 controls were traced and agreed to participate in a study which investigated self-esteem and classroom behavior through direct observation and teachers' reports. The children were now 6–8 years old and were mainly in Grades 1 and 2. It was found that the children designated "hyperactive" (both "true" and "situational") in their preschool years continued to manifest problems in elementary school, as measured by both classroom observations (more disruptive behaviors found) and teachers' reports. There was also evidence that the hyperactives already had lower self-esteem. The distinction made in the original study between "true" hyperactives and "situational" hyperactives appeared to have prognostic significance. "True" hyperactive preschoolers were rated higher than those whose hyperactivity had been "situational" on "out-of-seat" and "off-task" behavior. The study furthermore suggested that a hyperactive child in a classroom may negatively influence the interaction between the other children in the classroom and the teacher.

This 3-year follow-up study indicated that children referred for "true" (or pervasive) and "situational" hyperactivity in the preschool years continued to present similar problems in Grades 1 and 2, with the school behavior of the pervasive group being more disruptive than that of the situational group. This study compared group means and does not answer the question of how many children might have outgrown their difficulties in the preceding 3 years.

The most recent study evaluating preschoolers was carried out by Campbell and her associates in 1982.[8] They selected 46 2- and 3-year-olds whose parents identified them as having problems with restlessness, short attention, tantrums, difficulty playing alone, and defiance, together with 22 normal toddlers as a comparison group. Both groups were carefully evaluated. All children received a Stanford-Binet, during the completion of which they wore an actometer. They were also assessed by the ECMFFT, EFT, DALST, and the Cookie Delay Test. Their parents filled out the Behar Preschool Behavior Questionnaire and the Werry–Weiss–Peters Hyperactivity Scale. A home visit was made, and in addition children were observed during structured and free play, when the actometer was also worn.

Results of this study indicated that referred children shifted activities more during free play, were more active and inattentive during structured tasks, and made more impulsive responses on the Cookie Delay Test. Parents described these toddlers as having had a more difficult infancy than the controls. It is of interest that actometer readings (taken during psychometric testing or during free play) did not distinguish the groups. While these investigators feel that they may have identified a group of toddlers who are likely later to be diagnosed as ADD(H) and/or conductor disorder, they also felt that some of their parent-referred children may be within normal limits (terrible 2's) and may grow out of their problems.

Campbell and her group plan to follow these children, and a recent report (1984) describes the reassessment of this group 1 year later, when 35 of 46 problem children and 19 of 22 controls agreed to participate.[9] Mothers continued to rate problem children as more hyperactive and aggressive than controls, on the same scales used previously. Problem children continued to shift activity more during free-play observations and were more often out of seats in structured tasks. They continued to make more impulsive responses on the Cookie Delay Test. On the whole, however, both groups had improved over the year on many measures.

The data confirmed previous findings that symptoms of the hyperactive syndrome persisted over a year and that the syndrome can be identified in preschool children. The authors point out once again that the symptoms of the syndrome must be differentiated from difficult but typical toddler behaviors which are evanescent in nature. In a recent presentation Campbell[23] noted that children rated as more severely hyperactive at age 3 were more likely to be rated also as more aggressive. This suggests that both these complaints in early childhood are a measure of problem severity, that is, of more serious, rather than qualitatively different, problems.

TREATMENT OF HYPERACTIVE PRESCHOOLERS

Other than occasional reports of the behavioral treatment of single cases, few studies have been carried out which have systematically studied any form of treatment for this age group.

In the preschool study already described, carried out at the Montreal Children's Hospital by Schleifer and colleagues,[19] methylphenidate was compared to placebo in a double-blind crossover design in which each child acted as his or her own control and treatment order was randomized. After the first 3 weeks of nursery school, half the hyperactive children were given a 3-week trial of methylphenidate and the other half were given an identical-looking placebo. Three weeks later those on the active drug were changed to placebo and vice versa. Parents were informed that the two types of pills differed in potency, and that we did not know which would be more helpful. All children received an initial dose of 5 mg which was adjusted upward (except in one child, where it was decreased) until maximal therapeutic benefit was found with minimal side effects. The mean dose in this study was 5 mg b.i.d., and ranged from 2.5 mg to 30 mg daily.

After 14–21 days in each treatment condition, the hyperactive children were reevaluated by means of direct observations in the nursery. The laboratory tasks (ECMFFT, EFT, DALST, and auditory CPT) were repeated, and mothers rated their children on the Werry–Weiss–Peters Hyperactivity Scale.

Results indicated that methylphenidate was superior to placebo on the ECMFFT and on scores on the Werry–Weiss–Peters Hyperactivity Scale. Its effect was similar to placebo on all other measures including the nursery observations. No difference was observed in the way in which methylphenidate affected "true" and "situational" hyperactive preschoolers.

Side effects mitigated the therapeutic efficacy of methlphenidate for most children. In addition to the well-known side effects of reduced appetite and difficulty getting to sleep, we observed in several children the emergence of anxious clinging behavior. One child who had for 3 weeks looked forward to each nursery session developed acute separation anxiety while on the active drug and refused to enter the nursery. Others engaged in more solitary play, becoming more withdrawn and appearing sad. The two nursery teachers, who were initially blind as to which type of pill the child was receiving, began to guess the active treatment condition and to dislike the effects on the children. At the conclusion of the study only 3 children of 28 were continued on methylphenidate. Mothers generally felt they preferred the behavior of their child off medication.

Other treatment modalities as well as medication were built into this study. The nursery itself had two experienced teachers for only 6 children (3 hyperactive and 3 normal controls). The nursery teachers worked hard to channel overactive behaviors into sociably acceptable channels. They also attempted to teach children to comply with the rules of the "structured tasks" period of the nursery, and frequently succeeded.

Mothers of hyperactive children and mothers of normal children were placed together in mothers' groups (6 mothers in one group) led by a trained psychiatric social worker. These groups were perceived to be helpful by all the mothers. For the mothers of the hyperactive children the groups served to change their perceptions of the degree of abnormality of their children's behaviors, since many of the mothers of the normal youngsters talked about similar problems which their children had, (e.g., not obeying, not sleeping through the night, not listening). A psychiatrist was available to meet with each mother individually when this was requested.

The results of this treatment program indicated a gradual improvement in the children's behavior seen in the nursery observations and on the laboratory tasks over the experimental period, unrelated to drug condition.

We concluded from the treatment aspect of this study that the nursery, the mothers' groups, and the individual sessions for mothers were useful measures of treatment for hyperactive preschoolers. Methylphenidate was potentially useful, but its therapeutic effects were counteracted by unacceptable side effects. The study unfortunately did not assess whether behavioral improvements observed as occurring gradually during 3 months were maintained after the termination of the study. Nor is it possible to know which nonmedication treatment was most helpful.

A second study assessing the efficacy of methylphenidate on 56 hyperactive preschoolers was carried out by Keith Conners in 1975.[24] Children were randomly assigned to methylphenidate or placebo conditions for a period of 6 weeks. Parents filled out a 93-item behavior symptom list before and after treatment. Laboratory tasks included, among others, the Merrill–Palmer Intelligence Scale, the Beery–Buktenica Visual Motor Integration Test (VMIT), the Flowers–Costello Test of Central Auditory Abilities, a CPT, Kagan's ECMFFT, and recording of seat activity. On a neurological examination 80% of these children showed mild to moderate dysfunction and 63% had mild to moderate speech and language disorders. Over 80% of the parents reported that overactivity had begun in the first 2 years of life. Results indicated that on the parent questionnaire 4 of 18 items related to the hyperactive syndrome were significantly improved in the active-drug compared to placebo condition. Significant improvement was also seen on the intelligence test and on the test of visual–motor integration. There was no difference between methylphenidate and placebo in recorded activity, the CPT or the ECMFFT. Mean dose of methylphenidate in this study was similar to the study of Schleifer and colleagues, namely 1.5 mg/kg or 11.8 mg per day. In this study side effects were less of a problem, and the increase of solitary play or clinging behavior was not reported. The children did not gain as much weight on methylphenidate, but the difference was not significant. Conners[24] concluded, "it is the impression from the study that the results are more variable than in similar treatment of older children" (p. 74).

The two treatment studies described highlight the value of early intervention to improve the behavior of hyperactive preschoolers and to change the perceptions of mothers regarding the degree of deviance of their hyperactive youngsters. The presence of a trained nursery teacher with a high teacher-to-child ratio also appeared to be helpful.

The question of how many hyperactive preschoolers outgrow their problems without receiving any help is an important one. In a study carried out in Dunedin, New Zealand, 1037 babies were followed from birth to age 7. Chapel and coworkers[25] evaluated these children at age 3. Children identified by both parents and psychometrists who tested them as having poor concentration and/or overactivity were called "hyperactive," which was diagnosed in 56 of 1037 children (5.5%). Of these 56 children only 11% continued to show the problems at age 5, and 17% showed the problems at age 9. The prevalence rate at age 3 in this study is high, probably because some children were included who had only poor attention or only overactivity, and not the full syndrome. This would be likely to decrease the relative percentage of problems continuing into the later years. The authors concluded that their findings justified postponement of early intervention. It is our feeling that this conclusion is open to question, particularly for preschoolers in whom the full syndrome is present since their early years. In addition, we do not know to what extent being a "troublesome" young child affects self-esteem and parent–child relationships, even when the behavioral problems are only present for a few years but occur during a very important period for personality formation.

CHAPTER THREE

THE HYPERACTIVE CHILD IN ELEMENTARY SCHOOL

It would seem, Adeimantus,
That the direction in which education starts a man,
Will determine his future life.
—From *The Republic, IV*, by Plato, 429–347 B.C.

Most hyperactive children are referred for assessment in the first three grades of school. The pattern of behavioral and cognitive disorder described in Chapter 1 becomes most clearly delineated as an identifiable syndrome at this age period. For this reason the vast majority of the studies on the syndrome have concerned themselves with the 6-to-12-years age group; with only a minority of studies focusing on the preschooler or adolescent.

This chapter is, therefore, written for the purpose of facilitating the reader's sense of continuity in the manifestation of the syndrome at different ages, rather than undertaking the impossible task of summarizing the vast body of literature available related to this age group. The areas focused on are important in understanding the nature of the syndrome as it manifests itself during the elementary-school period.

Brief mention was made in the last chapter that some referrals for hyperactivity begin to be made in the preschool years. There are good reasons why the majority of referrals for assessment are delayed until the first grades of elementary school. It is not so much (or not at all) that the behavioral difficulties of the elementary-school child are "worse" than previously, but rather that the specific difficulties of the hyperactive child at that age make success at school from the point of view of behavior and achievement unlikely. Behavior which some tolerant parents and nursery teachers learn to cope with and hope children will "outgrow" cannot be tolerated in a classroom with 1 teacher and 30 children. Society's expectations have once again changed, and once again the hyperactive child will be unable to cope with the new demands placed on him or her.

At this developmental period cooperation in a structured group, compliance to disciplinary demands, the ability to sit still for longer periods, paying attention to tasks (which may be too difficult, too easy, boring, or repetitive) without constant adult intervention and, finally, the presence of certain cognitive and motor skills are all part of the expected norms. The lack of these skills, which enable the youngster to learn to read and write in the first grades of school, results in the child's sense of failure. Not only is the child expected to behave like the others in the class, but to learn at the normal rate in the normal way. Underachievement at school, a universal experience of the hyperactive child, is a source of great anxiety to parents and teachers alike and leads to feelings of inferiority and lowering of motivation in the child. It is, therefore, little wonder that referrals are common at this time.

Hyperactive children aged 6 to 12 years show several or most of the following:

1. Inappropriate activity unrelated to the task at hand.
2. Poor sustained attention.
3. Difficulties inhibiting impulses, resulting in attention-seeking behavior, calling out, being poor at waiting for their turn or losing games, and so on. Impulsivity is seen not only in behavior, but in cognitive style, that is, in an impulsive versus reflective approach to academic tasks. Low frustration tolerance is related to the difficulties in inhibitory impulses.
4. Difficulties in learning under conditions of partial reinforcement.
5. Poor school achievement, which may result from any of the above and/or from specific learning deficits or clumsiness affecting the acquisition of reading, arithmetic, or writing skills. In addition, many hyperactive children have difficulties with organizational abilities.
6. Poor self-esteem resulting in some hyperactive children being in actual states of clinical depression.
7. Difficulties in interaction with parents, sibs, teachers, and peers.

Each of these difficulties will be discussed under a separate heading.

PROBLEMS RELATED TO ACTIVITY

As Rutter[1] recently pointed out, ". . . 'hyperactivity' as a symptom is not a unitary variable, and the child who is fidgety is not necessarily the child who runs up and down all the time" (p. 27). Furthermore, Rutter pointed out that there was poor correlation between different measures of activity such as teachers' rating scales, parents' rating scales, and such direct activity measures as actometers (or more recently small microcomputers worn around the waist which measure 24-hour activity). It follows that these different measures are recording different aspects of activity; mechanical measures record quantity of activity, and rating scales record also or mainly quality of activity.

An anecdote will highlight the above distinction. Two trained observers came out of a classroom where they had been asked to observe and score blind the behavior of two children, one hyperactive and the other normal. The observers were puzzled because they noted that a third child in the classroom was much more restless than either of the two children they had observed. When they asked the teacher whether this child had also been referred for "hyperactivity," the teacher's reply was, "Oh, no, John [the child in question] is a restless kid, but he learns well and is no trouble." Obviously, the child who gets referred for assessment for "the hyperactive syndrome" has a constellation of symptoms, not only restlessness, and further, the quality of the behavior is seen as deviant.

What is labeled as "hyperactive" (possibly a misnomer) at this age may or may not be an actual increase in the quality of total daily activity, but rather is activity which is "off task," "out of seat," and disruptive for the whole class[2] as well as detrimental to the learning process for the child. Klein and Young[3] hold the view that it may be a combination of high activity with high disruptive behavior which distinguishes "hyperactivity" from high normal activity. However, a recent study by Porrino and coworkers[4] has demonstrated that when an actometer with memory, worn for a period of 7 days, is used, hyperactive children are indeed more active, including during their sleep, than are controls.

ATTENTIONAL DIFFICULTIES

This particular aspect of the syndrome has been considered its hallmark or cardinal feature, leading to a widely accepted change of nomenclature in DSM-III from "Hyperkinetic Reaction of Childhood" to "Attention Deficit Disorder with or without Hyperactivity" (ADD[H] or ADD). In a classic article, Virginia Douglas[5] wrote, "Hyperactivity is only one of a constellation of critical symptoms. I hope to convince you that the inability of these children to sustain attention and to keep impulse responding under control may be even more important symptoms" (p. 260).

There seem to be two main reasons for shifting emphasis toward attention-deficit symptoms of this complex syndrome:

1. The suggestion by Douglas that poor attentional and inhibitory mechanisms may be primary with respect to inappropriate activity (flitting from one goal to another) and form the cardinal symptoms of the syndrome.

2. Follow-up studies of adolescents who had been diagnosed as hyperactive when children[6] showed that "hyperactivity" as a symptom had begun to diminish, although the adolescents were still rated by their parents as more restless than normal adolescents. Hyperactivity, which had earlier been the major complaint together with difficulty paying attention, was still present but usually no longer the main problem. Chief presenting complaints in adolscence were poor school achievement, antisocial behaviors, and poor social relationships. It seemed that while serious difficulties continued, hyperactivity itself had decreased.

Clinicians who have evaluated and treated large numbers of hyperactive children have always known that "attention" was not a unitary dimension. It had always been a puzzle why hyperactive children who were described by teachers as having a concentration span of 3 to 6 minutes in the classroom could sit still and concentrate on certain TV programs for long periods of time or could spend a day fishing with father with excellent concentration. Clinically it always appeared as though the school-age hyperactive child had a "selective" attention deficit for school and homework. Perhaps a more sophisticated way of putting this is that concentration difficulties became apparent under certain environmental conditions which included elements of boredom, fatigue, repetition, low reinforcement levels, and low motivation. Certainly the complexity of the attentional problems of hyperactive children has been the focus of much empirical research and theoretical discussion. A thoughtful and comprehensive review of the area of attentional and cognitive problems has been written recently by Virginia Douglas.[7]

Donald Sykes, when a graduate student of Virginia Douglas, carried out a series of studies[8,9] aimed at delineating the nature of the attentional deficit of hyperactives. The attention task in which hyperactives had most difficulty was a vigilance task (the Continuous Performance Test, CPT).[10] The subject was required to make a response to visual stimuli which appeared on a screen (e.g., press a lever when the letter X follows the letter A) or auditory stimuli which were received through earphones. On both the visual and the auditory forms of this task, hyperactives made more errors of omissions and commission (i.e., they more often failed to respond or responded to the wrong stimuli) than normal children. The test took 15 minutes to complete, and the performance of hyperactives deteriorated more seriously over time than that of the normals. This deterioration was accompanied by increased physical activity as measured by the stabilometric cushion on which the subjects sat.

Sykes also studied the old adage that hyperactives were more "distractible" than normals, an observation originally made by Strauss and Lehtinen.[11] This observation, which had never been clearly confirmed, had resulted in many hyperactive children in the United States being placed by themselves in small rooms outside their classrooms. These small rooms were stripped of visual or auditory stimuli, and the hyperactive children were expected to be able to work without being distracted. Sykes attempted to "distract" hyperactives by piping intermittent white noise into the room while the subjects were doing the CPT. He also used a distracting color background in a "Choice Reaction Time Test." Neither type of distraction hindered the hyperactives' performance more than the performance of the normals. Sykes's work has answered some questions and raised others about the nature of the attentional deficit. While some hyperactives are described as being "distractible," this may not be true for the majority. Furthermore, it seems from Sykes's work that hyperactives do better when attention tasks are self-paced.

Rosenthal and Allen[12] confirmed Sykes's observation that relatively weak distractors did not impair the performance of hyperactive children more seriously than that of controls. This was not the case when the distracting stimuli were highly significant for the children, under which conditions the performance of hyperactive children was significantly more impaired than that of normals. (These conditions would be more likely to correspond to the type of "meaningful" distractors which tend to occur naturally in a classroom situation). Radosh and Gittelman[13] found that both high- and low-appeal distractors significantly impaired the performance of hyperactive children on arithmetic tasks, while only high-appeal distractors impaired equally the performance of normal and hyperactive children. The seeming contradictions of the last two studies are probably related to the use of different strengths of distractors as well as measurement on different performance tasks (e.g., timed classification vs. arithmetic problems).

In Douglas's recent review[7] she suggests that four primary deficits of hyperactive children, namely attentional, inhibitory, arousal, and reinforcement-mechanism deficits, can account for all the cognitive impairment of normally intelligent hyperactive children. She postulates that these primary deficits interact with secondary deficits such as diminished motivation, impaired metacognition, and the limited development of higher-order schemata (e.g., concepts, strategies) to produce the usual vicious cycle of poor learning and performance.

IMPULSIVITY

When the adult difficulties of the hyperactive child grown up are described in subsequent chapters, it will be apparent that the impulsivity problems (or series of problems) are the most serious and most sustained of the childhood clusters of symptoms. In adulthood it is rare that either hyperactivity or concentration problems are spontaneously complained about. This is not true for symptoms related to impulsivity (see Chapter 5). Unfortunately, the construct of impulsivity is even more difficult to define operationally and to consider as a unitary dimension than the other two core symptoms, although they also, as was suggested, are not simple unitary dimensions.

DSM-III gives the following operational criteria for impulsivity in childhood:

Impulsive behavior is manifested by at least three of the following:

1. Often acts before thinking
2. Shifts excessively from one activity to another
3. Has difficulty organizing work (this not due to cognitive impairment)
4. Needs a lot of supervision
5. Frequently calls out in class
6. Has difficulty awaiting turn in games or group situations

These criteria reflect many types of difficulties, including overlap with other core symptoms of the syndrome (e.g., needs a lot of supervision). With respect to the criterion "has difficulty organizing work (not due to cognitive impairment)" it is hard to know how to judge whether the poor organizational ability, if present, is or is not due to cognitive impairment such as poor cognitive strategies.

It was demonstrated by Campbell et al.[14] that hyperactive elementary-school children were more impulsive in their cognitive style. On the Matching Familiar Figures Test (MFFT), hyperactives and significantly shorter latencies and made more errors than matched normal children. The latter would seem to indicate their difficulty with inhibitory control. On the Embedded Figures Test (EFT), they isolated fewer embedded figures, indicating they were more field dependent. Campbell suggested that hyperactive children could be trained to delay response and to concentrate on essential components of a situation. In view of the seriousness of all aspects of impulsivity for the adult hyperactive, childhood training in these areas should be looked at very seriously once again (see end of chapter); however, the reader should note (although it is somewhat confusing) that impulsive cognitive styles as measured on cognitive-style tests such as the MFFT are not specific to hyperactive children and were demonstrated to occur also in children with other diagnoses.[15]

Various other laboratory tasks intended to measure aspects of impulsivity are maze tests and various self-control strategies.[15] These laboratory tasks may not correlate with one another or with systemic observation of the child. This difficulty, which is also evident with the other core symptoms, is not surprising since we are not dealing with unitary constructs.

For example, the CPT has generally been considered the best laboratory measure of sustained attention. Yet this test probably also measures impulsivity (or lack of inhibitory control). It is known that hyperactives do more poorly than matched controls on the CPT with respect to errors of omission (failing to press a button when a target stimulus appears) and errors of commission (pressing the button erroneously without the appearance of a target stimulus). Hoy et al.,[16] in an auditory version of the CPT, found that hyperactive adolescents were similar to controls on errors of omission, but made more errors of commission. The latter is likely to be the result of impulsivity rather than inattention and gives laboratory support to the clinical observation (see Chapter 5) that impulsivity is spontaneously complained of in hyperactive adults, while hyperactivity is complained about when probed. Difficulties with attention during work (see Chapter 9) could not be elicited even after probing.

It is apparent that less systematic research has focused on the various aspects of impulsivity than on the other two core symptoms. This is unfortunate, since, as mentioned above, symptoms of impulsivity seem to be the most enduring core symptoms of the childhood syndrome as seen in adult life. Also, symptoms of impulsivity may well respond to training procedures.

REINFORCEMENT ISSUES IN THE LEARNING OF HYPERACTIVE CHILDREN

Paul Wender[17] was the first to hypothesize that hyperactive children (whom he called children with Minimal Brain Dysfunction) have a primary defect in learning from praise and reward; that is, they have diminished sensitivity to positive and negative reinforcement.

Subsequently, this issue has been studied by several investigators, and the results raise doubts about Wender's hypothesis. Early work on this was done by Freiberg (at the time a graduate student of Virginia Douglas) on the issue of the effect of full and partial reinforcement on concept learning of hyperactives and normal controls.[18] Under conditions of full reinforcement, Freiberg found that hyperactives were able to learn concepts as well as normal children. Full reinforcement implied that every correct response was rewarded by the automatic appearance of a marble from a machine. However, under conditions of partial reinforcement when every other correct response was reinforced by a marble, while the performance of all children was lowered, the hyperactive children now learned the concepts significantly more slowly than did normals. It was difficult from Freiberg's work to sort out effects of motivational, attentional, and information feedback variables in decreasing speed of concept learning; it is likely that all three were involved.

While it is beyond the scope of this section to summarize the accumulating research on this important area, a few key studies will be cited.

Effects of reinforcement schedules on reaction time of hyperactives were demonstrated by Douglas and Peters.[19] Earlier work had indicated that positive reward on delayed reaction time was sometimes accompanied in the hyperactive children by more impulsive responding. In contrast, negative consequences did not lead to more impulsive responding but did improve reaction time. Douglas and Parry[20] showed that continuous reward reduced both mean reaction time and reaction-time variability in hyperactive and normal children. Most interesting was that extinction trials resulted in the hyperactives' reaction time dropping significantly more sharply than that of normals. This led Douglas[7] to conclude, "The results of these various studies do not support the notion that hyperactives are unresponsive to either positive or negative reinforcement. In fact, in case of rewards, the opposite appears to be true: the children seem to be unusually sensitive both to the presence of rewards and to the loss of anticipated rewards" (p. 302).

POOR SCHOOL ACHIEVEMENT

So much has been written about this area that only major clinical concerns will be addressed. Since poor school achievement in hyperactive children is a close-to-universal problem in both elementary and secondary schools,[21,22] whatever the multiple and interacting causes of this underachievement are its effects are very serious and manifest themselves in poor self-esteem and lower final occupational status (see Chapter 9). Certainly the causes are multiple and may not be identical for each child. The following are possible causes:

1. The core symptoms of the syndrome—hyperactivity, poor attention span, and impulsivity—interact to impair academic achievement.

2. Correlates of the hyperactive syndrome seen in many hyperactive children, such as (a) small decrements of overall IQ as seen in many studies[22]; (b) more subtest variability on IQ test[5]; (c) poor cognitive strategies and impulsive cognitive style; (d) motor clumsiness; (e) disorganization (impulsive or cognitive); (f) specific learning disabilities (e.g., language delays, perceptual difficulties, sequencing problems, auditory memory difficulties, auditory discrimination difficulties); and (g) hyperactives' worse performance on tasks done in a group versus an individual setting.

3. Secondary symptoms resulting from the above: (a) poor motivation; (b) the accumulated dearth of what should have been (but was not) learned (i.e., failure of past learning); and (c) mood depression.

These different deficiencies must interact to produce the proverbial vicious cycle of poor school achievement (see Figure 3-1).

POOR SELF-ESTEEM AND DEPRESSION

Campbell *et al.*[2] demonstrated that hyperactive children as young as 6 to 8 years already could be shown to have lower self-esteem than normal children. Some investigators have found that hyperactive children had concomitant depression.[23] These additional difficulties are probably present in all children who experience repeated failures in childhood and in this way are not specific to hyperactive children.

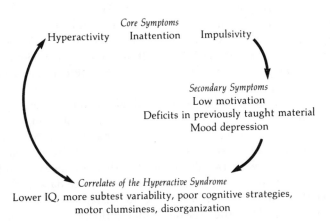

FIGURE 3-1. Vicious cycle of poor school performance.

However, while one may hope that early intervention could reduce these secondary problems, it is unlikely that any intervention, however early it is given, would altogether eliminate them.

DIFFICULTIES IN SOCIAL INTERACTIONS AT HOME AND AT SCHOOL

It was pointed out in Chapter 2 that from the beginning of life there is an interaction between the hyperactive infant and his or her mother which may be "good enough" even if the infant is difficult, provided the mother is not excessively perturbed and attachment proceeds normally. This interaction soon extends to include fathers, sibs, relatives, and other significant adults and peers. Studies pertaining to the hyperactive's social interactions have finally in the last few years received the interest they deserve. Interactions between the hyperactive child and his or her mother or parents will be described in Chapter 12. Here we will discuss interactions with peers and teachers.

PEER AND TEACHER RELATIONSHIPS

All workers who have systematically investigated the hyperactive child's peer relationships have concluded that this is a serious area of difficulty which begins before the school years but manifests itself most poignantly in elementary and secondary school. Other children very quickly, sometimes within hours, reject hyperactive children. The latter do not respond appropriately to social cues, have difficulty waiting their turn and losing in games, and tend to be bossy or irritable if they do not get their own way.[24,25] When this peer rejection is absent, it is likely that the prognosis is better. It has long been known from many studies that poor peer relationships are highly correlated with later poor outcome.[26]

The relationship of hyperactive children and teachers has recently begun to be studied. Thus Campbell et al. noted in their 3-year follow-up of hyperactive preschoolers[2] that hyperactive children in elementary school elicit more negative feedback from their teachers. Whalen and coworkers[27] demonstrated that this negative interaction decreased when the children received methylphenidate medication (vs. placebo). Campbell et al.'s study also suggested that the presence of a hyperactive child in the classroom may influence interaction patterns within the classroom as a whole, so that teachers of a class where there was a hyperactive child interacted more negatively not only with the child in question, but with other children in the class.

Observational studies in the classroom by Whalen et al.[28] indicated that disruptive and negative relationships with peers could be modified both by stimulants and by the nature of the classroom activity, for example, when hyperactive children had to engage in complex tasks which were not self-paced.

A recent study was that of Pelham,[29] which compared hyperactive children (5 to 9 years) to normal peers in both free play and structured cooperative tasks over five sessions. While the hyperactive children were more talkative, disruptive, and physically and verbally aggressive in the structured task, the aggressive interactions were most pronounced in the free play. In this study, contrary to others, stimulant therapy had little effect, except for the most aggressive hyperactive children.

We can conclude that hyperactive children in elementary school show aggressive interactions. While both the nature of the activity in the classroom and the use of stimulants will reduce the negative interactions, it is unlikely that these measures would altogether eliminate the interactional difficulties.

It is the opinion of the authors that further work is required to understand the complex nature of these social difficulties of the hyperactive child and to find ways of trying to ameliorate them. Poor social relationships may and probably do arise from the variety of behavioral problems of the hyperactive child, which are unacceptable to peers, siblings, parents, and teachers. Little attention has been given to the question of whether hyperactive children fail to perceive or misinterpret social cues, or whether their perception is accurate but they are unable because of their core difficulties to respond to them appropriately. Some investigators have begun to study the effect of social-skill training of hyperactive youngsters.[29] It is likely that in the future more studies will focus on the effect of this treatment. We have to keep in mind the profound cumulative effect, extending into the adult life, of poor social interactions.

TREATMENT

Medication

In the 1960s and '70s, many well-designed studies with placebo controls indicated that stimulant drugs (dextroamphetamine and methylphenidate) improved various symptoms in about 70% of hyperactive children. These controlled studies confirmed Bradley's findings[30] that Benzedrine improved the school performance and behavior of many of a group of disturbed children. With respect to behavior, aggression was said to decrease[31] and seemingly purposeless activity became more goal directed.[32-35] With respect to cognitive tasks, there was an improvement in sustained attention,[8,36] children became less impulsive, [14,37-39] learned rote material better,[37] had improved short-term memory,[38] did better on fine motor tasks,[39] and could better discriminate foreground and background.[14] While it is not generally believed that stimulants improve perception, motor ability, or higher cortical functions, but instead that these functions improve as a result of greater reflectivity and better attention, work on this question continues.

In an excellent review article, Kenneth Gadow[40] has summarized the effect of stimulants on learning, including reading, arithmetic, spelling, and handwriting. He points out that there is evidence of facilitation of academic performance with stimulant drugs, but that the effect is not very robust. Gittelman and coworkers,[41] from their study on the treatment of reading disorders, concluded that this effect pales by comparison to that of specific academic intervention.

The findings of Sprague and Sleator[42] indicate that for some hyperactive children the optimal dose for performance on a cognitive task (paired-associate learning) was 0.3 mg/kg of methylphenidate, while optimal dose for improving social functioning (Conners Brief Teacher Rating Scale) was 1 mg/kg. The ideal dose, however, for any target symptoms varies among children, and it has been demonstrated that a dose which is high enough to improve conduct problems may actually impair cognitive learning.

Long-term follow-up studies of drug effects,[43-48] have been very difficult to design for ethical reasons. For example, no child ethically or practically can be kept on "placebo" for 1 or more years. Even though these long-term drug studies leave much to be desired in their methodology, as a group they have failed to demonstrate long-term drug efficacy. In one of these studies,[43] where three treatments, chlorpromazine, methylphenidate, and no drug, were compared in terms of 5-year follow-up status on three matched groups of hyperactive children, no differences were found between the three groups. However, only in the methylphenidate group did a good home environment (good mother–child relationship) correlate with good outcome, implying a possible synergistic effect between a useful drug and the child's relationship to the mother.

The failure to demonstrate significant long-term drug effects may be due to the stimulants' relatively weak response in decreasing antisocial behavior, as a result of inadequate doses used, inappropriate schedules, too-crude measurements, failure of children to take the drug, or development of drug tolerance. Very likely this failure is due to the fact that other interventions (e.g., remedial teaching, social-skill training, counseling), in addition to medication, are required by these children. It is possible that these relatively negative results of long-term studies have resulted in fewer children being medicated and that there is a reduction in the initial enthusiasm generated by the success of stimulants in treating symptoms of hyperactive children in short-term studies.

Side effects from stimulants are well known. Reduced appetite and weight loss are frequent side effects at the beginning of treatment and are usually dose related. Medication is usually given at breakfast and lunch so that insomnia does not occur. Some children become irritable and weepy (particularly preschoolers, in whom stimulant therapy may not be useful). Headaches, stomachaches, and urticaria have been reported. Occasionally, children develop severe regressions and tactile hallucinations. This is rare and disappears with discontinuation of the drug. More recently, tics have been reported, but there is little evidence for what was thought to be the occurrence of Gilles de la Tourelle disease, since the coexistence of the latter with hyperactivity has been known for some time.

Suppression of growth, height, and weight was first noted by Safer, Allen, and Barr.[49] It was verified by some workers and found not to exist by others. In a review article requested by the FDA, Roche, Lipman, and Overall[50] concluded that "There is evidence of suppression of a moderate growth in weight. There may be some minor suppression of growth in stature during the same period but the evidence is less certain" (p. 849).

The work of Safer et al.[49] suggested that growth suppression was more marked with dextroamphetamine than with methylphenidate, that it was dose related (not seen in doses under 20 mg of methylphenidate daily), and that it did not wear off with time. They also noted a relatively small increase in heart rate and blood pressure. Neither effect seemed of sufficient degree (e.g., compared to exercise) to be likely to be detrimental to health.

It was once believed that the hyperactive syndrome was limited to childhood. Since this is not the case, and since it is known that drug effects wear off as soon as medication is discontinued, the notion that drugs can be administered until "maturation" has cured the problem is not true for those hyperactive children whose problems continue into adulthood. Some clinicians feel that these children require "stimulants" even in adult life (and a chapter is devoted to studies on stimulant-therapy effects in adults). Other clinicians suggest that other treatment modalities which may have more lasting effects should be looked for.

Behavior Modification

In two studies,[51,52] children were given positive reinforcement based on quality of schoolwork achieved in a given time rather than a reinforcement scheme based on unacceptable behaviors. Several single-subject studies have proven the efficacy of operant conditioning for reducing hyperactive behaviors.[53,54] Safer and Allen[55] in their textbook on hyperactivity devote one chapter to parent-management techniques and another chapter to behavior modification. Parent management techniques, in which parents are taught to improve their children's prosocial behaviors and become sensitive as to how they may unwillingly reinforce unwanted behaviors, are valuable in that parenting skills are improved for the hyperactive child as well as for his or her sibs. O'Leary et al. have pointed out that for optimal results in operant-conditioning techniques, both the home and the school must be involved.[56]

We know that positive drug effects generally disappear when the medication of hyperactive children is removed. We may ask the question whether the results of behavioral techniques are more enduring. There is as yet no satisfactory study which shows that the effects of behavior modification in hyperactive children are permanent or long lasting.

Gittelman-Klein and coworkers combined methylphenidate with behavior modification.[57] They found that children receiving methylphenidate alone or methylphenidate together with behavior modification (at home and at school) did better over 8 weeks than those who received behavior modification (at home and school) alone. For many children the combined approach is to be preferred.

Along with several investigators, Douglas and coworkers attempted to modify hyperactive behavior by means of a "cognitive training program" using self-reinforcement techniques to train children to use more effective strategies for cognitive tasks.[58] They report some degree of success, which was maintained for at least 3 months. This modality of training was applied by Barkley and coworkers to 6 hyperactive boys in a special classroom using a variety of self-control procedures.[59] Results were relatively minimal, although misbehavior was reduced and task attention during individual (but not group) work improved. No generalization of effect could be demonstrated and no change in activity level resulted.

The most positive note regarding therapy has come from the work of the Satterfields in California.[60] They conducted a prospective 3-year multimodality treatment study of 100 hyperactive boys. The treatment used was individual psychotherapy for the child and/or parent(s), group therapy, family therapy, and remedial education. All boys received stimulants. One therapy or several therapies were given as individually required. At 3-year follow-up the 50% of children who continued in therapy were more advanced educationally and less antisocial than those who had dropped out of therapy. The investigators found that compared to other outcome studies, the outcome of their comprehensively treated group was unusually good. The criticism of this study is that the families and children most motivated to continue in treatment may be nonrepresentative of the whole group and that their better outcome is a function more or as much of this variable as of the effectiveness of a broad range of treatment. Nevertheless, further follow-up of this "well-treated" group will be of great interest, and since the condition itself is one of many deficits in behavior, learning, social skills, and self-esteem, a broad approach to treatment is clearly indicated.

CHAPTER FOUR

HYPERACTIVES AS ADOLESCENTS

We are born so to speak twice over.
Born into existence and born into life,
Born a human being and born a man.
—From *Emile*, by Jean-Jacques Rousseau, 1712–1778

An understanding of the adolescence of hyperactives requires some reflections on our understanding of adolescence itself as a stage of human development. As far back as the writings of Aristotle, adolescence has been viewed as a period of inevitable turmoil which precedes maturity. At the turn of the century, Stanley Hall reinforced this point of view in his two volumes entitled *Adolescence: Its Psychology and Its Relation to Physiology, Anthropology, Sociobiology, Sex, Crime, Religion, and Education.*[1] Hall described adolescence as a period of "storm and stress" which in his opinion was a biological necessity. While Margaret Mead[2] was one of the first to challenge this point of view by describing the adolescence of Samoans as a relatively tranquil process, psychoanalytic writers reaffirmed the early view of inevitable chaos during puberty which resulted from a biologically determined upsurge of aggressive and sexual impulses confronting an immature ego. Anna Freud[3] went as far as to suggest that adolescents who remain symptom free and fail to show external evidence of inner conflict are at risk for normal adult development.

Daniel Offer[4,5] attempted by means of systematic empirical observations to test out these opposing views. He selected a typical group of 103 from 326 normal adolescents, using the concept of normality as a statistical average. Repeated interviews, psychological tests, self-rating scales, and family studies, as well as follow-up for 4 years to adulthood, confirmed that middle-class American adolescents experienced their adolescence with intermittent periods of mild anxiety and/or depression, but with otherwise only minimal signs of internal or external turmoil. Offer concluded that normal adolescents of today show little of the turmoil expected of them in the literature. Both Offer[5] and Rutter *et al.*[6] in their studies have, however, noted that in early adolescence arguments and disagreement with parents over insignificant issues such as hair styles, rules, etc., are common. We can conclude from the discrepancy between the early Greek view and the body of psychoanalytic theory on the one hand, and the contradictory observational findings of Offer and others on the other, that adolescence is a phase of human development which has a potential for conflict and turmoil, but is likely to be gone through without gross external signs of this in the average adolescent in the average family.

For a better understanding of how hyperactives fare in adolescence, we can draw on the theoretical considerations of Erik Erikson. In "Eight Stages of Man,"[7] Erikson puts forward a theory of personality development based on an epigenetic stage theory. While it is beyond the scope of this chapter to give details of his theory, one of his main themes is that human biopsychosocial development proceeds in a series of invariable epigenetic stages, each of which is characterized by a specific "normative crisis" which must be dealt with at that stage of development. Inadequate resolution of the stage-specific crisis will negatively influence the resolution of the crisis during the next stage of development. In the first year of life Erikson sees "basic trust versus mistrust" as the normative crisis and feels that adequate resolution of this is essential for the development of a healthy personality. This stage is followed in the toddler by "autonomy versus shame and doubt" and in the preschooler by "initiative versus guilt." For the school-age child, Erikson postulates that if previous stages have been relatively successfully accomplished, the child is emotionally free to leave home to attend school and will enjoy and focus his or her energies on the acquisition of the skills required in the culture. The normative crisis of the school-age child is viewed by Erikson as being "industry versus inferiority." He stresses the importance of both the child's readiness for school in terms of resolution of previous normative crises and the necessity for the child of a facilitating school environment. (We might add that the hyperactive child is emotionally and cognitively not ready for school and as a result frequently does not experience a facilitating school environment.)

Finally, having developed a sense of industry (i.e., a sense of mastery of the learning process) and therefore relatively successfully avoiding the ever-present potential (even in the normal child) of a sense of inferiority, the child is theoretically ready for the stage of adolescence. At this stage of development the adolescent must come to grips with a stable, enduring sense of ego identity, based on the experience of social health and cultural solidarity at the end of each major childhood crisis. Then there will be successful resolution of the normative crisis of this stage: a sense of "identity versus identity diffusion."

The previous chapter outlined the various social, emotional, be-havioral, and learning difficulties of the hyperactive child in elementary school. It was pointed out that already by Grades 1. and 2 there was evidence of the impairment of self-esteem, presumably because of the experience of failure in so many areas and the resulting criticism. It is not surprising that the hyperactive child enters the period of adoles-cence with severe preexisting difficulties such as gaps in learning and a lack of a sense of mastery of the learning process. He or she is ill prepared in many ways for the experience of secondary school.

Hans Huessy and colleagues[8] confirmed the theoretical concept that behavioral and academic problems of hyperactive adolescents are preceded by these same difficulties in elementary school. They evalu-ated and followed via teacher questionnaires 501 children attending several Vermont schools. The questionnaire tapped social maturity, academic performance, general attitudes and behavior, and neuromus-cular development. Children in the worst 20% were called "hyperac-tive." Those who fell in the worst 20% in Grades 2, 4, and 5 had a poor outcome in Grade 9, when 70% of them had severe antisocial and learning problems. In contrast, none of the children falling into the best 30% in Grades 2, 4, and 5 had any academic or social problems in high school. All children in this study who had academic and behavior problems in high school first showed these difficulties in elementary school.

In view of the obvious handicap with which hyperactive children enter their adolescence, it is surprising that historically the hyperactive child syndrome was considered to be a behavior disturbance limited to childhood.[9-11] Laufer and Denhoff,[12] who had extensive clinical expe-rience with hyperkinetic children, in an early paper wrote, "In later years this syndrome tends to wane spontaneously and disappear" (p. 646). Later, these investigators systematically followed 20 hyperac-tive children of normal intelligence into adolescence and found that they had a variety of psychopathological symptoms and that poor school performance was a complaint common to all.[13] In the same year (1962), Anderson and Plymate[14] also suggested that children diagnosed as having Minimal Brain Dysfunction (MBD) with hyperactivity devel-oped serious personality disorders in adolescence, which they called "Association Deficit Pathology." Little notice was taken of these earlier reports of the continuation of the syndrome into adolescence. It was not until the 1970s that several systematic and generally controlled studies were carried out.

These studies will be reviewed by dividing them into retrospective and prospective studies. In general, retrospective studies examine old records or charts of children seen in child psychiatry or guidance clinics several years previously. The diagnosis of hyperactive child syndrome is then made or confirmed by current diagnostic criteria retrospectively, and the investigators attempt to trace and interview all the subjects in whom the diagnosis could be clearly made. In prospective studies, children who are diagnosed to have the hyperactive syndrome are systematically followed and evaluated at various intervals of time for many years (e.g., 15–20 years).

RETROSPECTIVE STUDIES

Mendelson and coworkers[15] collected names of 140 children who had been evaluated 2 to 5 years earlier in the psychiatry clinic of St. Louis Children's Hospital or in the private practice of Mark Stewart, and had been diagnosed as having the hyperactive child syndrome. They were able to trace 108, but excluded 25 additional children because there was insufficient information in the chart. Eighty-three adolescents (mean age 13.4 years) were thus identified and their mothers were interviewed in their homes using a structured interview. Results indicated that 25% were in special classes, 2% in training schools, and 2% in psychiatric hospitals. The mothers reported that 70–80% of the adolescents were still having problems of restlessness and distractability, and 26% had long histories of antisocial behavior, with 17% having appeared before the juvenile court. The frequency of the complaint "overactivity" had decreased to 12%; it was replaced by the complaint "rebelliousness." This latter observation helps to explain why previously clinicians had believed that the syndrome was limited to childhood.

The above study was noteworthy in being one of the first systematic follow-up investigations of a large number of children diagnosed retrospectively as having the hyperactive syndrome. It nevertheless has some shortcomings, some of which are shared with all retrospective studies. One is the difficulty of making diagnoses by current criteria from old charts. The authors themselves pointed out, "We were not able to use uniform criteria for selection because the symptoms associated with hyperactivity had not been recorded systematically in the chart" (p. 273).[15] In addition, 25 patients had to be excluded because there was insufficient information in the chart for a diagnosis, and 35 children were not traced. Tracing "all subjects" is virtually impossible in all follow-up studies, whether they are retrospective or prospective. This study also did not use a control group.

In a later publication, Stewart and coworkers[16] reported on their interviews of the adolescents themselves. More than half reported that they were restless, impatient, irritable, impulsive, and found it hard to study. Forty percent of subjects had three or more of the following symptoms: chronic lying, frequent fighting, being difficult to raise, swearing, and being defiant; and 31% reported that they were stealing. Forty percent had low self-esteem, but this was not necessarily associated with conduct or antisocial behaviors. The subjects themselves agreed well with their parents' reports on them except in the area of getting along with peers and teachers, where the adolescents denied their problems. In evaluating this study, one must remember that an unspecified number of subjects had IQ's below 80, which would partially explain that 25% were in special classes.

Another retrospective study was carried out by Blouin and co-workers[17] in Ottawa, with certain specified aims. These investigators noted that previous follow-up studies had either been uncontrolled (as was the study cited above) or had employed normal adolescents as controls, thus not controlling for the experience of school (and other) failures. For this reason they used as comparison a group of adolescents who 5 years previously (when the diagnosis of hyperactivity of the hyperactive group had been made) had presented with "school difficulties," in the absence of mental retardation and hyperactivity. In addition the investigators, having noted the link described by others of alcoholism in the fathers of hyperactive subjects, did a careful survey of the drinking habits of both the 23 hyperactive and 22 nonhyperactive adolescents. They also attempted to evaluate the efficacy of methylphenidate treatment. Findings indicated that at follow-up the hyperactives had more conduct problems, were more impulsive and hyperactive, and scored higher on the Self-Injurious Behavior Scale. Since 90% of both groups reported that they had never used any drug other than alcohol or marijuana, only the use of these two drugs was investigated. Hyperactives reported that they used alcohol more frequently than controls (once a month or more), and they had used hard liquor more often than controls. There was no difference between the groups as to the use of marijuana, and the authors do not report that there was "alcohol abuse" or "alcoholism" in either group. No differences were found in the outcome of those who were treated with methlphenidate. Since it is possible that the "worst" hyperactives were treated with this medication, the finding requires further corroboration. The age range of subjects in Blouin's study is unfortunately not reported.

Feldman and coworkers[18] in Rhode Island carried out a 5-year retrospective follow-up study of 81 adolescents (mean age 15.5 years) who were originally diagnosed as having MBD. They found that about half of the subjects were now problem free. Ten percent had problems of an antisocial nature, and a third of the group required continued treatment and/or special education. It is not clear from this study whether all adolescents who had been diagnosed as MBD were also hyperactive. If some subjects were not "hyperactive," it would explain the more positive adolescent outcome in this study.

PROSPECTIVE STUDIES

The first controlled prospective study came from the Montreal group[19,20] and was a 5-year follow-up of 91 hyperactive adolescents who had been diagnosed as being pervasively hyperactive 4 to 6 years previously (1962–1965), when they were 6 to 12 years old. Children were admitted into the study if they met the following criteria:

1. Restlessness and poor concentration were the main complaints and were a major source of problems at home *and* at school. The condition was pervasive and had been present since the earliest years.
2. All children had Wechsler Intelligence Scale for Children (WISC) IQ's (Full Scale) above 85.
3. None of the children were psychotic, borderline psychotic, epileptic, or had cerebral palsy.
4. All children lived at home with at least one parent.

Initially 104 hyperactive children were included in the study and took part in a series of drug studies determining the efficacy of chlorpromazine[21] and dextroamphetamine.[22] While the presenting problems of these children were remarkably similar, they differed from one another with respect to family functioning; presence, absence, or degree and type of learning disability; and degree of conduct problems associated with hyperactivity. At that time DSM-III was not in use, but in retrospect it is our impression that all our subjects had ADD(H) and the majority had some degree of associated conduct problems. Of 104 subjects seen 4 to 6 years previously, 13 were not reevaluated, 11 had moved away and were not traced, and 2 refused to be interviewed. The loss represents only 11.5% of the original subjects.

The 91 adolescents of this study were 11 to 16 years of age (mean age 13.4) and had therefore probably not yet reached the age of peak risk for adolescent difficulties. Nevertheless, their outcome was disappointing. Despite a decrease of ratings of the initial symptoms of the syndrome (hyperactivity, distractibility, impulsivity, and aggression), they still scored worse on these symptoms than a matched (IQ, socioeconomic status, and sex) group of normal controls obtained at the time of the study from notices posted in various schools. The reduction of the severity of the original symptoms of the syndrome had also been observed by Mendelson, Stewart, and coworkers. Clinically the evaluators (G. W. and K. M.) found the subjects to be immature and to have difficulty maintaining goals, and they became sad during the interview as they recounted their failures and lack of plans for a future. (They were not considered to be clinically depressed because the mood change was transient.) The adolescents showed clear evidence of low self-esteem.[19,23] Their school records showed that they had failed more grades and received lower ratings on all subjects on their report cards when compared to matched normal controls in the same classroom.[24] They continued to use impulsive rather than reflective styles on cognitive tasks compared to normal controls[25] and showed no improvement on tests of intelligence and an actual decrement of performance on a motor task (Lincoln–Oseretsky).[20] Twenty-five percent had engaged in antisocial behavior, and the biggest difference between hyperactives and controls was on the factor of psychopathy of the Peterson–Quay checklist.

A shortcoming of the above study was the use of "normal" controls only rather than adding also a patient control group; thus there was no control for the fact of chronic failure. In addition, several measures used were designed for the study by the investigators, since more valid and reliable measures were not yet available. For example, the Werry–Weiss–Peters Hyperactivity Scale was used to measure hyperactivity since the Conners scales were not available, and our own Family Rating Scale, which has never been standardized, was also used.

Dykman and coworkers[26] in Arkansas avoided the problems posed by a "normal" control group. They carried out a follow-up study of 62 learning-disabled children and 31 normal controls. Twenty-three of the 62 learning-disabled children were hyperactive, 14 were hypoactive, and the remainder (25) were normoactive. The three learning-disabled groups of children, as well as a group of normal children, were reevaluated when they were 14 years of age. Almost half of the hyperactive learning-disabled group were found to have fairly severe problems of adjustment, mainly of an antisocial nature. In contrast, social deviancy was found to be rare among both normal controls and the nonhyperactive learning disabled. The hypoactive adolescents were considered more withdrawn, cold, and passive than controls, and all three learning-disabled groups were rated low on self-confidence. It is clear from this study that the presence of hyperactivity in learning-disabled children predicts poor social adjustment and conduct problems in adolescence.

The last prospective follow-up study to be reviewed is the most recent and differs in several respects from the other studies which have been summarized. This study was carried out on 110 adolescent boys diagnosed as ADD(H) and 88 normal adolescent boys in Los Angeles by Satterfield and coworkers.[27] Their aim was to study official arrests from childhood to adolescence on all of the subjects for whom arrest information was available, as recorded in the Los Angeles County Probation Department's automated juvenile index. The ages of the adolescents ranged from 13 to 21, and the mean age was 17 years. The two groups were not matched as to socioeconomic status; hence the classes were analyzed separately. Rates of single and multiple arrests were significantly higher in the hyperactives, as was institutionalization for delinquency. The percentage of hyperactive adolescents arrested at least once was 58% in the lower class, 36% in the middle class, and 52% in the upper class, compared to 11%, 9%, and 2% for the controls. The percentages of hyperactives who had more than one arrest in the three classes were 35%, 25%, and 28%. All the offenses were considered serious since minor offenses,—for example, running away, getting drunk, petty thefts, and possession of less than 1 ounce of marijuana—were excluded. This study is unique and differs significantly from all the other studies in both the number of arrests and the seriousness of the offenses for which the hyperactive subjects were arrested.

Taking all these studies together, there are several major areas of agreement and certain differences:

1. All studies measuring this found that the symptoms of the original syndrome had diminished in most of the adolescents, and were rarely the worst problems spontaneously complained about. (The latter were discipline problems, antisocial acts, poor school performance, and poor peer relationships.)

2. Low self-esteem, poor school performance, and poor peer relationships characterized all adolescent outcome studies which examined these problems.

3. The biggest difference between studies was seen in the percentage of adolescents who had repeated antisocial behavior. This varied from 10% in the Feldman[18] study to 25% in both the Mendelson[15] and the Weiss[19,20] studies and 45% in the Satterfield[27] study. In addition, the nature of the offenses was more serious in the Satterfield study.

What can explain these differences? The Feldman study is atypical in that it included children diagnosed as MBD, not all of whom were hyperactive. All were middle class and had had various therapies. These factors could explain the more hopeful outcome.

Satterfield himself suggests that his worse outcome may be the result of obtaining data from courts rather than from the subjects themselves, as well as of not losing any subjects. (It is known that those lost to follow-up represent a worse outcome group.[28]) It seems unlikely, however, that in other studies arrests were seriously under-reported, in that it would not be in parents' interest to lie about this since they were coming to the professional for help. Also, parents of juveniles have to attend court hearings with their adolescents, so that they would be aware of any arrests. Certainly not losing subjects may indeed have been one factor in the worse outcome of this study.

In addition, adolescents in the Satterfield study were older than the adolescents in the other studies, and the study is a more recent one. It is known that crime committed by youth is on the increase. It is also possible that more of the adolescents in Los Angeles carry lethal weapons, particularly handguns. The latter in the hands of antisocial and/or impulsive hyperactive adolescents is an unfortunate combination. Several of the major crimes committed by the adolescents in the Satterfield study were "assault with a deadly weapon." That the culture in Los Angeles is indeed different from the culture in many other areas can be seen from the relatively high percentage of serious arrests even in the normal control group. All this suggests that social factors are relevant as well as biological and psychological ones in determining adolescent outcome of hyperactivity.

Of course the question of why the hyperactive adolescent is vulnerable to antisocial acts is not possible to answer definitively. Besides a possible primary deficit in social learning, it has been emphasized that the parent–hyperactive child relationship tends to be a frustrating one, sometimes from the beginning. In addition, the constant experiences of failure and punishment, as described in Chapter 21, written autobiographically by a "hyperactive" adult, suggest the development of certain attitudes which could have turned the tide (but in his case did not) toward an antisocial kind of adjustment.

Loney and coworkers,[29,30] in their work on predictive factors, suggest that childhood hyperactivity is not the first link in the chain that leads to adolescent delinquency. In their model, childhood hyperactivity and specifically childhood aggressivity have different correlates both at referral and at follow-up. It seems that we still do not yet completely understand all the factors which contribute to an antisocial outcome.

ADULTHOOD

CHAPTER FIVE

THE ADULT HYPERACTIVE: PSYCHIATRIC STATUS

I say: fear not! Life still
Leaves human effort scope
But since life teems with ill
Nurse no extravagant hope.
Because thou must not dream,
Thus need'st not then despair!
—From *Empedocles on Etna*, by Matthew Arnold, 1822–1888

Are you sick or sullen?
—From letter to Boswell, by Samuel Johnson, 1704–1784

In the previous chapter outcome studies were reviewed which evaluated the hyperactive child when he had reached adolescence. The studies indicated that while the target symptoms of the syndrome (hyperactivity, distractibility, and impulsivity) had abated and were not usually the main problems complained about, they nevertheless continued to be present in most hyperactive adolescents. Main complaints from parents and adolescents now centered around poor school work, social difficulties with peers, problems related to authority figures (e.g., teachers), and low self-esteem.[1,2] The studies reviewed, while in agreement on most findings, differed from one another regarding the percentage of hyperactive adolescents involved in antisocial behavior, as well as the severity of the offenses committed by them.

Once hyperactive adolescents reach adulthood, from a theoretical point of view, it would be hard to predict whether their general functioning would now improve. Since adult life offers more varieties of life-styles and opportunities than does life in secondary school, one might predict that the "turbulent" hyperactive adolescent might settle down to a more productive and satisfying adult life. Alternatively, since as we know social skills, learning ability, and ability for reflection have been impaired since early childhood, it is equally possible that hyperactive adults would not be able to master the responsbilities of adult life. Some of the literature on hyperactives as adults will be selected and summarized, to help answer these questions.

In reviewing retrospective and prospective studies, we shall concentrate on those which included a control group. Only occasionally will a study be cited which lacked this important aspect of the design. In appraising the findings from the various investigations examining the outcome in adult life, we shall also try to assess whether the findings have sufficient agreement to support the concept of the predictive validity of the hyperactive syndrome.

There are two types of retrospective studies. The first type examines old charts of children seen in child psychiatry or child guidance clinics 2 to 25 years previously. The diagnosis of hyperactive child syndrome is made or confirmed retrospectively, and the investigators then attempt to trace and interview those subjects in whom the diagnosis could be clearly made. This methodology of retrospective studies was used to assess adolescent outcome as described in the previous chapter.

Another type of retrospective study starts by identifying a deviant adult population (e.g., psychiatry outpatients or alcoholics) and then makes a retrospective diagnosis of hyperactive child syndrome from the information obtained about the childhood history of these patients. We shall for convenience call these "follow-back" studies. While some of them will be reviewed in this chapter because of their inherent interest, follow-back studies have generally been uncontrolled. They also have the methodological difficulty of relying, for the childhood history, on the memories of the now-adult patients (or their parents), information which may go back as far as 20 years. We shall start by reviewing retrospective studies, then follow-back studies, and finally controlled prospective studies.

RETROSPECTIVE STUDIES

The oldest available retrospective study is that of Menkes *et al.* from Johns Hopkins in 1967.[3] It was the first study to assess outcome well into adult life (22 to 40 years) and is very frequently quoted, even though the study has certain methodological difficulties (including the lack of a control group), which will be discussed at the end of the chapter.

Menkes and coworkers traced and evaluated 14 of 18 subjects seen approximately 25 years earlier (1937–1946) in the Johns Hopkins Child Psychiatry Outpatient Clinic for problems of hyperactivity and learning difficulties. The diagnosis was established retrospectively from the charts. At the time of follow-up, the subjects were interviewed by one or more of the authors and were given a neurological examination.

Results indicated that 4 patients were in institutions where they were diagnosed as psychotic. Two patients were clearly retarded and were leading dependent lives with their families. Eight patients were currently self-supporting, but 4 of these 8 had spent some time in an institution. Three subjects complained that they still suffered from hyperactivity: "they felt restless and had a hard time settling down to anything . . ." (p. 396).[3]

Quite different results were obtained in a controlled 20- to 25-year retrospective study by Borland and Heckman.[4] These investigators traced 20 of 37 men who in their childhood had conformed to diagnostic criteria for the hyperactive child syndrome. Their mean age was 30 years. Nineteen brothers of these subjects were interviewed and served as a control group. Results indicated that the majority of men who had been hyperactive when they were children were now steadily employed and self-supporting. However, half of the subjects continued to show symptoms of the hyperactive syndrome. In addition, the hyperactive subjects had not attained as high a socioeconomic status as their brothers. Four of 20 subjects were antisocial and many were symptomatic, even though overall they had done well and had reached middle-class status.

Feldman and coworkers[5] in Rhode Island carried out a 5-year retrospective study of 81 adults whose mean age was 21 years, and, like Borland and Heckman, they chose 32 older brothers as the control group. These subjects were of middle-class status and had received various forms of therapy, including stimulants. They were originally diagnosed as having Minimal Brain Dysfunction or Hyperkinetic Impulse Disorder. Results indicated that about half of the group had no further symptoms or sequelae of the original syndrome. The use of stimulant medication was not associated with increased alcohol or nonmedical drug use in adulthood. A higher proportion of the subjects than of the controls had used marijuana. Their self-esteem was significantly lower than that of their brothers. Ninety-one percent were either at work or at school, and only 10% were considered to have serious emotional or behavior problems. In general, the findings of this study are similar to those of Borland and coworkers, but there is a lower percentage of antisocial problems in these subjects.

A recent retrospective study by Loney[6] will be reviewed in detail in Chapter 6 and only briefly referred to here. She evaluated 22 proband–brother pairs mainly with respect to (1) alcohol and nonmedical drug use; (2) carrying weapons; (3) aggressive acts; (4) antisocial behaviors including court appearances and sentences; and (5) Antisocial Personality Disorder (using modified Schedule for Affective Disorders and Schizophrenia, Lifetime Version, SADS-L, criteria). For the purpose of this chapter it is of interest that 45% of hyperactive subjects versus 18% of their brothers were diagnosed as having an antisocial personality disorder.

FOLLOW-BACK STUDIES

Wood and coworkers[7] selected from a psychiatric outpatient clinic 15 adults whose predominant symptoms were impulsivity, poor attention, restlessness, and emotional lability. The parents of these patients completed the Abbreviated Conners Parent Rating Scale based on their memory of their children when they were 6 to 10 years of age. Two-thirds of these parent ratings placed the adult patient in the 95th percentile for hyperactivity during the middle-childhood years. The implication of this finding was that these adult psychiatric patients were still manifesting continued problems of the hyperactive child syndrome. The limitation of this interesting study is the lack of a control group such as psychiatric patients with different presenting problems and the uncertain validity of parents scoring the childhood behaviors of their now-adult children.

A second follow-back study was carried out by Shelley and Riester[8] on 16 young adults serving in the U.S. Air Force. The subjects experienced difficulty in performing certain routines expected of them, such as marching properly, learning judo, and other tasks requiring fine and gross motor skills. As a result, they experienced anxiety and self-depreciation and reported difficulties in impulse control and concentration. On a neurological evaluation, most were found to be clumsy, and half of the group had dysdiadochokinesis or finger apraxia. Their mean Performance IQ on the Wechsler Adult Intelligence Scale (WAIS) was 22 points below their Verbal IQ. The parents of these men revealed that as children most had been regarded as overactive and had experienced difficulties at school. Subsequently these men had improved, until on entering the Air Force they were required to perform tasks which they found difficult. The implication of this study is similar to that of the study of Wood and coworkers, namely that the symptoms of the childhood syndrome continued into adult life. However, the subjects in this study did not become symptomatic until they were required to carry out tasks which they could not master. The methodological difficulty with this study is similar to that of the previous one, namely that there was no control group and that the childhood syndrome was diagnosed many years later from the memories of the parents.

In another study of similar methodology, 133 Danish adoptees were carefully evaluated as to current psychiatric status. The investigators, Goodwin and coworkers,[9] diagnosed 14 of the adoptees as alcoholic and compared the childhood histories of those who were alcoholic to the remainder of the group, who acted as controls. They found that 43% of the alcoholics (compared with 15% of controls) had below-average school performance; 50% were hyperactive, compared to 15% of controls; 21% were antisocial, compared to 2% of controls; 64% were shy, sensitive, insecure, compared to 20% of controls; 50% were aggressive and impulsive, compared to 18% of controls; and 29% were "often disobedient," compared to 4% of controls. This study suggests that alcoholics are more likely to have a childhood history resembling the hyperactive syndrome than are normal controls (nonalcoholic adoptees).

The final follow-back study to be described is also the most recent and comprehensive. Gomez and coworkers in 1981[10] evaluated 100 psychiatric inpatient veterans and compared them with 28 normal controls. The patients were divided into four categories: psychotics (26), affective disorders (25), alcoholics (24), and character disorders (15). Only organic brain disorders were excluded. The investigators derived a screening instrument to evaluate a childhood history of the hyperactive syndrome by utilizing 12 of 61 behavioral items from the Wender Utah Personality Inventory. Sixteen items were selected from the Utah Personality Inventory current-behavior questionnaire to screen for the adult hyperactive syndrome. Each item, scored on a 5-item scale, related to attention deficit, hyperactivity, or impulsivity.

The overall percentage of patients reporting a childhood history of the hyperactive syndrome was 32%, versus 4% of controls ($p < .0005$). Furthermore, 20% of patients reported both a childhood history and adult symptoms of hyperactivity, compared to none in the control group. Character-disorder patients reported the greatest prevalence of a childhood history of the hyperactive syndrome.

These follow-back studies all indicate that symptoms of the hyperactive child syndrome may continue into adult life[7,8] and predispose to alcoholism[9] and psychiatric illness, most particularly to character disorders.[10] They do not give us a clear idea as to the specificity of the adult psychiatric status of hyperactive children. The question therefore arises as to whether there is any predictive validity to the syndrome's outcome in adult life, or whether the childhood condition predisposes the individual to all types of psychopathology in adult life.

In order to get a clearer idea of these possibilities we will review the 15-year prospective controlled follow-up studies carried out by the current authors at the Montreal Children's Hospital. The first of these studies, the 5-year follow-up, has already been described (see Chapter 4, pp. 55–56) and was carried out when the subjects were adolescent. The findings of both the 10-year follow-up (when the mean age of the subjects was 19 years) and the 15-year follow-up (when the mean age of the subjects was 25 years) will now be described in some detail. In this chapter we shall focus on the psychiatric status and biographical information of the subjects, omitting aspects such as their antisocial behavior, alcohol and nonmedical drug use and abuse, work record, self-esteem, social skills, and physiological parameters, which will be dealt with in subsequent chapters.

TEN-YEAR PROSPECTIVE CONTROLLED FOLLOW-UP STUDY FROM THE MONTREAL CHILDREN'S HOSPITAL[11-15]

The methodology of this follow-up study will be described in detail here; it will not be repeated in subsequent chapters.

Originally, in 1962–1965, 104 hyperactive children were included in the study and took part in a series of acute drug studies determining the efficacy of chlorpromazine[16] and dextroamphetamine[17] on their behavior and intellectual functioning. At the time of assessment, all children were 6 to 12 years of age, and they were admitted into the study if they met the following inclusion and exclusion criteria:

1. Restlessness and poor concentration were their main complaints and had been present since their earliest years.
2. The complaints were a major source of problems at home and at school (i.e., condition was pervasive).
3. All children had WISC IQ's (Full Scale) of above 85.
4. None of the children were psychotic, borderline psychotic, epileptic, or had cerebral palsy.
5. All children were living at home with a least one parent.

Although there was a marked similarity in the presenting complaints of these children, they differed from one another with respect to socioeconomic status; personality characteristics; family functioning; presence, absence, degree, and type of learning disability; degree of severity of presenting complaints; and degree of conduct disorder associated with hyperactivity. Although DSM-III was not available at that time, it is our impression in retrospect that all our children had ADD(H) and the majority had associated conduct problems (mild to severe).

Loss of subjects is a problem for most follow-up studies, since there exists good evidence that those lost to follow-up represent not a random group but a group with poorer outcome.[18,19] While we did all we could to trace subjects, using every method possible, and offered every conceivable realistic reward to avoid refusals, nevertheless in the 10-year follow-up we did not succeed in interviewing more than 76 of 104 subjects. The 28 subjects not seen included 19 not traced and 9 refusals. One subject was dropped from the analysis because he had become "retarded" from glue sniffing. The 28 subjects not seen were compared on initial measures to the 75 subjects who took part in the analysis. There was a trend for those lost to follow-up to have higher initial ratings of aggressivity, but no differences were seen in initial socioeconomic status, WISC IQ, or severity of target symptoms.

Treatment Received by the Hyperactives during Their Elementary-School Years

Ten children in the group had received individual psychotherapy or family therapy (defined as more than 25 regularly scheduled visits). The remainder of the group had been seen for 10 to 25 interviews, mainly for crisis intervention and drug management. The 75 hyperactive subjects had received varying lengths and types of drug therapy during their first 5 years of treatment. None had received methylphenidate, but 6 had received dextroamphetamine for 6 to 48 months. Nine subjects had a mixed drug history, 27 subjects had received chlorpromazine only for 6 to 48 months, and 35 subjects had received no drug for longer than 6 months. In general, the group represented a relatively untreated group, with few receiving adequate counseling or drug therapy.

Seventeen subjects who had received chlorpromazine for 18 to 48 months were compared on all the outcome measures with 21 subjects who had received no drug for longer than 6 months. The two groups were matched on age, IQ, sex, and socioeconomic status. No differences related to treatment were found.

The Control Group

Forty-five normal subjects were selected for the control group, but one of these was later dropped for the purpose of matching the groups. Thirty-five of these were selected in 1968 at the time of the 5-year follow-up study of hyperactive children. At that time, notices were posted in three high schools, asking for volunteers who would participate in some studies on adolescents in which they would be required to talk with a psychiatrist and do some pencil-and-paper tasks. Payment was offered for volunteers who were selected. The three high schools were selected to represent a range of socioeconomic statuses. Many students volunteered, and we included those who met all the following criteria: (1) they matched individually with a hyperactive subject on age, WISC IQ, socioeconomic status, and sex; (2) they had never failed a grade; and (3) neither teacher nor parents complained that they were or had been a behavior problem.

At the beginning of the 10-year follow-up (1974), we decided to enlarge our control group from 35 to 45 subjects. Accordingly, 10 additional subjects were included, generally referred to us by another control subject as being someone they knew at work or school (high school, college, or university). The inclusion criteria already described were used to select these additional volunteers.

Results

BIOGRAPHICAL DATA

Fewer hyperactive subjects than controls were still living with their parents (76% vs. 95%), and hyperactives made more geographic moves than controls (mean 2.8 vs. 1.2, $p < .01$). They had a significantly higher number of *car accidents* than controls (mean 1.3 vs. 0.07, $p < .05$) although the number of subjects who had car accidents was not significant. Their *school history* indicated that they had completed less education. Significantly more hyperactives were still in high school at follow-up evaluation. Their average marks were lower, and they discontinued high school for this reason more often than controls. They failed more grades in elementary and high school than controls, and they were expelled significantly more frequently. No one school subject was found to be responsible for their failure.

PSYCHIATRIC ASSESSMENT

There was no significant difference between the two groups with respect to their ability to relate to the examiner, their verbal ability in the interview, and the number or type of spontaneous complaints. The two groups were significantly different in the number of problems of adjustment elicited by probing during the psychiatric interview, although the types of problems were not different. There was a trend for the hyperactives to have fewer friends. Significantly more hyperactives felt restless during the interview, and significantly more hyperactives were observed to be restless (although actually getting off the chair was rare). Personality-trait disorders were diagnosed significantly more often in the hyperactive subjects than in controls. The two most frequent types of trait disorder in the hyperactives were "impulsive" and "immature–dependent," compared to "depressive" and "obsessive–compulsive" in the control group. Two hyperactive subjects were diagnosed as borderline psychotic (this did not reach significance), and no subjects in either group were psychotic.

Personality-trait disorders were considered to be less severe with respect to deviance in functioning than borderline personality disorders. The personality-trait disorders (impulsive, immature, obsessive–compulsive, and depressive) were diagnosed when these traits were apparent in many life situations and over several years. These traits were considered to be "characterological" rather than clinical states. They did not prevent the subject from functioning socially, attending school, or holding jobs.

In contrast, each of the 2 hyperactive subjects diagnosed as borderline psychotic had had one or more psychiatric hospitalizations, one for attempted suicide and the other for severe anxiety and depression. Both suffered from chronic anxiety and depression severe enough to prevent them from holding jobs or attending school. One was socially isolated, and the second had a number of casual acquaintances who were engaged (like him) in drug dealing. On being interviewed, the level of anxiety of these 2 subjects resulted in disorganized thinking; a history was obtained with difficulty. However, neither subject had a schizophrenic type of thought disorder or had ever had hallucinations or delusions, and so neither could be diagnosed as schizophrenic.

BRIEF PSYCHIATRIC RATING SCALE. Of the 16 items on this scale,[20] anxiety, tension, grandiosity, and hostility were significantly higher in the hyperactive group. The sum of all scores was significantly worse in the hyperactive group. No differences were found in somatic concern, emotional withdrawal, conceptual disorganization, guilt feelings, mannerisms, depressive mood, suspiciousness, hallucinatory behavior, motor retardation, uncooperativeness, or unusual thought content.

PERCEPTION OF CHILDHOOD. As part of the psychiatric interview, hyperactive subjects were asked "what had helped them most during their childhood." The commonest responses recorded were that someone, usually the mother, believed in their final success, or that a teacher seemed to turn the tide of failure. Also, they discovered that they had some special talent. When asked "what made things worse," the commonest responses were family fights (usually concerning the hyperactive subject), feeling different (inferior, "dumb"), and being criticized. Significantly more hyperactives than controls rated their childhood as unhappy.

SELF-RATING SCALES. Subjects rated themselves on the California Psychological Inventory (CPI),[21] which was originally designed to tap cultural ideals of self-esteem and social interaction, and on the SCL-90,[22] which was designed to measure classical psychopathology such as that found in psychiatric outpatient clinics. On the CPI hyperactive subjects rated themselves significantly worse than controls on 9 of 18 items and had worse scores (not statistically significant) on the other 9 items. The SCL-90 did not, at 10-year follow-up, differentiate the hyperactive and control groups.

The conclusion drawn from this study of hyperactives as young adults was that compared to controls they were having difficulties in several areas:

1. They had more impulsive personality traits, more accidents, and made more geographic moves.

2. They achieved a significantly lower level of education and left school because of low marks and expulsion.

3. They rated themselves lower on a personality inventory designed to measure self-esteem and social integration.

4. They rated themselves as more pathological on the brief psychiatric rating scale.

5. While 2 subjects had severe borderline personality disorders and were not functioning (too few to be significant statistically), none were diagnosed as schizophrenic.

6. The subjects could be divided into three groups.[23] First are those who had in terms of their functioning outgrown the symptoms of the syndrome (this healthy group has been found by several other investigators.[4,5] Second is a group (about 50% or more of the total) who continue to have significant problems of the original syndrome, particularly problems of impulsivity and hyperactivity.[4,5] These continuing problems interfere to varying degrees with their work and interpersonal functioning and are associated with low self-esteem and various psychiatric symptoms of anxiety. The third group is small and is made up of hyperactive adults who have severe psychopathology (borderline personality disorders) or are chronic severe offenders of the law. (For further details of these groupings, see Chapter 13.)

FIFTEEN-YEAR PROSPECTIVE FOLLOW-UP STUDY FROM THE MONTREAL CHILDREN'S HOSPITAL

This study, which has recently been completed,[24] was undertaken because we felt that the subjects at 10-year follow-up (mean age 19 years) were too young for either hyperactives or controls to have reached the maximum age of risk for psychiatric disorders.

Of the 75 subjects evaluated for the 10-year follow-up, we were able to interview 63 for the purpose of the 15-year follow-up, that is, 83% of the group. However, if we consider the 104 subjects who were originally included in the study, 35 subjects (33.6%) were for various reasons lost to the 15-year follow-up: 23 were untraced, 9 refused, and 3 have died (2 in accidents and 1 from suicide).

In addition, 6 subjects only agreed to be interviewed by telephone, and whenever possible, their parents were seen instead. Because of the lower reliability of this information, it was not included in the analysis which was finally carried out on 61 subjects (the results from 2 subjects not being ready for inclusion in the statistical analysis).

Of 45 controls seen originally, 1 could not be traced, 2 refused to be seen again, and 1 lived too far away. Hence the results of 41 controls were analyzed, together with the results of 61 hyperactive adults.

Evaluations

Psychiatric status was evaluated in several different ways:

1. A semistructured interview given by one of two qualified psychiatrists (G. W. or L. H.), from which the diagnosis was made jointly according to DSM-III[25] criteria. Neither of the two psychiatrists was blind as to which subjects were hyperactive.

2. The SADS-L[26] was administered by a qualified psychiatrist (T. M.) who had not previously participated in the study and who was blind as to which subjects were hyperactive. He was assisted at each interview by a research assistant (T. P.). The SADS-L was modified from a lifetime version to the past 5 years, except for the category of Antisocial Personality Disorder.

3. Self-rating scales: the SCL-90[22] and CPI.[21]

In addition to the above, histories of alcohol use and abuse, nonmedical drug use and abuse, court and police records of antisocial behavior, and work record were obtained in separate interviews by one of two research assistants (T. P. or D. T.), who also administered tests of social skills and self-esteem. All tests and interviews were administered in the same order (as far as possible) to both controls and hyperactives.

At the conclusion of the data collection of this study, all four authors met regularly for the purpose of reviewing all sources of information for each individual hyperactive or control subject in turn. At this time not only was all information summarized but a DSM-III diagnosis was made jointly by the two psychiatrists. Where agreement was not immediately present (which was rare), the mass of material was gone over until a consensus was obtained on the diagnosis.

In addition, each subject was discussed by the four investigators in order to assign a number (1–99) on the Global Assessment Scale (GAS) of the SADS-L.[26] This scale measured the general level of everyday-life adjustment.

Results

BACKGROUND INFORMATION

The hyperactive subjects and controls were not different with respect to socioeconomic status, age, or sex, but there was a trend for the control group to have a higher IQ on the WAIS (see Table 5-1). There was a significant difference between the years of education completed,

TABLE 5-1. Background Variables: 15-Year Follow-Up

	Controls (n = 41)	Hyperactives (n = 61)	Significance
Age (years)	25.2	25.1	
Range (years)	21–32	21–33	
IQ (WAIS Full Scale)	108.5	105.2	$p < .09$ (trend)
Number of subjects in socioeconomic status (Hollingshead Scale)			
1	1	4	
2	6	5	
3	14	24	
4	13	24	
5	7	2	
Number of males	38 (90%)	58 (90%)	
Number of females	4	6	
Education completed			
University degree	17	3	
High school	20	37	$p < .01$
Never completed high school	4	19	
Mean number of children	0.12	0.76	$p < .04$
Number of geographic moves			
Past year	0.65	0.83	
2 years ago	0.65	0.50	
3 years ago	0.63	0.37	
Living arrangements			
Living alone	8	12	
Living with opposite sex (not married)	3	11	
Married	12	18	
Separated or divorced	1	2	
Living with parents	15	16	

with the hyperactives completing less education. The hyperactives had significantly more children, but there was no difference between the percentage of subjects in each group who were married, divorced, separated, living alone, or living with a member of the opposite sex.

CONTINUING SYMPTOMS OF THE SYNDROME

This was measured in three different ways (see Table 5-2):

1. Sixty-six percent of the hyperactives on probing complained of at least one symptom (restlessness, poor concentration, impulsivity, explosiveness) of the syndrome, versus 7% of the controls. In addition, the problem was less severe in those controls who complained of a symptom. Items on the SCL-90 directly related to the hyperactive syndrome were included if the subject rated himself or herself as having the problem to a moderate or severe degree (i.e., 3 or 4 on a scale from 0 to 4 where 4 indicated the problem was present "extremely").

2. Significantly more hyperactives than controls complained that they *"felt* restless." This was systematically probed for all subjects.

3. The two psychiatrists, while completing the history and psychiatric-status interview (which lasted 1–1½ hours), rated the amount of movement of the subject on a 3-point scale where 1 represented normal; 2 represented repeated, usually small muscle movements (e.g., foot or finger tapping or frequent changes of position); and 3 represented getting up from the chair and moving around at least once during the interview. (Movements connected with smoking were excluded.) Significantly more hyperactives than controls were found to be

TABLE 5-2. Continuing Symptoms of the Syndrome

	Controls (n = 41)	Hyperactives (n = 61)	Significance
Presence of one or more mildly to severely disabling symptoms (restless, distractible, impulsive)	3 (7%)	39 (66%)	$p < .0001$
Severity of above			
Mild	2	17	
Moderate	1	13	
Severe		9	
Number who complained of feeling restless (question probed)	14 (29%)	38 (64%)	$p < .01$
Number observed to be restless during interview	4 (9.7%)	26 (44%)	$p < .0001$

restless (44% vs. 9.7% of controls), and the quality of restlessness related more to small muscle movements or changing positions frequently than to getting up and moving around at least once.

PSYCHIATRIC HISTORY (see Table 5-3)

Fewer hyperactive subjects than controls were "normal." Here "normal" was defined as having no psychiatric diagnosis, functioning well in all areas, and having no significant symptoms. This "supernormality" was seen in 33% of controls and in 11% of hyperactives, and is obviously rare even in the control subjects.

There was a trend for more hyperactives than controls to have a higher number of symptoms unrelated to the hyperactive syndrome. Significantly more hyperactives than controls complained of sexual problems (homosexuality, premature ejaculation, occasional impotence).

When the complaints or symptoms of all subjects were categorized into neurotic, psychotic, somatic, interpersonal, or autonomy-related problems, no difference was found between the two groups on somatic symptoms, psychotic symptoms, or symptoms related to autonomy. However, significantly more hyperactives complained of neurotic and interpersonal problems, and the number of "symptom groups" per subject was higher for the hyperactives. There was a trend for the hyperactives to have more acts of physical aggression "in the past 3 years," but they did not report more verbal aggression (e.g., severe arguments). There were significantly more suicide attempts in the hyperactive group (6 compared to 0), and 1 hyperactive died from suicide.

DIAGNOSIS (see Table 5-4)

From Table 5-4 it can be seen that on the semistructured, nonblind interview there was a trend for a higher percentage of hyperactives to be given a DSM-III diagnosis, and significantly more hyperactives than controls were given more than one diagnosis. The hyperactives scored significantly worse on the GAS, which measured overall functioning. Final scores for each subject on this scale were arrived at following joint discussion by all four investigators, who took into account the subject's total record. The only single DSM-III diagnosis which distinguished the two groups was Antisocial Personality Disorder, which was found in 2.4% of controls and 23% of hyperatives (see Table 5-5).

The 12 subjects who refused to take the SADS-L interview were diagnosed for Antisocial Personality Disorder according to the criteria

TABLE 5-3. Psychiatric History

	Controls ($n = 41$)	Hyperactives ($n = 61$)	Significance
Normal (no spontaneous complaints; doing well; no diagnosis)	14 (33%)	7 (11%)	$p < .0008$
Number of subjects spontaneously complaining of symptoms not directly related to hyperactive syndrome	26 (63%)	50 (82%)	$p < .07$ (trend)
Number of subjects complaining of sexual problems	1 (2.4%)	11 (20%)	$p < .03$
Number of subjects complaining of neurotic problems	21 (51%)	48 (79%)	$p < .01$
Number of subjects complaining of psychotic problems	1 (2.4%)	5 (8.2%)	
Number of subjects complaining of interpersonal problems	22 (54%)	46 (75%)	$p < .05$
Number of subjects complaining of somatic symptoms	16	27	
Number of subjects complaining of symptoms related to autonomy, self-esteem, and direction	28	41	
Number of above 5 symptom groups per subject (possible 5)	3.5	4.5	$p < .002$
Suicidal thoughts in past 3 years	11	24	
Suicide attempts in past 3 years	0	6	$p < .04$ (1 died)
Deaths from accidents or suicide during 15 years of follow-up	0	3	(no analysis done)
Period of alcohol abuse in past 3 years (months)	11	27	
Problems with physical aggression	2	12	$p < .07$ (trend)

TABLE 5-4. Psychiatric Interview (Nonblind, Semistructured)

	Controls (n = 41)	Hyperactives (n = 61)	Significance
Number of subjects given a DSM-III diagnosis	14	32	$p < .09$ (trend)
Number of subjects carrying more than one DSM-III diagnosis	2	22	$p < .01$
Global Assessment Scale	3.7[a]	4.4[a]	$p < .0007$

[a]Percentile means.

TABLE 5-5. Psychiatric Interview (Blind, Structured) Diagnosis of Antisocial Personality Disorder

	Controls	Hyperactives	Significance
	(n = 37)	(n = 51)	
Strict SADS criteria for Antisocial Personality Disorder	0	1	
Modified SADS criteria for Antisocial Personality Disorder (omitting necessity of having "no one they feel close to")	1	11	$p < .05$
Modified SADS criteria for Antisocial Personality Disorder as well as adding information more accurately obtained elsewhere	1	1	$p < .01$
	(n = 41)	(n = 61)	
DSM-III diagnosis of Antisocial Personality Disorder	1 (2.4%)	14 (23%)	$p < .01$

of this scale, and any subjects scoring as fitting into this diagnosis were included. While only 1 of 61 subjects fitted strict SADS-L criteria for this diagnosis, the number was increased to 23% of the group (14 subjects) when the criteria were modified by omitting the necessity of "having no one they felt close to" and by adding information more accurately obtained elsewhere (Table 5-5).

It should be noted that the DSM-III diagnosis requires "clinical judgment." For example, Section D in the DSM-III diagnosis of Antisocial Personality Disorder states that "the rights of others must be violated through chronic antisocial acts." In 5 of our 14 subjects thus diagnosed the rights of others were violated by the following possibly *minor* antisocial acts:

- Derek: "drunk almost nightly in bars while not working and using common-law wife's money against her will."
- Wayne: drunken driving leading to an accident without carrying insurance; failure to pay back money borrowed, and no specific plan for this; physical fights (usually but not always when drunk).
- James: physical fights in bars while drunk; intermittent shoplifting (not caught).
- Barry: no plans to pay debts; failure to pay parking tickets (arrested for this); physical fights (usually but not always when drunk).
- Jennifer: drinks heavily, often drunk; difficult to live with when drunk; abuses drugs; gets into physical fights.

These subjects clearly met DSM-III criteria A, B, C, and E.

In general, one-third of our DSM-III antisocial personalities were mild, and might have been excluded from the diagnosis by some investigators.

SELF-RATING SCALES (see Tables 5-6 and 5-7)

CPI (Table 5-6). This self-rating inventory seemed to tap differences between hyperactives and controls very sensitively. As seen from the table, out of 18 possible items, hyperactives scored themselves significantly more negatively on 8 items, there was a trend for hyperactives to score themselves more negatively on 5 items, and no differences between the two groups were seen on 5 items. On no items did the control group score itself more negatively.

SCL-90 (Table 5-7). On this self-rating scale of classical psychopathology, hyperactives scored themselves worse on somatization, phobic anxiety, and overall scores of psychopathology. They did not score themselves different from controls on psychoticism, paranoid ideation, hostility, anxiety, depression, or interpersonal sensitivity. On this same

TABLE 5-6. California Psychological Inventory

	Controls (n = 33)	Hyperactives (n = 42)	Significance
Dominance	48.9	46.0	
Capacity for status	48.0	43.8	$p < .06$ (trend)
Social ability	51.6	46.9	$p < .06$ (trend)
Social pressure	56.0	54.5	
Self-acceptance	56.0	53.7	
Sense of well-being	48.2	37.5	$p < .001$
Responsibility	43.1	32.7	$p < .001$
Socialization	47.7	35.4	$p < .001$
Self-control	48.0	40.8	$p < .01$
Tolerance	48.4	38.9	$p < .001$
Good impression	45.8	41.7	$p < .1$ (trend)
Community	50.3	46.4	$p < .1$ (trend)
Achievement conformance	48.6	39.5	$p < .003$
Independence	53.7	46.5	$p < .002$
Intellectual efficiency	50.4	40.0	$p < .001$
Psychological mindedness	53.6	49.7	$p < .09$ (trend)
Flexibility	51.1	51.7	
Feminine–masculine	49.6	50.8	

TABLE 5-7. SCL-90 (Means on Scale of 0–4)

	Controls (n = 39)	Hyperactives (n = 60)	Significance
Somatization	0.4	0.6	$p < .04$
Obsessive–compulsive	0.7	0.9	
Interpersonal sensitivity	0.7	0.8	
Depression	0.7	0.7	
Anxiety	0.5	0.7	
Hostility	0.5	0.6	
Phobic anxiety	0.1	0.3	$p < .03$
Paranoid ideation	0.8	0.9	
Psychoticism	0.3	0.4	
Global	0.5	0.8	$p < .004$

scale 5 years earlier, no differences were obtained between hyperactive young adults and controls,[14] indicating some increase in symptomatology over the years.

Certain aspects of our methodology require further discussion. It has been shown in other studies that subjects lost to follow-up, rather than representing a random sample of the whole group, represent those whose outcome is worse.[18,19] It was also our own impression that the subjects who were hard to trace, and who were interviewed near the end of the study for this reason, sometimes had more psychopathology. This was somewhat mitigated by our impression that those who refused completely to be interviewed (9 subjects), and those who were interviewed on the telephone (6 subjects) but whose results were not included in the analysis, represented a healthier group whose reasons for not wanting to come in were generally that they were doing well and did not want to be reminded of the past. In some cases this was confirmed by their parents. In summary, we cannot know how our findings were affected by our inability to interview all subjects seen initially. It is possible that some of the subjects not traced (33.6%) may have died or been in jail. We could say that the findings represent a minimal estimate of the degree of psychopathology, personality disorders, and continuing symptoms of the syndrome in adulthood of children who were diagnosed as hyperactive 15 years previously.

The diagnosis of Antisocial Personality Disorder requires further comment. We diagnosed this according to three different diagnostic criteria which gave us three different results. Using DSM-III criteria, 23% of the hyperactive subjects were given this diagnosis compared to 2.4% of the normal subjects. Using the SADS-L criteria, only 1 hyperactive subject and no controls were diagnosed Antisocial Personality Disorder. The difference was due to the section on the SADS-L requiring seriously impaired personal relationships to be present for the diagnosis to be made. The question asked of the subject is, "Is there one person you feel very close to?" and the majority of our subjects answered this in the affirmative. When we left out this section of the SADS-L (as was done by Loney and coworkers[6] in their recent follow-up study), 11 hyperactive subjects were given the diagnosis, a figure which corresponds more closely to the figure obtained with the DSM-III. When information was included which was given more accurately in other interviews, the number of Antisocial Personality Disorders on the modified SADS-L increased to 14 (23%). This highlights the importance of the specific diagnostic criteria used for this personality disorder and may account in part for different results between different investigators.

One may ask whether the fact that we relied on the subjects' own information resulted in gross underestimate of various types of deviance. However, after the study was completed, we collected official court records for all subjects, including those lost to the follow-up. Of the latter, 3.7% had known criminal records. Of those interviewed, only 1 subject (who later suicided) failed to give us accurate information on criminal offenses. (Traffic offenses were omitted from the above correlation.) If we take criminal court records as one measure of whether subjects were honest with us, it seems that this was not a problem.

Our results regarding the percentage of Antisocial Personality Disorder (23%) are below those obtained by Loney et al. in 1981 (45%).[6] In addition, the severity of offenses in our group was less serious than for the subjects in both Loney's and Satterfield et al.'s[29] studies. (The latter is reported in detail in both Chapters 4 and 6).

These discrepancies with other studies may be partially explained by the likelihood that fewer of our hyperactive subjects carried weapons. Unfortunately, unlike Loney, we did not systematically explore this at the time of the study. After, we recalled 10 of the more severe subjects, and of these none carried or had carried guns or weapons. It is likely that weapons carried by people with impulsive personality traits, such as adult hyperactives, result in violent crimes. Another reason for the discrepancy may have been differences in the types of children originally included in the study. Most of our group had initially at intake what would now be termed ADD(H) *with* conduct problems. The degree of the latter may have been less severe in our subjects.

Gittelman and her coworkers[30] have recently completed a controlled prospective follow-up study of 113 hyperactive children who at follow-up evaluation were 16–23 years old. Her intake criteria were similar to ours, as was the percentage of her subjects who at follow-up had antisocial behaviors. Of particular interest was her finding that there was a marked degree of overlap at follow-up between the presence of ADD(H) (i.e., continued core symptoms of the syndrome) and antisocial behavior. Those subjects who had outgrown the syndrome had no more antisocial behaviors than were found in matched normal controls.

To summarize our results:

1. More than half of the hyperactive adults—66% compared to 7% of normal controls—still had at least one disabling symptom of the hyperactive child syndrome. Almost half of the hyperactive group (44%) were observed to be restless (mostly by fidgeting or changing sitting position frequently) during the psychiatric interview, compared

to 10% of the normal controls. (These observations were not made blind.) In general, the findings indicate that about half of our hyperactive adults had not outgrown all aspects of the syndrome.

2. Two subjects in the hyperactive group and 1 subject in the control group were diagnosed as schizophrenic on the SADS-L and DSM-III. This difference was not significant, indicating that in this study, unlike the early findings of Menkes et al.,[3] there is no evidence that hyperactivity in childhood predisposes to psychosis in adulthood. There was no evidence that adult hyperactives abuse alcohol more than controls. (For details of alcohol use and abuse, see Chapter 8.)

3. Using DSM-III criteria for the diagnosis, 23% of our subjects had an Antisocial Personality Disorder. The figure for the modified SADS-L criteria was similar. No other single diagnosis distinguished the hyperactives from the normal group.

4. On a variety of different measures and on the history, there was evidence that hyperactive adults were doing less well than normal controls. They had less formal education and more symptoms unrelated to the hyperactive syndrome than did normals—for example, symptoms of phobic anxiety, somatization, and sexual problems. They were given more "diagnoses" than normals and scored significantly worse on all items of the CPI, which was designed to measure folkloric ideals of social living and interaction. On the GAS, they scored as functioning much more poorly than normal controls.

5. Hyperactive subjects made significantly more suicide attempts than controls, and 1 subject successfully suicided. Altogether 3 subjects have died, 2 in accidents and 1 from suicide. Although the number does not reach statistical significance, verbal reports from other investigators indicate that this is also true for the hyperactive group in other studies. Only collaborative evaluation could assess the significance of this finding.

SIMILARITIES AND DIFFERENCES OF THE VARIOUS STUDIES OF ADULT OUTCOME

1. In all studies about half of the subjects had a fairly good outcome. This might include some continuing symptoms, but they were not present to a degree that made them significantly disabling. Most subjects were working and self-supporting. The subjects in the Feldman et al. study[5] perhaps had the most optimistic outcome. This may have been because they were middle class and had received more adequate treatment. In addition, it is possible that not all subjects in

Feldman's study were hyperactive. It was shown in Dykman and Ackerman's study[27] that learning-disabled children without hyperactivity have a better outcome than those with hyperactivity. The poor outcome of the subjects in Menkes et al.'s study[3] is at variance with other studies, and the possible reason for this will be discussed.

2. In all studies about 50% of the subjects had mildly or severely disabling continuing symptoms of the syndrome, as well as other symptoms of psychopathology.

3. In all studies reviewed a significant percentage of hyperactive adults compared to controls had Antisocial Personality Disorders or committed antisocial acts. Both the percentage of subjects and the severity of their antisocial acts varied between studies. In two studies[4,24] the percentage was about 23–25%.

4. That there may be a risk for psychosis, as suggested by Menkes et al.'s and Gomez et al.'s studies,[3,10] was not borne out by the main body of studies reviewed.

5. The finding that hyperactives as adolescents consume more alcohol[28] did not in any study reviewed indicate that hyperactive adults had a higher incidence of alcohol abuse or alcoholism.

It seems that Menkes's study is at variance in its finding to the other studies, which show a fair degree of similarity of outcome in spite of their different methodologies. Reasons for this may include the following aspects of the Menkes study:

1. Lack of control group

2. Lack of clear exclusion criteria and the inclusion of the mildly retarded and possibly prepsychotic children

3. The very low socioeconomic status and degree of chaotic family relationships

One may conclude that the hyperactive child syndrome is a pervasive condition in childhood, affecting behavior, social functioning, learning, and self-esteem. While about half of hyperactive children seem to outgrow the symptoms of the syndrome, half continue to be disabled to a varying extent by continuing symptoms. The childhood condition predisposes to various psychiatric diagnoses (but not to schizophrenia or alcoholism) and to increased symptoms of psychopathology. It leads to Antisocial Personality Disorder in a significant minority of the subjects.

While, as mentioned above, the childhood condition predisposes to various kinds of maladjustment in adult life, there is clearly some specificity and predictive validity to the syndrome.

The findings of this 15-year controlled follow-up study, carried out when the subjects were in their mid-20s or older—an age of high risk for adult psychiatric conditions—show some increase of psychiatric morbidity in the subjects compared to 5 years earlier, but in general the findings of the earlier 10-year follow-up study are confirmed.

CHAPTER SIX

ANTISOCIAL BEHAVIOR

Violence is here
In the World of the sane
And violence is a symptom
I hear it in the headlong weeping of men
who have failed
I see it in the terrible dreams of boys.
whose adolescence repeats all history.
—From *The Face of Violence*, by Jacob Bronowski, 1908–1974

There has long been concern about the adult outcome of people diagnosed as hyperactive in childhood. This concern has been particularly marked with regard to adult antisocial behavior. Studies linking these two conditions and thus addressing this concern generally fall into the following types of groupings:

1. Adolescent outcome studies: prospective and retrospective
2. Studies of families of hyperactives.
3. Studies of adult psychiatric and/or antisocial subjects with histories suggesting childhood hyperactivity
4. Adult outcome studies of hyperactive children: prospective and retrospective.

In this chapter we will briefly review only those aspects of the various groups of studies that link hyperactivity in childhood to later antisocial behavior. Results of our prospective 10- and 15-year follow-up studies of hyperactives as adults which pertain to antisocial behavior will be presented, as will some findings related to moral development of these subjects.

ADOLESCENT OUTCOME STUDIES: PROSPECTIVE AND RETROSPECTIVE

Mendelson and coworkers[1] carried out a retrospective study of 83 children diagnosed as hyperactive from initial chart reviews. Mothers were interviewed when the children were 12 to 16 years of age. Some

22% had long histories of antisocial behavior which included lying, stealing, fighting, and destructiveness. Fifteen percent had set fires, and 7% had carried weapons. Fifty-nine percent had had some contact with police, and for 17% this contact occurred three or more times. Twenty-three percent had been taken to the police station one or more times, and 18% had been before the juvenile court. The behavior problems for the group as a whole were so severe that 40% of the parents had seriously considered having their child live away from home, and the authors were concerned that 22% of the sample would become adult sociopaths. In direct interviews with these subjects, Stewart et al.[2] reported that 37% admitted to truancy and 25% to stealing. Unfortunately, no control or comparison group was available.

Weiss[3] and Minde[4,5] and associates (see Chapter 4), in a comprehensive 5-year prospective controlled follow-up study of 91 subjects, age 10–18 (mean age 13.3 years), found that some 25% of the hyperactives had a history of significant antisocial behavior. Ten subjects had court referrals, and 2 had been placed in reform schools.

Ackerman et al.[6] compared four groups of 14-year-old children: 23 hyperactive learning-disabled boys, 25 normoactive learning-disabled boys, 14 hypoactive learning-disabled boys, and 31 controls. All had IQ's of at least 80. The authors found that 6 of the 23 hyperactive learning-disabled adolescents (about 23%) had had recent trouble with school authorities and 3 were in serious trouble with the law—for example, one was an inmate in a state training school, having been caught breaking and entering to support his drug habit, while another had been caught breaking into cars. In contrast, only 4% of the normoactive learning-disabled group and 3% of the controls displayed socially deviant behaviors. This led the authors to conclude that at age 14, hyperactive learning-disabled boys showed academic *and* behavior adjustment problems, whereas normoactive learning-disabled boys showed only academic problems.

The study which shows the clearest and strongest association between hyperactivity and antisocial behavior in adolescents is that of Satterfield et al.[7] The authors studied official arrest records of 110 boys, age 14–21 (mean age 17.3 years), who were diagnosed in childhood as suffering from Attention Deficit Disorder (ADD[H]) and 88 normal control subjects, age 13–20 (mean age 16.9 years). The two groups were matched for socioeconomic status, and most subjects were white. The authors found that the percentage of hyperactives arrested for serious offenses (e.g., robbery, burglary, car theft, and assault with deadly weapon) was significantly greater when compared to controls. For example, the percentages of hyperactive subjects arrested at least once for a serious offense in the lower, middle, and upper socioeconomic statuses were 58%, 36%, and 52%, compared with 11%, 9%, and 2% for the controls. (These figures were significant at the $p < .05$ to $p < .001$ level.) Findings were even more striking for multiple serious arrests, for which percentages for the hyperactives in the lower, middle, and upper socioeconomic statuses were 45%, 25%, and 28%, compared to 6%, 0%, and 0% for the controls. (These figures were significant at the $p < .01$ to $p < .001$ level.)

Again, 25% of the hyperactive group was institutionalized for delinquent behavior compared to 1% of the control group. This outcome was not related to socioeconomic status or length of psychopharmacotherapy. Satterfield stresses the strong relationship between juvenile delinquency and adult arrest found by others[8,9] and suggests that a sizable number of the delinquent hyperactives will become adult offenders.

All the studies of adolescent hyperactives cited thus far indicated a higher rate of antisocial behavior in this group as opposed to control or comparison groups. However, Kramer and Loney[10] and Loney et al.[11] followed 135 boys who 5 years earlier had been diagnosed as hyperactives and were then 12–18 years of age. Measures of delinquent behavior at follow-up were obtained from independent structured interviews with the boy, the mother, and the father. The behavior was then categorized in one of four groups and rated for frequency on a 4-point scale ranging from no involvement to chronic or continuous involvement.

The four categories of behavior were:

1. *Offenses against Persons.* This included a variety of aggressive and sexual acts (e.g., assault, intimidation, rape, peeping). Twenty-one percent of the hyperactive subjects reported behavior in this category. These behaviors were primarily fighting. By way of comparison, 50% of a general-population Illinois sample of 14- to 18-year-olds[12] admitted to fighting.

2. *Offenses against Property.* This category included such acts as shoplifting, vandalism, setting fires, and breaking and entering. Twenty-nine percent of the hyperactive group admitted to acts against property, usually shoplifting or minor vandalism. In contrast, 56% of the subjects in the Rivera study had committed minor thefts (less than $20 in value), and 13 percent admitted to more serious property offenses (e.g., breaking and entering).

3. *Drug Offenses.* This included using, giving, or selling illegal substances such as marijuana, amphetamines, and hallucinogenics. Nineteen percent of the hyperactives admitted to drug offenses. Two Iowa drug surveys[13,14] suggest that this level of involvement is at or below expected norms for the state.

4. *Alcohol Offenses.* This included possession and use of alcohol while a minor (without parental consent); having given or sold it to a minor; and drunkenness at any age. Twenty-eight percent of the sample had such offenses. However, between 30% and 35% of Iowa 14- to 17-year-olds at large said they used alcohol at least once per week.[14] Even though the hyperactives had a fairly high incidence of antisocial behavior during adolescence, this was not greater than similar age and area population norms. Methodological differences involving subject selection, socioeconomic status, and measures of antisocial behavior, and differences in when the studies were conducted may, in part, account for this surprising finding.

Blouin *et al.*,[15] in a 5-year follow-up study of adolescent hyperactives, compared 23 hyperactive subjects to 22 subjects matched for age, sex, and IQ who had school difficulties but were not hyperactive. Even though hyperactives had greater alcohol intake and were rated as having more conduct disorders by their parents, police contacts and times in jail were infrequent in both groups and not significantly greater among hyperactives.

Another study which suggested low rates in antisocial behavior in hyperactive adolescents was by Feldman *et al.*[16] The authors followed 81 adolescent hyperactives retrospectively and gave them comprehensive physical, emotional, and psychiatric evaluations. They found that 57% of their subjects showed no evidence of Minimal Brain Dysfunction (MBD) or its sequelae. Thirty-five, or the remaining 43%, had adjustment problems needing intervention, but of these, only 7% or 8% of the total sample had serious problems (e.g., 3 were drug abusers, 3 were under court custody for delinquent behavior, and 1 was a chronic runaway).

It is not totally clear why some studies find high rates of antisocial behavior in hyperactive adolescents and others find that the rates are not significantly higher than in various comparison and control groups. Methodological differences and differences in where and when the various studies were carried out, as well as population differences (e.g., socioeconomic status), are all factors possibly accounting for the discrepancy. (This is further discussed in Chapter 4.) Nonetheless, the various studies did raise concern about the possible future outcome of hyperactives becoming adult offenders.

STUDIES OF FAMILIES OF HYPERACTIVES

Another group of studies that have given rise to apprehensions that hyperactive children may become adult sociopaths involves the families of the hyperactives. (These studies are discussed at greater length in Chapter 12.)

Morrison and Stewart[17] interviewed parents of 59 hyperactives and 41 control children and discovered a high prevalence of alcoholism, sociopathy, and hysteria in fathers and mothers of hyperactive children. Cantwell[18] had similar findings when he gave a systematic psychiatric examination to parents of 50 hyperactive children and 50 matched controls. There were increased prevalence rates for alcoholism, sociopathy, and hysteria, but not for affective disorders, in the parents of the hyperactive children.

In an attempt to clarify whether genetic or environmental factors were at work, Morrison and Stewart[19] interviewed the legal parents of 35 adopted hyperactives. The children had had almost no contact with their biological parents, having been cared for by hospital nurseries, adoption agencies, or foster homes prior to placement at an average age of 15.7 weeks. The high prevalence of hysteria, sociopathy, and alcoholism found in biological parents of hyperactive children was not found in adopting parents.

Stewart et al.[20] pointed out several shortcomings of these studies. One problem was that they used normal children as controls, rather than children attending a psychiatric clinic for reasons other than hyperactivity.

Morrison[21] addressed this criticism by comparing the family history of 140 children and adolescents with hyperactive child syndrome with those of 91 age- and sex-matched patients with other primary psychiatric diagnoses. Again, parents of hyperactive children were more likely to have Antisocial Personality Disorder and hysteria than parents of nonhyperactive children. Some 11% of hyperactives had a parent with such a diagnosis. Parents of nonhyperactive children were more likely to have endogenous psychosis. However, unlike previous findings,[17,18] alcoholism was not more prevalent in the families of the hyperactive children.

Thus family studies have suggested an association between hyperactive children syndrome and adult Antisocial Personality Disorder, thereby contributing to the concern about the adult outcome of the syndrome.

ADULT PSYCHIATRIC DISORDERS IN PATIENTS WITH HISTORIES SUGGESTING CHILDHOOD HYPERACTIVITY

A third group of studies attempting to link childhood hyperactivity with adult disturbances, including antisocial behavior, involved looking retrospectively into the childhood histories of disturbed adults to see if they might be compatible with the patient having been hyperactive as a child. There are obvious limitations to this type of approach. One of the most significant drawbacks is the memory distortions in patients and their families produced by a 20-year time lapse and current psychiatric difficulties. However, Morrison[22] compared 48 adult psychiatric patients who gave childhood histories of hyperactivity with two groups of patients who did not give such histories. Both comparison groups were matched for age and sex, and the second group was also matched for socioeconomic status. Subjects who presented childhood histories of hyperactivity showed more personality disorders (of all types), more sociopathy, more alcoholism, and less affective disorders than the comparison groups.

In a more detailed study, Morrison[23] showed that three times as many adult psychiatric patients with a history of childhood hyperactivity had violent behavior directed against people when compared to matched adult psychiatric patients with no such histories. Arrests and convictions were also more frequent in the adult patient with childhood hyperactivity. In fact, two-thirds of the "hyperactive child syndrome" group had a history of either crime or violence, compared to one-third of the "nonhyperactive child syndrome" group.

However, the way in which the retrospective diagnosis of "hyperactive child syndrome" was made may account for these results. To be considered to have had hyperactivity, subjects needed to report high activity levels and short attention spans, as well as symptoms suggesting a severe degree of impairment socially, for example, repeated truancy, suspension or explusion from school, frequent fighting, scholastic failure with repeating at least one grade, dyslexia, acalculia, and dysgraphia. It can be seen that subjects selected may have been primarily conduct disordered, which would account for the adult picture.

A number of authors[24-30] have all tried to make a case for the adult diagnosis of Attention Deficit Disorder. Even though antisocial behavior is not necessarily part of the picture in the adult diagnosis of this entity, predominant symptoms such as problems with impulse control and emotional lability are common and often result in antisocial behavior. Perhaps the most graphic description of this combination is given by Morrison and Minkoff,[27] who present a number of case histories in an attempt to present explosive personality as a sequel to the hyperactive child syndrome. However, few of these studies have shown a significant proportion of their adult Attention Deficit Disorder population to be "antisocial." For example, in the Wood[25] study, only 7% of the subjects had "trouble with the law." In the Mattes[30] study, only 2 of 29 of his attention-deficit subjects had the diagnosis of Antisocial Personality Disorder. This was comparable to his comparison group.

It is thus important to distinguish between certain behaviors which can be termed "antisocial" (e.g., fighting, lying, impulsive steal-ing) and more formal diagnosis of Antisocial Personality Disorder. It appears that "antisocial" behavior is much more prevalent in adult Attention Deficit Disorder patients than is Antisocial Personality Dis-order. These types of studies therefore give rise to some degree of concern about hyperactive children becoming adults with Antisocial Personality Disorder.

ADULT OUTCOME STUDIES OF HYPERACTIVE CHILDREN: PROSPECTIVE AND RETROSPECTIVE

The last group of studies that will be discussed involve the follow-up (prospectively or retrospectively) of children thought to have been hyperactive into adulthood.

Retrospective Studies

In Menkes et al.'s[31] 25-year retrospective study of 14 subjects first referred for hyperactivity and learning difficulties, the relative negative outcome centered on the fact that at follow-up 4 subjects were psy-chotic. Eight subjects who at follow-up were self-sufficient had spent time in institutions for delinquent boys, and 1 had been in jail. Thus psychosis, not antisocial behavior, was a primary concern for adult outcome in the results of this study. Other retrospective studies that have followed hyperactive children into adulthood have found neither psychosis nor serious antisocial behavior to be particularly prevalent. Thus, Laufer,[32] in a 12-year questionnaire follow-up of 66 subjects 15–26 years of age, found that although 30% had problems with police, none of the subjects was in jail. Borland and Heckman[33] compared 20 men (mean age 30 years) whose childhood medical records conformed to diagnostic criteria for hyperactive child syndrome 20–25 years ago with their brothers (mean age 28 years). The authors found that men diagnosed as hyperactive in childhood were not experiencing severe social or psychiatric problems at follow-up. Most had completed high school and were steadily employed and self-supporting. They did, how-ever, have more work difficulties, lower socioeconomic status, and more problems of a psychiatric nature when compared to their broth-ers. Some of these problems may have resulted from the persistence of symptoms of hyperactive syndrome, for example, hyperactivity, ner-vousness, impulsivity, inclination to becoming upset, and problems with temper. Four of these 20 men with childhood hyperactivity were "sociopathic." The authors described them as restless, often impulsive, and easily frustrated by work they considered unexciting and repetitious. They changed jobs more frequently and had more social and marital difficulties. However, they had not had problems with antisocial behavior in recent years.

The findings of Feldman *et al.*[16] were similar. These authors carried out a 10- to 12-year retrospective follow-up study on 48 young adults (mean age 21 years) previously diagnosed as hyperactive and found that 91% were either in school or working. Only 10% had significant adjustment problems, which included drug use, lack of direction and/or motivation, and schizoid personality disorders. Antisocial behavior was not prevalent in this group at this age.

Loney *et al.*'s[34] study of 22 formerly hyperactive subjects and their brothers (both at age 21 years) had somewhat different findings using modified Schedule for Affective Disorders and Schizophrenia, Lifetime Version (SADS-L)[35] criteria for diagnosing Antisocial Personality Disorder. The authors found 10 of 22 (45%) formerly hyperactive subjects could be diagnosed as having Antisocial Personality Disorder compared to 4 of 22 (18%) of the brothers. The first category of criteria included antisocial behavior in childhood (such as truancy, expulsion from school, persistent lying, stealing, vandalism, repeated running away, involvement with juvenile court, academic underachievement, early or aggressive sex, early drug use, and chronic violation of rules). Three of these behaviors before age 15 were required. The second category of criteria required poor occupational performance, as characterized by frequent job changes, significant unemployment, or serious absenteeism. One of these behaviors was required. The third category of criteria involved adult antisocial behavior such as two or more serious arrests, two or more divorces/separations, physical fights, being drunk weekly or more, frequent default on debts, and periods with no permanent residence. At least two of these behaviors were required. Loney modified the last category of criteria, Impaired Interpersonal Relationships, by not requiring them for the diagnosis because she felt these behaviors were not well measured in the direct SADS-L interview and because they were not required in the DSM-III diagnostic criteria.

In addition, Loney and her coworkers[34] obtained a more detailed examination of self-reported acts and official sanctions via the Iowa Crime and Punishment Survey (CAPS),[36] which was constructed by these authors. This survey is divided into categories which include: moving traffic violations, crimes against persons, crimes against property, and contacts with police. There were significant differences between formerly hyperactive subjects and their brothers predominantly in the area of crimes against persons. Significantly more of the hyperactive group had concealed a gun or knife, been in a fight where weapons were used, and threatened to hurt or almost hurt someone. For those subjects who had been in a fight where weapons were used, significantly more hyperactives than their brothers (54% vs. 15%) reported that bodily injury which had resulted required a physician's attention. There was also some suggestion that formerly hyperactive subjects committed more offenses in general, though this did not reach statistical significance.

In the punishment section of the survey, hyperactives and their brothers did not differ significantly in the total number of police contacts; however, the hyperactives had more serious consequences from their contacts. Nine of 22 (41%) formerly hyperactive subjects had been convicted and spent time in jail or prison, compared to 1 of 22 (5%) of the brothers. The authors suggest that the greater severity of the sanctions given probands was related to their increased rate of offenses against persons. Loney also deals extensively with drug and alcohol use (which will be addressed in Chapter 8) and with predictive factors for adult antisocial behavior and drug and alcohol abuse (which will be discussed in Section IV, Predictive Factors). However, this study, unlike those of Feldman et al.,[16] Laufer,[32] and Borland and Heckman,[33] does suggest serious concerns about adult antisocial behavior in subjects who were diagnosed hyperactive in childhood.

Prospective Studies

There are few studies that have followed hyperactive children prospectively into adulthood. Most have been predominantly clinical, with no control groups.

Thus Huessy et al.[37] did an 8- to 10-year follow-up study of 84 subjects he had seen in childhood for behavior disorders and treated with medication. At the time of follow-up, 5–11 years later, the subjects were 9–24 years of age. Guidance counselors and parents were interviewed by phone, and records of schools, hospitals, social agencies, and departments of corrections were surveyed. Fifteen of the 84 subjects had serious antisocial behavior requiring contact with the Department of Corrections (i.e., Probation and Parole, State Correctional School, or New Hampshire Jail). The authors point out that while expected institutionalization for unmanageable or delinquent behavior was 0.5%, 13% of the study group had been thus institutionalized. The absence of any control or comparison group and the uncertainty of other factors (e.g., socioeconomic status, IQ) limit the interpretations one can place on these findings. However, the suggestion that some of these subjects have serious problems with the correctional department certainly exists.

Another uncontrolled prospective study by Milman,[38] followed 73 patients diagnosed in childhood as having MBD and further classified as either Developmental Lag (38%) or Organic Brain Syndrome (62%). They were followed some 9–15 years later when they were 15–23 years of age (mean age 19.4 years). At follow-up some 14% of the subjects were thought to have Antisocial Personality Disorder. Again, no comparison group existed, and factors such as socioeconomic status and organicity may have influenced the results.

Gittelman and coworkers,[39] in a prospective follow-up of 103 hyperactive and 100 control subjects age 16–23 (mean age 18.9 years), found an increased prevalence of antisocial disorders in the hyperactive group compared with the control group of about 20%. This is not surprising, since a history of conduct disorder was found in 45% of the hyperactive child and 16% of the controls. However, the authors stressed that if cases with persistent Attention Deficit Disorder were disregarded, there was no significant difference between former patients and controls with regard to antisocial disorders. Conduct disorders usually preceded or coincided with onset of Substance Use Disorder. There was also a trend for the antisocial hyperactives to have a somewhat more serious pattern of antisocial behavior than similarly diagnosed controls. The difference in severity did not reach statistical significance but tended to be seen in excessive fighting, small thefts, and weapon use.

TEN-YEAR PROSPECTIVE CONTROLLED FOLLOW-UP STUDY

As part of the comprehensive 10-year follow-up study of hyperactives as young adults described in Chapter 5, we examined in some detail the history of antisocial behavior of young-adult hyperactives (mean age 19 years) and their matched normal controls.[40]

Assessments

Subjects had comprehensive psychiatric,[41] physiological,[42] psychological,[43] electroencephalographic,[44] and biographical assessments, reported on elsewhere.

Details of antisocial behavior, particularly drug use, alcohol abuse, and court/police involvement, were obtained during a semistructured, openended psychiatric interview only after a fairly good rapport had been established with the subjects and confidentiality was assured.

Data on age, type, extent, duration, and effects of nonmedical drug use (which will be addressed in Chapter 8), as well as on age, frequency, and reasons for court or police involvement, were obtained. Acts which did not result in court or police involvement were also explored. Stealing behavior during elementary school, high school, and currently was examined with respect to the reasons for stealing, circumstances under which stealing took place, frequency and severity of the thefts, and consequences. Also, the affective state of the subjects before, during, and after the stealing episodes was explored. Finally, if subjects stopped stealing at a particular point in time, the reasons for this were also addressed.

Unfortunately, the interview was the main source of information available to the research; all juvenile records are destroyed when the patient turns 18. Adult court records were later consulted for confirmation. The details of drug abuse and undiscovered antisocial behavior were usually unknown to the parents, so they were not a reliable source of information even though they were interviewed as part of the family studies.[45]

Moral Development

A small subgroup of 18 matched pairs of hyperactives and controls was randomly selected from the overall group of 75 hyperactives and 44 controls. Subjects were required to match for sex (male), age (within 12 months; mean age 22.1 years for hyperactives, 21.8 years for controls), IQ (WAIS, within 10 points; mean 112 for both); socioeconomic status[46] (mean 3), and educational level (within 1 year; completed 12–13 years of schooling), and were given moral development tests.[47] The test consisted of hypothetical situations involving moral dilemmas. Subjects were asked to respond to a series of questions which tapped their moral judgment, and in each case the reasoning behind their response was probed. The interview was recorded in audiotape, transcribed, and then scored by an experienced scorer. The scores reflected the stage of moral development of the subjects. For example, reasons such as avoiding personal punishment or gaining personal rewards put a person in a lower moral development stage than altruistic, humanitarian reasons.

Court Referrals

More hyperactive subjects than controls had court referrals in the 5 years prior to evaluation (47% vs. 32%, $p < .07$). There was no significant difference between the two groups, however, in the number of subjects who had court appearances within the year before evaluation. A separate analysis of the number and seriousness of individual offenses indicated no significant difference between the two groups with respect to disturbing the peace, theft, aggression, or drug or traffic offenses committed within the 5 years prior to the 10-year follow-up.

Aggression

Aggression was described as a problem at one time in the subjects' history by 31% of control subjects and 55% of hyperactive subjects.

Significantly more hyperactives fell into the moderate category with regard to the severity of this problem ($p < .05$) when compared to controls. Mean age at which aggression stopped being a problem (16.5 years for controls and 15.1 years of hyperactives) was not significantly different for the two groups. This problem with aggression (as reported by the subjects) seems to have peaked in the high-school period and did not constitute a significant problem in young adulthood.

Details of Stealing History

Controls and hyperactives were compared on various aspects of their stealing histories at different stages of development: during elementary school; during high school; and currently.

We see that there was an overall decline in the number of subjects who stole as they got older, and few (4 controls and 6 hyperactives) stole currently. There were also no significant differences between the two groups in the number of subjects who stole at any of the three stages. Wanting the object or money and excitement tended to be the main reasons given for stealing at all three stages and, again, no significant differences were seen in the controls and hyperactives.

No significant differences were seen in the two groups with respect to the circumstances of the stealing (i.e., whether it was premeditated or impulsive or both) at any of the three time periods. It is interesting that hyperactives did not report their stealing as being more impulsive. We find that most of the thefts at all three time periods fell into the minor category, that is, objects with a value of less than $50. However, during the high-school period, more hyperactives were involved in more severe thefts. For example, 6 subjects had stolen items with a value higher than $500, compared to 0 controls ($p < .003$).

For both hyperactives and controls at all three time periods the most frequent consequence was nothing or parental reprimand. However, more hyperactives than controls had police or court involvement, particularly in high school, and hyperactives often claimed that this was a deterrent to continuing this behavior. Differences in consequences for the two groups did not reach statistical significance.

There was generally no significant difference in the various affective states of the groups before, during, or after stealing. However, in the high-school period, significantly more hyperactives described fear during stealing than did controls ($p < .007$).

Looking at the reasons hyperactives and controls gave for stopping stealing, we see that significantly more hyperactives than controls stopped stealing in the high-school period because they feared the consequences ($p < .05$). The main consequence feared was the adult court system when they were no longer minors. No differences were seen between the two groups during the elementary-school period, nor did the groups differ on whether or not they thought stealing was wrong during the three time periods.

The suggestion that there is a more negative subgroup exists. Three hyperactive subjects were known to have been or were currently in adult jails. None of the controls had similar histories.

Moral Development

The 18 matched pairs of hyperactives and controls showed no significant differences in the mean score on the moral development test,[47] indicating that both controls and hyperactives had reached similar levels of moral development. This is not surprising, since most of the antisocial behavior of adolescence seems to have subsided, and so we are not dealing with the significantly delinquent young-adult group whose moral development may be affected.

The 18 hyperactives who constituted the matched-pair subgroup were compared to the whole group of hyperactives on all the parameters outlined above (nonmedical drug use, court referral, aggression, and stealing). No significant differences between the two groups were found on any of the parameters. Similarly, the 18 matched-pair control subjects were compared to the whole group of 44 controls, and again no significant differences were found on these parameters.

One can thus conclude that the nonmedical drug use and "antisocial" (aggression, court referrals, stealing) histories of the matched-pair subgroup were not significantly different from the overall group of hyperactives and controls. They were, therefore, a representative sample with respect to nonmedical drug use and "antisocial" histories.

In Summary

Generally speaking, the 10- to 12-year follow-up of hyperactives as young adults suggests that: (1) as young adults, hyperactives had less "antisocial" behavior compared to their adolescent period mainly because of their fear of the adult court system; (2) hyperactives as young adults did not differ significantly from normal controls on levels of moral development as measured by the Kohlberg[47] test; (3) only a small subgroup of hyperactive subjects are, as young adults, more heavily involved in drug abuse and antisocial behavior.

These findings may be affected to some extent by the Canadian setting, where the degree of drug abuse and antisocial behavior may not be as severe as in some large urban settings in the United States. However, the results are, on the whole, encouraging for a more positive outcome for these patients than was previously anticipated.

FIFTEEN-YEAR CONTROLLED PROSPECTIVE FOLLOW-UP STUDY[48,49]

The 15-year controlled prospective follow-up study described in detail in Chapter 5[48] was undertaken because the authors felt that at 10-year follow-up, where the age range was 17–24 years (mean age 19 years), the outcome was still in a state of flux. For example, the 10-year follow-up study showed that young-adult hyperactives had more court referrals and nonmedical use of drugs in the last 5 years but not in the last year when compared to their matched normal controls. Therefore, a clearer, more stable outcome picture could be gained by continuing to follow the group for another 5 years. The comprehensive assessment described in detail in Chapter 5[48,49] included interviews which focused on past (in the last 3 years) and current alcohol and nonmedical drug use and antisocial behavior. Some subjects were also given the SADS-L,[35] modified (i.e., last 5 years as opposed to lifetime). Computerized court records were consulted to verify subjects' reports. These records included all criminal charges as well as highway offenses falling under the criminal code since age 18.

Results

ANTISOCIAL BEHAVIOR (Table 6-1)

In the last 3 years there was a trend for more hyperactive subjects to have to appear in court for various offenses compared to control subjects (11 vs. 2, $p < .09$). The total number of court appearances was also higher for the hyperactive group (24 vs. 2, $p < .07$). Most of the hyperactives had to appear in court for highway offenses which fell under the criminal code—for example, speeding. A small minority of subjects (3 or 4) were involved with criminal offenses such as theft, drug possession, or dealing.

TABLE 6-1. Antisocial Behavior: Subjects' Reports

	Controls ($n = 41$)	Hyperactives ($n = 60$)	Significance
Court appearances			
Number of subjects (total 3 years)	2	11	$p < .09$
Total number of court appearances (in last 3 years)	2	24^a	$p < .07$
Police involvement (only)			
Number of subjects (total 3 years)	22	31	
Number of police involvements	65^b	118^c	
Offenses (thefts): no police or court involvement			
Number of subjects (total 3 years)	4	10	
Number of offenses	42^d	89^e	
In last 3 years			
Number of subjects with other offenses	4	8	
Number of other offenses	8	174^f	$p < .05$
Number of subjects with any offenses with or without court or police involvement	24	41	

^{a}15 of the 24 court appearances were made by 2 subjects.
^{b}31 of the 65 police involvements involved 3 subjects.
^{c}51 of the 118 police involvements involved 3 subjects.
^{d}40 of the 42 offenses were committed by 2 subjects.
^{e}72 of the 89 offenses were committed by 2 subjects.
^{f}160 of the 174 offenses were committed by 4 subjects.

However, it must be stressed that court appearances are but the tip of the iceberg and many more hyperactives and controls are involved in antisocial behavior which only involves the police or has no police or court involvement. This last category often reflects frequent shoplifting, traffic offenses, and possession and/or selling of nonmedical drugs. There were no significant differences in the number of hyperactives and controls who had offenses which involved the police only or did not come to the attention of either the police or the courts.

When thefts were eliminated and other offenses not involving police or the courts were explored, hyperactives had significantly more such offenses ($p < .05$). Many of these were speeding. It is also striking that in most categories 2 or 3 particular individuals committed most of the offenses. This was true in both the hyperactive and control groups but particularly in the hyperactive group (e.g., 160 of 174 offenses were committed by 4 hyperactive subjects).

TABLE 6-2. Aggression

	Controls (n = 41)	Hyperactives (n = 61)	Significance
Subjects with physical aggression (last 3 years)	2	12	$p < .07$
Severity of physical aggression[a]			
Mild	1	3	
Moderate	1	5	
Severe	0	4	
Subjects' verbal aggression	8	18	

[a]Mild: infrequent outbursts (less than once/month), physical damage to objects only; moderate: between mild and severe; severe: frequent outbursts (more than once/week), police or court involvement, physical injury to someone.

AGGRESSION (Table 6-2)

A larger number of hyperactive subjects tended to have problems with physical aggression in the last 3 years when compared to control subjects (12 vs. 2, $p < .07$). The severity of the physical aggression appeared somewhat greater, though this did not reach statistical significance. Nor were any statistically significant differences seen in subjects' reports of verbal aggression.

GLOBAL ASSESSMENT SCALE (Table 6-3)

On the basis of combined information obtained from subjects in interview, the SADS,[35] and the SCL-90,[50] the research team formulated a global assessment. The number of hyperactives and controls with

TABLE 6-3. Global Assessment Scale: Combined Information from Subjects' Verbal Reports, SADS, and SCL-90

	Controls (n = 41)	Hyperactives (n = 61)	Significance
Antisocial behavior			
Total	11	22	
Mild	8	5	
Moderate	3	10	$p < .01$
Severe	0	7	
A period of drug or alcohol abuse (last 3 years)			
Alcohol	11	27	
Nonmedical drug	1	10	$p < .07$

antisocial behavior did not differ significantly. However, the severity of the antisocial behavior was much greater in the hyperactive group ($p < .01$). (See severity scale in Table 6-4.)

ANTISOCIAL DIAGNOSIS (Table 6-5)

One is left with the question, "Do hyperactives become Antisocial Personality Disorders as adults, and if so how often?" The answer largely depends on how one defines Antisocial Personality Disorder, as well as on the instruments, sources, and criteria one uses to make the diagnosis. Thus when one employs a purely clinical definition, namely that of chronic antisocial behavior, and when the source of the information is the subject himself, we find that 1 of the 41 controls and 14 of the 61 hyperactives are judged to be antisocial ($p < .01$). In contrast, employing strict SADS criteria for Antisocial Personality Disorder, none of the controls and 1 of the hyperactives receive this diagnosis. However, when one modifies the strict SADS criteria by eliminating the Impaired Interpersonal Relationships requirement—

TABLE 6-4. Categories of Antisocial Behavior

Category "0"
  No antisocial acts reported
  One minor theft
  One traffic infraction (parking excluded) in 3 years
  Possession of hash once
Category "1" (mild)
  Two minor thefts in 3 years
  Possession of hash not more than once
  Buying stolen goods
  Two to three traffic violations (parking tickets excluded)
  Nonpayment of child support
Category "2" (moderate)
  Three or four minor thefts with no major thefts in the last 3 years
  Four traffic violations (parking tickets excluded)
  Possession of drugs at least twice, or more
  Selling drugs, but no longer doing this
  Assault without injury requiring medical attention and not more than once
Category "3" (severe)
  A major theft or more
  Four or more minor thefts in 3 years
  Drug dealing continuous
  More than four serious traffic violations
  One or more break-in and entry
  Assault with significant physical injury

TABLE 6-5. Antisocial Diagnosis (Depending on Instrument, Criteria, and Source)

	Controls (n = 41)	Hyperactives (n = 61)	Significance
Chronic antisocial behavior since age 18 (subjects' reports)	1	14	p < .01
Strict SADS	0	1	
Modified SADS omitting close relationship	1	11	p < .05
Modified SADS plus other source information	1	14	p < .01
DSM-III	1	14	p < .01
Court record (last 3 years)			
Criminal	0	3	
Highway offenses under criminal code (e.g., speeding)	0	7	p < .07
Court record since 15-year follow-up			
Criminal	0	7	
Highway	0	4	

which, as Loney et al.[34] pointed out, is not well tapped by direct questions such as "Is there anyone you really feel very close to?" or "Do you keep the same friends for a long time?" and is not a criterion in the DSM-III—we find that 1 control and 11 hyperactives receive an antisocial diagnosis. When one uses the modified SADS criteria and information obtained from the subject, 1 control and 14 hyperactives received the diagnosis (p < .01). Interestingly, DSM-III criteria yield the same numbers. Thus the clinical ratings, the modified SADS criteria using all available data, and the DSM-III all yield the same number of antisocial subjects: 1 control and 14 hyperactives.

Verifying these findings by going into court records showed that no controls and only 10 hyperactives had court records in the past 3 years. Seven of the 10 hyperactives with court records had highway offenses falling under the criminal code (e.g., speeding), and only 3 had true criminal offenses (e.g., breaking and entering). Court records were also used to see if subjects not seen at 5-, 10-, or 15-year follow-up had significant legal problems (Table 6-6). This was not the case; only 1 hyperactive of the 14 not seen at 15-year follow-up had a court record, and 2 of the 25 not seen at 5- or 10-year follow-up had criminal court offenses while another 2 had highway-code offenses. It may well be that some subjects have left the area, and therefore their legal problems are not reflected in Montreal court records.

TABLE 6-6. Court Records of Subjects Lost

	Controls (n = 4)	Hyperactives (n = 14)
Not seen at 15-year follow-up		
Criminal	0	1
Highway	0	0
		(n = 25)
Not seen at 5- or 10-year follow-up		
Criminal		2
Highway		2

DISCUSSION

VALIDITY OF FINDINGS

One is always concerned in follow-up studies as to whether the subjects followed are a representative group and valid conclusions can therefore be drawn from the data obtained. Cox et al.[51] have stressed that the group of subjects lost to follow-up often constituted a more negative outcome group. However, we were able to get some view of this through telephone contacts with the subject or his or her family on all subjects lost between 10- and 15-year follow-up. Most were functioning adequately. Furthermore, review of court records on the lost subjects revealed that only 1 hyperactive had a court referral. Nonetheless, it would be safest to assume that the group followed reflects a more positive outcome group.

ANTISOCIAL BEHAVIOR

Generally the hyperactive group did not have significantly more antisocial behavior when compared to the matched control group. This was similar to our[40] 10-year follow-up finding and Loney et al.'s[34] report of hyperactives and their brothers on the CAPS. However, there was a trend for more hyperactives to be selling nonmedical drugs, and to have more court appearances ($p < .09$). As in Loney's sample, these hyperactives also tended ($p < .07$) to have more problems with physical aggression. Most importantly, the severity of antisocial behavior was significantly greater for the hyperactive group.

LIMITATIONS OF SPECIFIC DIAGNOSTIC CRITERIA SCALES

It is important to stress that the antisocial personality diagnosis will vary with the source of information and criteria employed. However, the comparability of results from the various instruments and sources has been outlined. The limitations of the various instruments in making the diagnosis of Antisocial Personality Disorder are more fully discussed in Chapter 5.[48]

However, perhaps the greatest limitation is that the diagnostic criteria do not really differentiate the person with Antisocial Personality Disorder who has marked criminal behavior and populates adult jails from the individual with the same diagnosis who has no criminal history but functions marginally. The following case vignettes will illustrate the point.

Paul was first referred at age 11 for hyperactivity, poor school performance, and some behavior problems. He was the youngest of five children being raised by a single mother; father had deserted the family when Paul was an infant. Shortly after the desertion, mother had to be hospitalized for depression and appeared somewhat overwhelmed by the task of raising her five children. However, she was employed as a housecleaning supervisor and supporting the family as best she could.

Throughout adolescence, Paul continued to have problems. He was failing in school despite good normal intelligence and no learning disabilities. He was involved in a number of delinquent behaviors such as theft, vandalism, and breaking and entering, and was known to the juvenile detention authorities. When interviewed in his early 20s during the 10-year follow-up study, he was in jail and had a long history of drug abuse, drug dealing, breaking and entering, and robbery with violence. He had had many arrests for these various crimes and had spent more time in jail than out of jail. When seen at 15-year follow-up, Paul was not currently in jail and was planning to be married, but his behavior patterns and life-style had not changed significantly. Paul met the criteria for Antisocial Personality Disorder on the various scales.

James was referred at age 7 for hyperactivity, school failure, eneuresis, and behavior problems. At time of referral, he was being cared for by a woman in a boardinghouse which housed 12 other people, because his mother was hospitalized for psychiatric conditions and his parents were separated. He had normal IQ but some coordination problems.

Throughout high school, James continued to do poorly academically, was absent a good deal, got into occasional fights, and had relatively few friends. He finally dropped out of school at age 16 when the law no longer required that he attend. James then made some half-hearted attempts to get work. He would find the occasional short-term or part-time menial job, for example, selling plants, maintenance, cleaning. When seen at 10-year follow-up, in his late teens, he was unemployed most of the time, had few friends, was very tense, and had extremely poor self-confidence and self-esteem.

When seen at 15-year follow-up, James now had, in addition to his significant unemployment, a substantial drinking problem which often resulted in numerous brawls in which individuals were injured. However, most of these fights did not result in arrests or court hearings, and he has never been to jail. James also smokes marijuana and sells the drug sometimes to acquaintances. He was living with father and step-mother, and there were some problems with this arrangement. James shoplifts occasionally but has not been caught. He continues to be nervous and have low self-esteem and wishes he could find a job and drink less. However, he has no specific plans that would help him in that direction.

James too, meets diagnostic criteria for Antisocial Personality Disorder. However, as one can clearly see, we are in fact dealing with very different types of pathology in these two people with the same diagnosis.

SIMILAR AND DIVERGENT FINDINGS

The few studies that have looked at young-adult hyperactives give divergent findings. Some report quite negative outcomes,[7,31,37,38] while others[16,32-34,49] suggest a less pessimistic picture.

These divergent findings can have a number of explanations. The *time* when the studies were carried out may significantly affect findings. We are well aware that the crime rate has generally increased in the last 20–25 years, and so a follow-up study conducted in the 1960s[31] may have different findings than one carried out in the 1980s.[7] The *geographical location* of the patient population may also affect the divergent findings. Thus carrying weapons is much less prevalent in Canada[49] than it appears to be in California[7] or Iowa,[34] resulting in less serious offenses in our group when compared to the others. The use of control and comparison groups growing up at the same time and in the same area would help, but would not totally eliminate the problem of comparison of studies conducted at different times and places. A third factor which accounts for discrepancies involves methodological differences. Thus, whether studies are prospective or retrospective, whether they use court records, subject reports, parental interviews, old charts, or questionnaires—all methods have their particular biases and short-comings. This affects the findings and conclusions. Furthermore, the ages of the subjects at time of follow-up (even for those describing long-term follow-up and adult functioning,[37,38]) may range from 14 to 30 years. Many studies have shown that adolescents function, on the whole, less well than adults. Thus studies with younger subjects, such as Satterfield et al.[7] (mean age 17), may show more negative results.

It is perhaps most important to stress that outcome of hyperactive children is not uniformly good or bad but distributes into roughly three categories:[52] (1) those hyperactive young adults whose functioning in many spheres is fairly normal; (2) those hyperactive young adults who continue to have significantly more social, emotional, and impulsive problems than matched controls but whose difficulties are not suffi-ciently severe to reflect marked psychiatric or antisocial pathology; (3) and finally, those hyperactives who clearly constitute a signifi-cantly disturbed group requiring psychiatric hospitalization and/or adult jails.

The various studies may reflect a difference in the proportion of subjects who fall into these different outcome groups. Thus, a study that has included a high proportion of subjects who are both hyperac-tive and conduct disordered[7] as well as aggressive[34] would have more subjects in the negative outcome group than one that did not.[16] Factors which influence outcome are discussed at length in Section IV. How-ever, IQ, socioeconomic status, and family structure and pathology may all influence outcome. Studies vary greatly in these factors. As pointed out by Loney et al.,[11] Milman,[38] and Hechtman,[53] often not one factor affects outcome in itself, but rather the cumulative effect of a number of factors acting synergistically results in positive or negative picture in adulthood. It is our challenge to try to identify and treat the more negative outcome group and pinpoint the factors which contrib-ute to this picture.

SUMMARY

We have reviewed the various adolescent and adult studies which have given rise to concerns of antisocial adult outcome in hyperactive chil-dren. We have presented our own long-term prospective follow-up study as well as studies of other workers[16,33] which suggest that the concern may be exaggerated and that few hyperactives grow up to be serious adult offenders. The possible reasons for these different find-ings are discussed.

In summary our study suggests that hyperactives as adults are not *significantly* different from controls on measures of current drug and alcohol use (see Chapter 8) and antisocial behavior. However, one sees *trends* of greater drug, alcohol, and antisocial involvement in the hyperactive group. Even though a significantly greater number of hyperactives were diagnosed as having Antisocial Personality Disorder in accordance with DSM-III and modified SADS criteria, the limitations of these diagnoses, in that they represent greatly varying levels of functioning and pathology, was pointed out. These trends do not generally reflect a high proportion of seriously malfunctioning individuals. They may represent mild disturbance in a fair number and/or a small subgroup of subjects who have more negative outcomes with significant greater antisocial and psychiatric difficulties. It is this subgroup which we need to identify early and successfully treat.

CHAPTER SEVEN

VALUES AND BELIEFS

When I hear the people
Praising great ones,
Then I know that I too
shall be esteemed.
I too, when my time comes
shall do mightily.
—From "Song of Greatness,"
by Mary Austin (née Hunter), 1868–1934

As part of the comprehensive 15-year follow-up described in Chapter 5, we questioned subjects on their beliefs, values, and ideals. We wished to determine whether these differed in hyperactive adults compared to controls, and more particularly, if antisocial subjects—hyperactives or controls—were different in these measures when compared to nonantisocial subjects. We also wished to clarify whether the subjects' antisocial behavior was impulsive and whether or or not they had a clear view that they were behaving wrongly.

It was hypothesized, with condierable tentativeness, that these beliefs, values, and ideals may be reflections of superego and/or ego-ideal development. We could thus gain some impression of whether hyperactives and controls differed in ego-ideal or superego development, and whether these psychic entities could be shown (via beliefs, values, and ideals) to be different in antisocial and nonantisocial individuals. We are defining ego ideal as the internalized image of a person's ideals and aspirations with respect to the kind of person he or she would like to be and the kind of things he or she would like to do.

RESULTS

Antisocial Subjects

Subjects with a history of substantial antisocial *behavior* (e.g., breaking and entering, drug dealing and possession, assault, stealing, and numerous serious traffic offenses) were categorized as antisocial. Unlike the more strict time (last 3 years) and scale (SADS,[1] DSM-III[2]) criteria which were used in Chapter 6 to define antisocial subjects, here a longer time-frame and less stringent criteria were used to distinguish the groups. As expected, a significantly higher proportion of hyperactives fell into the antisocial behavior category than controls (27% vs. 7%, $p < .05$).

Generally, for all areas explored, openended questions were asked, which were further clarified by more detailed questions. Responses were then later categorized to permit comparison. Subjects were asked a very openended question; for example, "Is there anything you strongly believe in?" The beliefs of the subjects were then categorized as: religious, political, parental values, belief in oneself, or other.

Strong Beliefs (Table 7-1)

Generally, a significantly larger proportion of control versus hyperactive subjects had any strong beliefs (78% vs. 51%, $p < .01$). There is no significant difference between the proportion of nonantisocial and antisocial hyperactives having any strong beliefs (47% vs. 59%). The number of antisocial control subjects was small (3) when compared to nonantisocial controls (38).

For both hyperactives and controls, the most frequent type of beliefs fell in the "other" category (39% and 45% respectively). This category included such statements as "I believe in the value of the family unit" or "I believe that people should be kind, decent, and respectful of each other." Subjects denied that these values or beliefs derived from their religious or parental values. In this regard, it is interesting to note that antisocial hyperactives described a higher proportion of their beliefs as reflecting parental values when compared to nonantisocial hyperactives (30% vs. 8%, $p < .01$). On the other hand, nonantisocial hyperactives attributed a higher proportion of their values to their religious teachings.

View of Own Behavior (Table 7-2)

Subjects were asked whether they had done anything in the past year *that they felt was ethically or morally wrong.* There is no significant difference between hyperactives and controls in the number of subjects who felt they had done something morally wrong (32% vs. 37%). Although more antisocial hyperactives felt that they had done something wrong in the past year than nonantisocial hyperactives (47% vs. 27%), this did not reach statistical significance.

TABLE 7-1. Strong Beliefs

	Hyperactives			Controls		
	Nonantisocial	Antisocial	Total	Nonantisocial	Antisocial	Total
Number of subjects	45	17*	62	38	3*	41
Subjects with beliefs (%)	47	59	51**	82	33	78**
Total number of beliefs	25	13	38	36	2	38
Type of belief (%)						
Religious	36	15	29	19	0	18
Political	4	0	2	11	0	10
Parental values	8**	30**	16	19	0	18
Self	12	15	13	8	0	8
Other[a]	40	38	39	42	100	45

[a] For example, family unit; value of human relationship; money; natural environment.
*$p < .05$.
**$p < .01$.

TABLE 7-2. View of Own Behavior

	Hyperactives			Controls		
	Nonantisocial	Antisocial	Total	Nonantisocial	Antisocial	Total
Number of subjects	45	17	62	38	3	41
Subjects who felt some behavior wrong (%)	27	47	32	39	0	37
Total number of wrong acts	14	10	24	14	0	14
Types of wrong behavior (%)						
Interpersonal[a]	64*	37*	54	78	0	78
Antisocial	14	12	14	7	0	7
Physical aggression	14	25	18**	0	0	0**
Other[b]	7	25	14	14	0	14

[a]For example, hurt others' feelings; unfaithful; verbal aggression.
[b]For example, drinking, not working.
*p < .05.
**p < .02.

With respect to the type of reported behavior which the subject viewed as being morally wrong, hyperactive and control groups cited more deeds in the interpersonal area. This included such things as doing or saying something which hurt someone's feelings, being unfaithful, and/or being verbally aggressive. Both groups of hyperactives, however, reported more acts which they considered morally wrong related to antisocial and physically aggressive behavior when compared to controls. The greater physical aggression is particularly striking: 18% for hyperactives, 0% for controls ($p < .02$).

In the comparison of antisocial hyperactives with their nonantisocial counterparts, the antisocial groups reported significantly fewer interpersonal transgressions (37% vs. 64%, $p < .05$) but more misdeeds involving physical aggression (25% vs. 14%). The latter was not statistically significant. There was no difference in the two groups regarding reports of antisocial behavior (12% vs. 14%). It would appear that hyperactives in general report more difficulty controlling their physical aggression, and that this is particularly marked in the antisocial subgroup. These differences suggest that antisocial hyperactives do have an internalized sense of right and wrong but do not perceive some of their antisocial acts as "being wrong."

Admired Characteristics of Ideal Fantasy Person (Table 7-3)

Subjects were asked to describe an imaginary ideal person, stressing the admired and valued qualities of such a person. These qualities were then grouped under one of four categories. These included:

1. Worldly success (e.g., money, job, education)
2. Personal qualities (e.g., intelligence, dependability, generosity)
3. Social qualities (e.g., friendliness popularity)
4. Physical qualities (e.g., attractive, strong)

Hyperactives and controls both stressed personal qualities most frequently (77% vs. 68%). The personal qualities included such things as intelligence, dependability, kindness, sensitivity, caring, generosity, courage, and honesty. However, worldly success in terms of job, education, and money was somewhat more important to the antisocial hyperactive and control groups than to their nonantisocial counterparts (e.g., for hyperactives, 19% vs. 7%). (This was not significant.)

The antisocial hyperactive group also tended to value social qualities and physical qualities more than the nonantisocial hyperactive group. Thus we see the increased emphasis on external values in the antisocial group.

TABLE 7-3. Admired Characteristics of Ideal Fantasy Person

	Hyperactives			Controls		
	Nonantisocial	Antisocial	Total	Nonantisocial	Antisocial	Total
Number of subjects	45	17	62	38	3	41
Total number of characteristics	44	26	70	54	5	59
Type of characteristic (%)						
Worldly success	7	19	11	13	20	14
Personal qualities	86	61	77	69	60	68
Social qualities	5	12	7	7	20	8
Physical qualities	2	8	4	11	0	10
Other	0	0	0	0	0	0

Admired Characteristics of Real Admired Person (Table 7-4)

Subjects were asked to describe a real person they admired, stressing the qualities they valued in this person. Responses were again grouped under worldly success, personal qualities, social qualities, and physical qualities. Again, both hyperactives and controls stressed personal qualities (72% and 82% respectively). The external values of worldly success and social qualities were again only slightly more pronounced in the antisocial hyperactive group compared to the nonantisocial one, but this difference was not significant.

Relation to Real Admired Person (Table 7-5)

Subjects were asked to identify the real person they admired most and their relationship to this person. The responses with regard to the nature of the relationship with the real admired person were categorized as follows:

1. Public figures, for example, entertainers, sports personalities, politicians, community leaders (teacher, boss, priest)
2. Family members, including immediate or extended family
3. Friends.

Both hyperactives and controls identified a family member most frequently (46% and 43% respectively) as their admired person. Friends were a close second (29% and 32%), while public figures were third (23% and 22%). There was no significant difference in these findings in the two groups.

The antisocial hyperactive group selected family and friends more often than the nonantisocial group. The nonantisocial hyperactive group selected public figures more often than the antisocial group (29% vs. 12%, $p < .01$).

DISCUSSION

It must be stressed that these results reflect only conscious aspects of the superegos and ego ideals of the subjects. They represent group findings rather than intensive in-depth work with an individual subject. Therefore, the comments which follow need to be seen in a tentative, hypothetical light.

The findings suggest that hyperactives, in general, have more immature superegos than the matched control group. This is seen in the fact that a larger proportion of the hyperactive group had signifi-

TABLE 7-4. Admired Characteristics of Real Admired Person

	Hyperactives			Controls		
	Nonantisocial	Antisocial	Total	Nonantisocial	Antisocial	Total
Number of subjects	45	17	62	38	3	41
Total number of charac-teristics	48	23	71	41	4	45
Type of characteristic (%)						
Worldly success	15	17	15	10	0	9
Personal qualities	75	65	72	83	75	82
Social qualities	10	17	13	5	0	4
Physical qualities	0	0	0	2	25	4
Other	0	0	0	0	0	0

TABLE 7-5. Relation to Real Admired Person

	Hyperactives			Controls		
	Nonantisocial	Antisocial	Total	Nonantisocial	Antisocial	Total
Number of subjects	45	17	62	38	3	41
Total number of responses	35	17	52	34	3	37
Relation to real admired person (%)						
Public figure	29*	12*	23	24	0	22
Family	43	53	46	41	67	43
Friends	26	35	29	32	33	32
Other	2	0	2	3	0	3

*p < .01.

cant antisocial behavior (27% vs. 7%, $p < .05$) and themselves reported more antisocial and particularly physically aggressive behavior (18% hyperactives vs. 0% controls, $p < .02$) The difficulty in controlling physical aggression seems to be most marked in the antisocial hyperactive group, suggesting particular superego weakness in this group. This superego immaturity is not absolute, since antisocial hyperactives do recognize many of their antisocial and aggressive acts as being morally wrong. However, at times superego lacunae are evident, and some of these acts are not seen by the antisocial hyperactive subject as being wrong (e.g., institutional vs. personal theft).

Immaturity of the ego ideals can be postulated from the fact that fewer hyperactives than controls have strong beliefs. This immaturity appears to be more pronounced in the antisocial hyperactives than in the nonantisocial group. One sees suggestions of externalization and environment dependence of ego-ideal elements in this antisocial hyperactive group. For example, they are more likely to identify their values as parental values, in contrast to the more abstract religious values of the nonantisocial group. The antisocial group also tended to stress more external, reality-based, concrete qualities such as worldly success, sociability, and physical attractiveness in their ideal person when compared to the nonantisocial group. The need for concrete external presence of the idealized object is again seen in the fact that fewer of the antisocial hyperactives than of their nonantisocial counterparts selected more distant public figures as their real admired people. We thus see a superego which inadequately controls antisocial and aggressive behavior and an ego ideal which lacks internalization, abstraction, and autonomy.

The immaturity in the superego and the ego ideal may have resulted from the fact that the handicap these patients were presumably born with (i.e., hyperactivity, poor attention span, increased impulsivity) made it more difficult to establish adequate early significant relationships. Their ego development similarly may have been affected because interpretation of, integration in, and accommodation to the environment would be more difficult with such a handicap. It is, therefore, not surprising that when early relations to parents and ego development are compromised, ego-ideal and superego structures will thus be affected. In addition, these patients may have more difficulty inhibiting impulsive drives (particularly aggressive ones), which further stress and overwhelm the immature superego, resulting in inadequate neutralization and control of these drives.

Lampl-de-Groot[3] and Murray[4] have suggested that arrested ego-ideal development may interfere with the internalization of social values, resulting in delinquency. There is a graphic example of this in one subject who was involved in breaking and entering but did not think he was doing anything wrong. (However, most hyperactives who committed antisocial acts did view them as wrong).

The antisocial hyperactives seem to have an immaturity in super-ego development which has resulted in what Anna Freud[5] referred to as "failed socialization." This deficiency may sometimes result in an impulsive character. There may also be disruption in identification with parents or identification with the antisocial part of the parent. Cant-well[6] and Stewart and Morrison[7] found an increased incidence of alcoholism, sociopathy, and hysteria in the parents of hyperactive children. The fact that more antisocial hyperactives had beliefs which they identified with parental values suggests the possibility of such a delinquent parental identification.

The study thus presents an interesting example of the interrelationship between constitutional factors, early parental relations, environmental accommodations, and subsequent internal psychic structures. These psychic structures (superego and ego ideal) in turn influence later self-concept, interpersonal relationships, and environmental accommodations.

CHAPTER EIGHT

DRUG AND ALCOHOL USE
AND ABUSE

If on my theme I rightly think
There are five reasons why men drink
Good wine, a friend, because I'm dry
or least I should be, by and by,
or any other reason why.
—From "Alcoholism" by Henry Aldrich, 1648–1710

Interest in adult drug and alcohol use and abuse and its association with childhood hyperactivity has been less intense and less widespread when compared with interest in childhood hyperactivity and its association with adult antisocial behavior. This is somewhat surprising in view of the significantly larger number of adults who have problems with alcohol and substance abuse as compared to those having problems with antisocial behavior. Often drug and alcohol abuse are closely linked with antisocial behavior and adult criminal offenses and, therefore, are simply included under the umbrella of "antisocial behavior" rather than dealt with separately. For example, Weiss et al.[1] in the 5-year follow-up of hyperactives as adolescents, mentioned that 25% had significant antisocial behavior but not how many subjects had any drug or alcohol abuse. Similarly, Satterfield[2] in their follow-up of hyperactive adolescents, grouped alcohol intoxication and possession of less than 1 ounce of marijuana under nonserious offenses, together with running away from home, vandalism, and petty theft. They then investigated only serious crimes such as robbery, burglary, grand theft, and assault with a deadly weapon, and there was no further discussion of drug and alcohol abuse.

However, interest in this area increased with the increased use of stimulant medication to treat hyperactivity. There were concerns that children who receive stimulant medication during childhood may be more prone to solve future adult problems via drug (e.g., amphetamine) or alcohol abuse. In addition, various types of studies, such as adolescent and adult follow-up studies, family studies, and adult-patient

118

studies (all of which will be discussed in greater detail later in this chapter), suggested that the condition itself may result in adult drug or alcohol abuse. Thus, either the condition or the treatment (possibly both) could make hyperactive children more vulnerable to adult drug and/or alcohol abuse.

In an attempt to elucidate this issue, we will review the various studies that have linked childhood hyperactivity with adult drug and alcohol abuse. Generally these studies fall into four categories:

1. Follow-up studies of adolescent hyperactives: prospective and retrospective.
2. Studies of adult psychiatric patients (including alcoholics) with possible histories of childhood hyperactivity.
3. Studies of families of hyperactive children.
4. Follow-up studies of adult hyperactives: prospective and retrospective.

FOLLOW-UP STUDIES OF ADOLESCENT HYPERACTIVES: PROSPECTIVE AND RETROSPECTIVE

The study often quoted to show increased alcohol use in hyperactive adolescents is that by Blouin and his colleagues.[3] They did comprehensive evaluations on 23 hyperactives (approximately 14 years of age) and 22 subjects with school difficulties but without hyperactivity. Both groups were initially matched for age, sex, and Full Scale IQ. In addition to various psychological tests, both parents and the adolescent were interviewed with regard to health, school progress, social and behavioral difficulties, and drug treatment. A drug/alcohol-abuse questionnaire was also given after the subject was reassured of the confidentiality of responses. The authors found that 90% of the subjects in this sample reported that they had never used any drug other than alcohol or marijuana. The hyperactive subjects used (not abused) alcohol to a greater extent than the school-difficulty control group. They reported that they used alcohol once a month or more, more frequently than the controls. Hyperactives used hard liquor significantly more than controls, and there was a nonsignificant trend toward greater beer and wine use. There was no difference in the reported marijuana use in the two groups, and no differences in alcohol or marijuana use existed between the two groups 3 years prior to follow-up. The authors also compared drug and alcohol use between stimulant (Ritalin)-treated hyperactives and nontreated group matched for age, IQ, and academic achievement. There were no significant differences between the groups in terms of drug abuse, but there was a trend toward greater beer and wine use among the treated group. There were no similar trends for alcohol (hard liquor) or marijuana use.

In a less well-controlled study (described in detail in Chapter 6), Mendelson et al.[4] interviewed mothers of 83 hyperactives age 12–16 years. Some 15% were reported as drinking excessively, and 5% had a history of drug abuse. There was no control or comparison group, so the significance of these findings cannot adequately be assessed.

Similarly, Feldman et al.[5] (see details in Chapter 6) followed 81 hyperactive adolescents retrospectively. The age range was 12–20 years with a mean of 15.5 years. Subject interviews revealed that 3 of the 81 hyperactive adolescents were drug abusers, and it is uncertain if any had problems with alcohol abuse. This small number is reassuring and contrasts with Blouin's et al.[3] finding, but again no control or comparison group exists.

Beck et al.[6] in an attempt to determine if stimulant treatment in childhood contributed to drug abuse in adolescent hyperactives, compared 30 hyperactive subjects who had received at least 6 months of stimulant treatment during childhood (though not currently) with 30 subjects matched for age, sex, and socioeconomic status. (Socioeconomic range was from ghetto poverty to lower middle class.) The control subjects were drawn from medical and surgical inpatient units but did not have chronic disabilities or previous psychiatric histories. The sample was 14–19 years of age, with a mean of 17.8 years. Most hyperactives (28 of the 30) were not currently using any nonmedical drugs and had not used any for more than 6 months before the interview (27 of the 30). However, only 22 of the 30 control subjects were not using drugs currently, and only 19 of the 30 had not used them in the last 6 months. It appears that the control group used nonmedical drugs to a greater extent than the hyperactive group.

Another study which suggested that drug and alcohol use in hyperactive adolescents was not significantly greater than in age-matched population-survey controls was that of Kramer et al.[7,8] These authors evaluated 124 hyperactive boys aged 12–18 years in a 5-year follow-up study. The subjects were originally selected from initial referral records if their histories suggested they were not retarded, had Minimal Brain Dysfunction (MBD), and had been given stimulant medication in the first 6 weeks after referral. At follow-up comprehensive assessments included interviews with the boy and the parents; behavioral rating scales from the boy, the parents, and teachers; and an extensive battery of cognitive, personality, and achievement tests.

Drug and alcohol use was discussed under delinquency variables. Drug involvement included possessing, furnishing, selling, or using one or more of a variety of illegal substances (e.g., marijunana, stimulants, sedatives, hallucinogens). Involvement with illegal drugs was reported by 19% of the sample, with 16% of the subjects themselves stating that they had smoked marijuana. By way of comparison, two Iowa drug surveys suggested that this level of involvement was at or *below* norms for the state. In one survey, Hays[9] showed that of 6th-, 8th-, 10th-, and 12th-graders 2%, 11%, 22%, and 33% respectively had used marijuana at least once and 6–17% had tried other drugs. In another survey, Chambers[10] questioned 14- to 17-year-olds and found that 23–35% of the subjects claimed to use marijuana and 4–13% said they had tried hallucinogens, heroin, and cocaine. Involvement with alcohol included any possession, furnishing, selling, or use (without parental consent) while a minor or to a minor, and drunkenness at any age. Twenty-eight percent of the subjects revealed such involvement. By comparison, Hays[9] reported 37% of Iowa 6th-graders and 84% of 12th-graders had some alcohol involvement. Chambers[10] similarly showed that 30–36% of Iowa 14- to 17-year-olds used alcohol at least once a week. Thus, drug and alcohol use in the Iowa study was either at or below matched-age survey norms for that state.

Henker et al.[11] broached the problem of drug use in hyperactive adolescents and its association with stimulant treatment in childhood from a general-survey point of view. Nearly 500 junior-high-school boys (12–15 years of age, mean age 13 years) were assessed with anonymous questionnaires. The "drugs" included both over-the-counter and prescribed medication as well as illicit substances. Information was also obtained on current and earlier treatment with stimulant medication. Those subjects who had received stimulant medication were designated as the "hyperactive" group. The authors thus compared 17 stimulant-medicated boys to 466 boys who had never received stimulant medication. There was no evidence that the "hyperactive" group had any increase in use of illicit or nonmedicinal substances. In fact, the comparison group seemed to use alcohol slightly more than the hyperactive group. Only 2 of the 17 subjects in the "hyperactive" group had used illicit drugs and showed more frequent drinking. The remainder, the large majority of the group, had no experience with illicit drugs and intended none. Current alcohol consumption was low and restricted largely to special occasions.

We thus see that most studies of hyperactive adolescents[5-7,11] do not show significant drug or alcohol use. Blouin et al.'s[3] study showed increased alcohol use (though not necessarily abuse), while Mendelson et al.'s[4] had no comparison group. However, the second category of studies to be discussed has given rise to concerns regarding the link between childhood hyperactivity and adult drug and/or alcohol abuse.

STUDIES OF ADULT PSYCHIATRIC PATIENTS (INCLUDING ALCHOLICS) WITH POSSIBLE HISTORIES OF CHILDHOOD HYPERACTIVITY

Goodwin et al.[12] compared alcoholics and nonalcoholics in a sample of 133 Danish adoptees, mean age 30. He found that the alcoholics, as children, were more often hyperactive, truant, antisocial, shy, aggressive, disobedient, and friendless. The adoptive parents of the two groups did not differ with regard to socioeconomic status, psychopathology, or drinking histories. However, 10 of the 14 alcoholics had biological parents who were alcoholic, with no known alcoholism among the biological parents of nonalcoholics. The connection between alcoholism and the hyperactive child syndrome suggested by this study is weak. The subjects who were alcoholic in adulthood had many difficulties (e.g., genetic predisposition, social problems), in addition to their hyperactivity, which may have contributed to their alcoholism.

In a more recent study on male alcoholic patients Wood and his associates[13] estimated that 33% of the 27 alcoholic male subjects (all less than 40 years) met criteria for Attention Deficit Disorder, Residual Type. This diagnosis was made by questioning subjects about their childhood, giving their parents a parental rating scale which tapped behavior of their children at age 8–10, and seeing if adults met various adult behavior requirements for this syndrome. This retrospective aspect of the diagnosis is a shortcoming, as is the fact that two-thirds of the 27 subjects were in the two lower socioeconomic statuses and none were in the two upper ones. However, as the authors themselves point out, no conclusions can be drawn without studying the prevalence of Attention Deficit Disorder in nonalcoholic subjects (patients and nonpatients) in this same socioeconomic status.

Some control for socioeconomic status was attempted by Morrison,[14] who compared 48 adult psychiatric patients who retrospectively reported symptoms compatible with childhood hyperactivity with two groups of patients who gave no such histories. Both comparison groups matched the "hyperactive" group on age and sex and the second group was also matched for economic status. The authors felt that Substance Abuse was the most frequent primary diagnosis in the "hyperactive" group, as compared to Affective Disorder in the comparison groups. Twice as many subjects in the hyperactive group received a primary diagnosis of Alcoholism when compared to the other two groups. However, this did not reach statistical significance. The authors concluded that formerly hyperactive subjects showed significantly more personality disorders of all types, more sociopathy, more alcoholism, and less affective disorders than controls. Schizophrenia and drug abuse occurred no more often in these subjects than in the comparison groups.

The connection between childhood hyperactivity and adult alcoholism was also made by Tarter et al.,[15] who reported more symptoms of childhood hyperactivity in individuals with severe primary alcoholism than in those with milder, secondary alcoholism, other psychiatric patients, and normal controls.

We thus see that several studies[12,13,15] have looked at adult alcoholics and sought childhood hyperactive histories in their subjects. Other authors have looked at adult psychiatric patients with childhood histories of hyperactivity and found some increased alcohol use in this group compared to a matched comparison group.

The final group of studies[16,17] have sought to diagnose adult Attention Deficit Disorder, Residual Type, and to see if these subjects are responsive to stimulant medication. In Wood et al.'s[16] study some 27% of the 15 subjects (mean age 28 years) reported drinking problems and 7% reported drug use. However, no control or comparison group was used, so the significance of this frequency is difficult to assess. Is it greater or less than a matched patient or population comparison group?

Mattes et al.[17] did use a comparison group, and patients with current drug or alcohol addiction were excluded, although drug or alcohol abuse without evidence of physical addiction was not an exclusion criterion. Most of Mattes's patients were 18–45 years of age and were referred from a psychiatric outpatient clinic. To be included in the study patients had to meet age and questionnaire (for adult Attention Deficit Disorder symptomatology) criteria. Three of the 27 such patients with childhood hyperactivity met DSM-III criteria for alcoholism compared to 4 of the 37 similar patients without such childhood history. Likewise, 10 of the 29 subjects in the "childhood hyperactive" group met DSM-III criteria for drug abuse, while 6 of the 37 patients without childhood hyperactivity met these criteria. These differences were not statistically significant. We thus see that no significant increase in drug or alcohol abuse existed in adult patients with childhood histories of hyperactivity compared to a patient group without such childhood histories.

In summary, one can say that adult studies examining alcoholics who give histories suggestive of childhood hyperactivity attempt to link childhood hyperactivity and adult alcoholism. These studies need to be regarded with caution because they often lack suitable control or comparison groups and they rely too heavily on the subjective recall of the alcoholic subjects themselves. Studies that have looked at adult Attention Deficit Disorder, Residual Type, are also handicapped by retro-spective diagnosis. However, with suitable comparison groups[17] the link between childhood hyperactivity and adult alcoholism/drug abuse appears weak.

STUDIES OF FAMILIES OF HYPERACTIVE CHILDREN

The other group of studies which have linked childhood hyperactive syndrome with adult alcoholism and/or drug abuse involve the families of hyperactive children. Thus, Morrison and Stewart[18] interviewed the parents of 59 hyperactive and 41 control children and showed a higher prevalence of alcoholism, sociopathy, and hysteria in the parents of the hyperactive children.

Cantwell[19] had similar findings. Systematic psychiatric examina-tions of parents of 50 hyperactive children and 50 matched controls showed increased prevalence rates for alcoholism, sociopathy, and hys-teria, but not affective disorder, among the parents of the hyperactive children. This was particularly true for those parents who were thought to have been hyperactive children themselves.

The biological link between childhood hyperactivity and adult dis-orders, including alcoholism, sociopathy, and hysteria, was further strengthened by Morrison and Stewart,[20] who showed the high preva-lence of these conditions in biological but *not* adoptive parents of hyper-active children. However, the careful prescreening of potential adoptive parents would probably eliminate individuals showing any psychiatric disturbance and so adoptive parents represent a preselected, well-functioning group.

Stewart et al.[21] sought to show that the alcoholism and antisocial disorders seen in parents of hyperactive children are really associated with children who are unsocialized–aggressive rather than hyperactive. He tried to distinguish between these two groups of children. Indeed, Antisocial Personality Disorder and alcoholism were more frequent in fathers of unsocialized–aggressive boys. However, 27 of the 38 subjects classified as unsocialized–aggressive were also hyperactive, so it may well be the combination of these two conditions which is important.

Morrison,[22] in a more recent study, sought to correct the limita-tions of previous family studies[18,19] that had used normal children as controls rather than children attending a psychiatric clinic for reasons other than hyperactivity. Thus, the increased psychopathology seen in parents of hyperactive children may be seen in all families whose children have emotional problems and may not be particularly linked to hyperactivity. Morrison compared family histories of 140 children and adolescents with hyperactive child syndrome with the family histories of 91 psychiatrically ill children matched for age and sex but who did not have ADD(H). Parents of hyperactives were more likely to have Antisocial Personality Disorder and hysteria but *not* alcoholism when compared to parents of nonhyperactive psychiatrically ill children. The incidence of alcoholism in both groups of parents was fairly high, casting doubt on the specific link between alcoholism and hyperactivity.

This lack of specific connection between alcoholism and hyperactivity was further shown by Offord et al.,[23] who compared 31 delinquent children who were hyperactive with 35 delinquents who were not hyperactive. The two groups did not differ in socioeconomic status, IQ, school performance prior to onset of antisocial behavior, number of broken homes, and frequency of parental mental illness, including alcoholism. The hyperactive delinquent group had 16 parents (5 mothers, 11 fathers) who were definitely and probably alcoholic compared to 19 parents (2 mothers and 17 fathers) for the nonhyperactive delinquent group.

We thus see the link between childhood hyperactivity and adult alcoholism suggested by the earlier family studies[18-20] has not been borne out by later, somewhat better-controlled studies.[22,23]

FOLLOW-UP STUDIES OF ADULT HYPERACTIVES: PROSPECTIVE AND RETROSPECTIVE

Laufer[24] reported on a 12-year questionnaire follow-up of subjects 15–26 years of age who had initially been referred for hyperkinesis and treated with stimulants. The questionnaires were sent to parents of subjects, and 66 of 100 were returned. This methodology may constitute a positive bias: those returning mailed questionnaires may be a more positive outcome group. Further, parents of young adults are rarely fully aware of the extent of nonmedical drug or alcohol use by their children. However, 5 of 66 reported experimenting with marijuana or LSD, 3 of 56 reported nonprescription use of stimulants, and none reported habitual use of any drugs except alcohol. Four of 50 reported excessive drinking. The absence of a comparison group and the possible methodological bias outlined previously make it unclear what significance these findings carry.

In a somewhat better-controlled study Feldman et al.[5] evaluated 48 subjects referred in childhood for hyperactivity and 32 of their siblings. The mean age at referral was 9 years and at follow-up 21 years. A comparison of nonprescribed drug use was carried out between the young-adult hyperactives, their siblings, and 200 normal population-survey controls. Fifty percent of the adult hyperactives had tried marijuana, compared to 37% of their siblings and 33% of the normal survey controls. This finding was of only borderline significance ($p = .10$). Only one of the adult hyperactive subjects reported using marijuana daily. The use of psychostimulants (speed and cocaine) was less in the hyperactive group than in the normal survey group (20% vs. 26%). Generally there was no evidence that use of stimulant drugs in childhood is associated with drug abuse in young-adult life, since no statistically significant differences were detected among young-adult hyperactives, siblings, and normal survey controls.

Feldman et al.'s[5] results, however, focused more concern on alcohol use. Sixteen percent of the 48 young-adult hyperactive subjects reported being drunk before school or work compared to none of the 32 siblings ($p < .02$). There was also a trend for the young-adult hyperactive group to have greater frequency of drunkenness when compared to their sibling comparison group ($p < .01$). Some 15% reported being drunk more than one time per week. Other items such as having blackouts, using alcohol to relieve anxiety, tension or depression, and whether or not alcohol use was a problem for the subject did not differentiate young-adult hyperactives from their siblings. However, as the authors point out, as many as 15% of students under the age of 25 in their state may be problem drinkers or potential abusers of alcohol. Therefore, the figure for alcohol abuse for the young-adult hyperactive group is not significantly different from that of students of similar age in that state.

In another retrospective study of a slightly older group, Borland and Heckman[25] compared 20 men (mean age 30 years) whose childhood medical records conformed to diagnostic criteria of hyperactive child syndrome 20–25 years ago with their brothers (mean age 28 years). No hyperactive subjects or their brothers met the criteria for a diagnosis of alcoholism, and only 1 hyperactive subject met the criteria for drug dependence. Again, no marked evidence of drug or alcohol abuse was seen in the adult hyperactives.

In one of the few prospective follow-up studies, Milman[26] followed 73 patients diagnosed in childhood as having MBD. At follow-up, 9–15 years after the initial assessment, subjects were 15–23 years of age with a mean of 19.4 years. None of the subjects in the study used alcohol pathologically, although a few had experimented with drugs, and 1 was a confirmed marijuana user. The author cites the white, largely Jewish, middle- and upper-class population as being partly responsible for these results. However, these findings are in keeping with those of others.[24,25]

The importance of comparison groups and particularly different types of comparison groups in interpreting one's findings was clearly illustrated by Loney and coworkers.[27] The authors are conducting an extensive follow-up study of 200 subjects treated in childhood for hyperactivity and 100 of their full brothers. All follow-up assessments take place when the subjects are 21–23 years of age. The data on 22 proband–brother pairs have been analyzed thus far. In addition to the brother comparison group, the authors used the data from the National Survey on Drug Abuse[28] as another comparison source. The Schedule for Affective Disorders and Schizophrenia, Lifetime Version (SADS-L)[29] was used in making the diagnosis of alcoholism, drug abuse, and Antisocial Personality Disorder. Hyperactive subjects and their brothers did not differ significantly on any of the 19 individual criteria for alcoholism. Six of the 22 hyperactive subjects met criteria for definite and probable alcoholism, while 5 of the 22 brothers met these same criteria. This figure was thought to be high compared to normal males. At the time of the interview, 3 of the 22 hyperactive adults and none of their brothers currently met criteria for alcoholism. However, this did not reach statistical signficance even at the $p = .10$ level. Similarly, there were no differences between the hyperactive adults and their brothers in either current or lifetime diagnosis of drug abuse. However, when the responses of hyperactives and their brothers were compared individually to normative data from the national survey, it appeared that more hyperactives have had experiences with inhalants, cocaine, opiates, and nonmedical sedatives and stimulants than the average 18- to 25-year-old in the survey. Thus hyperactives have experimented with a greater range of illegal substances. In a supplementary analysis of the national survey which involved extent of current use, hyperactives used marijuana to a greater extent. They, more than their brothers, considered themselves to be regular users of both cocaine and opiates.

All this suggests some increased involvement with drugs by the hyperactives when compared to the national survey and possibly their brothers as well. As the authors point out, a clearer view of the significance of these findings will emerge when the larger sample is evaluated, when a more current (1981) national survey is completed, and when a subgroup from the national survey which matches the subjects on age, sex, race, and region can be extracted and compared.

In a prospective follow-up study of 103 hyperactives age 16–23 (mean age 18.9), Gittelman[30] showed that at follow-up hyperactives had about a 12% increased prevalence of Substance Abuse Disorder when compared to normal controls. Drug as opposed to Alcohol Use Disorder accounted for most of this increase. The rate for alcohol abuse was very similar in the two groups. The drug abuse often preceded the alcohol abuse. The substance abuse was often linked to conduct disorder or antisocial life-style, which was also much more prevalent in the currently hyperactive group. In fact, if cases with persistent ADD are disregarded there was so significant difference between former patients and controls with regard to antisocial disorders and substance abuse disorder. Furthermore, in all cases, the conduct disorder preceded or coincided with the onset of substance abuse disorder and almost all cases of substance abuse occurred among probands with an antisocial disorder. The authors thus stress that continuing symptoms of ADD into young adulthood are strongly linked to antisocial and substance abuse disorder. This is particularly true of those hyperactives with concurrent conduct disorder.

In contrast, Lambert,[31] in an 8-year follow-up of some of the subjects in the Berkeley Hyperactivity Studies, showed that at 17 and 18 years of age children initially diagnosed as hyperactive generally show more use of substances. However, their use of substances is not significantly different from random controls, with the exception of cigarettes. Lambert points out that self-concept measures and evidence of positive peer relationships are critical predictions of hard-drug use. In turn, children who report conduct disorder at age 17 and 18 also report less successful relationships with peers. Thus again, the important link of conduct disorder and substance use is seen.

We thus see that some studies support the link between childhood hyperactivity and adult alcoholism or drug abuse, while others do not. Generally, studies which look at adult alcoholics and try to identify childhood hyperactivity,[12,13,15] and some family studies[18,19] support this link. However studies which have followed hyperactives into adolescence[5-7] and young adulthood[24-26] have not shown a strong connection between childhood hyperactivity and adult drug and alcohol abuse. Stimulant treatment in childhood seems to have little influence on adult drug or alcohol use.

However, some studies hinted at concerns. For example, Feldman et al.[5] suggested some increased alcohol use in the young-adult group, although not significantly higher than state norm surveys. Loney et al.[27] showed fairly high alcohol use though no greater than the brother comparison group. National survey comparison data, although they have serious limitations of comparability, also suggested greater drug use (though not *abuse*) in the hyperactive group. Gittelman et al.[30] clearly linked persistent hyperactivity with substance abuse disorder (particularly drugs) and conduct disorder.

With these concerns in mind, we carried out detailed assessments of past and current alcohol and drug use in our 10- and 15-year follow-up studies. For details regarding subjects and methodology, see Chapter 5.

DRUG AND ALCOHOL USE AND ABUSE AT TEN-YEAR FOLLOW-UP[32]

Scales of Severity of Nonmedical Drug Use (Table 8-1)

The scales of severity of use for the various nonmedical drugs were constructed by the research team after consultation with colleagues in the department and questioning similar-aged controls not in the study. This was done because data from the 10-year follow-up study indicated that the level of use generally was too mild to be tapped by existing abuse scales. Normative scales for a Canadian population of this age group were not available. This does limit comparability with other studies; however, the stages in the scales were very specifically and operationally defined so comparisons would be possible.

Results

NONMEDICAL DRUG USE (Table 8-2)

A significantly greater percentage of hyperactive subjects had used nonmedical drugs in the 5 years preceding 10-year follow-up (75% vs. 54%, $p < .04$), but there was no difference between the groups with respect to nonmedical drug use in the year before the follow-up. There was no difference between the groups with regard to type of nonmedical drug used in the previous 5 years. However, significantly more controls than hyperactives had used hallucinogens (38% vs. 9%, $p < .02$) within the year before the follow-up. There was no difference between the two groups with respect to severity of drug use (mild, moderate, or abuse) in the 5 years or in the year prior to follow-up. However, there was a trend for more hyperactives than controls (17% vs. 4%, $p < .08$) to have been involved in selling nonmedical drugs in the last 5 years.

ALCOHOL USE (Table 8-3)

Most subjects, controls and hyperactives, used alcohol. However, currently (in last 3 months) most used it to a mild extent, and no significant differences existed between hyperactives and controls.

When one examines maximum use, that is, the period of time during the past 5 years when subjects used alcohol most heavily, one finds that significantly more controls than hyperactives fall into the moderate category ($p < .05$). However, when one combines the abuse and addiction categories and compares them with the mild and moder-

TABLE 8-1. Scales of Severity of Nonmedical Drug Use

	Alcohol	Marijuana/hashish	Hallucinogens (LSD/mescaline)	Stimulants (amphetamines/speed)	Cocaine	Heroin	Barbiturates/ Mandrax
Mild	Average one to three drinks/week Drunk once/month socially	One to three times/ week	One time/month	One time/month	One time/month	Use one to three times *ever*	One time/week
Moderate	Four or more drinks/ week Drunk two to three times/month socially	Three times/week to three or four times/ day	One time/month to three times/week	One time/month to three times/week	One time/month to three times/week	Between Mild and Abuse	Two times/week
Abuse	Eight drinks every weekend Drunk every weekend Two to four drinks/ day	More than four times/day Impaired functioning for at least 24 hours/ week	More than three times /week	More than three times/ week, injecting, or impaired functioning	More than three times/week	One time/week	Three times/week or impaired functioning
Addicted	Four or more drinks/ day Drunk two or more times/week Drinks in the morning	Psychological and/or physical dependence	Psychological and/or physical dependence	Psychological and/or physical dependence	Psychological and/or physical dependence	Psychological and/or physical dependence	Psychological and/or physical dependence

TABLE 8-2. Nonmedical Drug Use and Abuse at 10-Year Follow-Up

	In the past year			In the last 5 years		
	Controls (%)	Hyperactives (%)	Sig.	Controls (%)	Hyperactives (%)	Sig.
	(n = 44)	(n = 74)		(n = 44)	(n = 74)	
Used nonmedical drug	45	59		54	75	$p < .04$
Sold nonmedical drug	2	8		4	17	$p < .08$ (trend)
	(n = 21)[a]	(n = 42)[a]		(n = 23)[a]	(n = 53)[a]	
Used hashish or marijuana	95	95		100	96	
Used barbiturates	None	4		None	11	
Used narcotics	None	4		4	13	
Used hallucinogens	38	9	$p < .02$	52	45	
Used stimulants	14	14		26	29	
	(n = 20)[a]	(n = 44)[a]		(n = 24)[a]	(n = 55)[a]	
Severity of drug use						
Mild	65	66		54	52	
Moderate	20	22		33	29	
Abuse	15	11		12	18	

Note. Four subjects had used cocaine periodically (usually for less than 1 year) and 4 subjects tried heroin three to four times. One subject thought he might have been addicted to heroin for a few months at age 19.
[a]These are the numbers of subjects within each sample who used any nonmedical drug.

TABLE 8-3. Details of Past Drug and Alcohol Use at 10-Year Follow-Up

	Ever used (not in last 3 months) (n)	Mean age started (years)	Mean age max. use (years)	Duration of max. use (months)	Extent of max. use			Mean age stopped (years)
					Mild (n)	Moderate (n)	Abuse/ addiction (n)	
Alcohol								
Controls	9.0	14.8	18.4	16.3	12.0	13.0	10.0	
Hyperactives	20.0	16.0	18.1	10.5	14.0	6.0	27.0	
Sig.	p < .01	p < .035				p < .05		
Hashish and marijuana								
Controls	13.0	16.5	17.7	17.0	18.0	7.0	0	19.7
Hyperactives	26.0	15.7	17.5	13.5	17.0	11.0	7.0	18.1
Sig.	p < .01	p < .07					p < .05	
Hallucinogens								
Controls	6.0	16.4	16.6	4.1	6.0	7.0	2.0	17.0
Hyperactives	10.0	16.7	17.1	13.8	16.0	5.0	4.0	18.6
Sig.				p < .004				p < .024
Stimulants								
Controls	6.0	16.3	16.3	2.0	4.0	1.0	1.0	17.6
Hyperactives	10.0	16.9	17.8	9.8	6.0	1.0	5.0	18.5
Sig.								
Cocaine								
Controls	2.0	20.6	20.6	12.0	1.0	1.0	0	21.0
Hyperactives	7.0	18.1	18.8	3.2	5.0	0	2.0	18.6
Sig.		p < .019	p < .02					p < .015
Heroin								
Controls	0	0	0	0	0	0	0	0
Hyperactives	5.0	17.8	19.4	3.7	3.0	0	3.0	20.5
Sig.								
Barbiturates								
Controls	3.0	16.6	16.6	6.5	3.0	0	0	17.0
Hyperactives	6.0	18.0	18.7	6.3	4.0	0	2.0	17.7
Sig.								

ate categories, one finds that significantly more hyperactives ($p < .01$) fall into the abuse or addiction categories.

The findings suggest that more hyperactives than controls had periods of maximum use of alcohol that were serious (bordering on abuse). However this was not the case currently. Evidently, controls also started drinking earlier—at a mean age of 14 compared to 16 years ($p < .035$). The age at which both groups consumed the most alcohol was 18.

HASHISH AND MARIJUANA

The majority of both hyperactives and controls had used marijuana in the 3 months prior to evaluation, but most used the drug only to a mild extent. However, significantly more hyperactives had tried hashish or marijuana at one time (20 compared to 9, $p < .01$) though there was no difference between the groups in the 3 months prior to evaluation.

During the period of maximum use, significantly more hyperactives than controls fell into the abuse category—7 compared to 0 ($p < .05$)—and there was a trend for them to start using marijuana slightly earlier (15.7 compared to 16.5 years, $p < .07$). There was no difference in the mean duration of maximum use (17 and 13.5 months), mean age of maximum use (17 years), and mean age when the subjects stopped (19 years for controls, 18 years for hyperactives).

HALLUCINOGENS (LSD, MESCALINE)

Few of our subjects used either drug in the 3 months prior to evaluation (1 control and 3 hyperactives). However, though not statistically significant, slightly more hyperactives than controls had used hallucinogens in the past.

No differences appeared in the extent of maximum use; most subjects were in the mild or moderate category. However, hyperactives had a longer duration of maximum use when compared to controls (13.8 months compared to 4.1 months, $p < .004$). The mean age at which subjects first started using these drugs and mean age of maximum use were not different for the two groups. However, mean age stopped was significantly older for the hyperactives (18.6 compared to 17.0 years, $p < .024$).

STIMULANTS (AMPHETAMINES, SPEED)

Again, we see that few subjects (no controls and only 2 hyperactives) were currently using stimulants. Relatively few had any history of using this type of drug in the past (6 controls and 10 hyperactives). The extent of maximum use for those few who had used it was usually mild. There appears to be no difference between the hyperactive and control groups in the age at which the drug was first used (16 years), age of maximum use (16 and 17 years), age stopped (17 and 18 years), or the mean duration of maximum use (2 to 9.8 months). No significant differences whatever were seen between hyperactives and controls with regard to use of this drug.

COCAINE

Few subjects (1 control and 4 hyperactives) were currently using cocaine. A few, too, had used it in the past (2 controls, 7 hyperactives). The extent of maximum use was usually mild. No significant differences with regard to cocaine use as described above were seen in the two groups. However, when one examines the mean age started, the age of maximum use, and mean age when stopped, we see that hyperactives were significantly younger in all these measures: 18 years compared to 20 years ($p < .02$).

HEROIN

Interestingly, none of our control subjects had ever tried this drug. One hyperactive had used it in the 3 months prior to evaluation and only 5 others had ever tried it. In the last 5 years the maximum extent of use was usually mild (3 subjects); however, 2 subjects were in the abuse category and 1 in the addiction category. Even though these numbers did not reach statistical significance, it is important to note that 3 hyperactives had at one time fallen into the abuse or addiction category compared to 0 controls. None of these were currently addicted to or abusing herion, although 1 continued to use it to a mild degree. The 2 other subjects who had abused the drug in the past had stopped using it altogether for 4 years and 1 year respectively at the time of the interview.

BARBITURATES, MANDRAX

None of the subjects (hyperactives or controls) were currently using barbiturates or Mandrax. However, 3 controls and 6 hyperactives had histories of having used these drugs in the past. Most had used it to a mild extent, though 2 hyperactives fell into the abuse category.

No significant differences in the two groups on the above measures were seen. The groups also did not differ significantly in the mean age they started use of these drugs (controls 16.6 years; hyperactives 18.0 years). The mean age of maximum use was 16.6 years for controls and 18.7 years for hyperactives and the mean age at which subjects stopped using the drugs was 17.0 years for the controls and 17.7 years for the hyperactives.

REASONS FOR DISCONTINUING NONMEDICAL DRUG USE

The most common reason given by both controls and hyperactives for discontinuing the use of any drug (with the exception of cocaine) was that they did not like the side effects or physical consequences of the drugs. Cocaine use was usually discontinued because of lack of funds. Legal or social consequences played a minor role, usually with regard to marijuana or hallucinogens. No significant differences were seen between controls and hyperactives in their reasons for discontinuing nonmedical drug use.

Discussion

There has been concern that prolonged stimulant treatment of hyperactive children would predispose them to increased general drug use and possible abuse. Furthermore, the difficulties hyperactives have with school failure, familial stresses, poor self-esteem, and poor peer relationships would also perhaps predispose them to drug abuse. Generally, we have not found this to be the case. Hyperactives as young adults, when compared to controls, may have had more nonmedical drug use in the last 5 years, but not currently.

Alcohol and marijuana are the only substances which large numbers of subjects in both groups continue to use to any significant extent. Current use of other drugs (hallucinogens, stimulants, cocaine, and heroin) was slightly higher by hyperactives but by and large not significantly different from the matched control group. Both groups generally started using drugs between 16 and 17 years, had a maximum period of use between 17 and 18 years, and stopped between 18 and 19 years. The main reasons for discontinuing drug use seem to be physical consequences and side effects. It is interesting that legal and social consequences or shifts in life-style are not reported by the subjects to be main reasons for stopping the use of drugs.

It must be pointed out that a small subgroup of hyperactives seem more heavily involved in nonmedical drug use. This is reflected in the consistently higher (though not statistically significant) numbers of hyperactives involved in the use of marijuana, hallucinogens, stimulants, cocaine, and heroin. Heroin is particularly striking in that 5 hyperactives in our study have tried it, 3 falling into the abuse or addiction category, compared to none of the controls. It may well be this subgroup that is picked up by the follow-up studies of Robins[33] and others that suggest a more negative adult outcome.

There was a general view that at 10-year follow-up, when the subjects were 17–24 years of age (mean age 19 years), outcome was still in a state of flux. For example, a significantly greater percentage of hyperactive subjects had used nonmedical drugs in the 5 years preceding 10-year follow-up, but there was no significant difference between the groups in this regard in the year prior to follow-up. Furthermore, there was some concern regarding the small subgroup that appeared to have greater drug and alcohol involvement. Was this a function of the times, their particular age and stage of life, or did it suggest a small but stable poor-outcome group who would become long-standing abusers of drugs or alcohol? To clarify these issues and, hopefully, to obtain a clearer, more stable outcome picture, the 15-year follow-up was undertaken when the subjects had a mean age of 25 years.

DRUG AND ALCOHOL USE AND ABUSE AT FIFTEEN-YEAR FOLLOW-UP[34]

For details regarding subjects and methodology please refer to Chapter 5.

Scales of Severity of Nonmedical Drug Use

The scales of severity of use of alcohol and the various nonmedical drugs that were constructed by the research team (as described earlier in this chapter; see Table 8-1) at 10-year follow-up were used again at 15-year follow-up to enable comparison over time.

Results

ALCOHOL USE (Table 8-4)

Most subjects, both controls and hyperactives, had used alcohol currently (in the last 3 months) and had done so to a mild or moderate extent with no significant differences between the two groups. There was a trend ($p < .08$) for more hyperactives than controls to fall into the abuse category when the *average* use of alcohol in the last 12 months was assessed. In looking at the last 3 years of alcohol use together and separately, no significant differences between controls and hyperactives were found.

TABLE 8-4. Current Alcohol Use at 15-Year Follow-Up

	Controls (n = 41)	Hyperactives (n = 61)
Any alcohol use (last 3 years)	39	56
Severity of use (last 3 months)		
None		
Mild	18	29
Moderate	15	10
Abuse	5	14
Addiction	1	3
Times drunk (last 3 months)	7.3	7.8
Extent and frequency of average use (last 12 months)		
None		
Mild	21	30
Moderate	13	9
Abuse	4	16 (p < .08)
Addiction	2	2
Extent and frequency of heavier use (last 12 months)		
Moderate	2	1
Abuse	4	3
Addiction	1	6

Note. In looking at last 3 years together and separately, no significant differences were found.

NONMEDICAL DRUG USE (Table 8-5)

Approximately 50% of subjects in both the control and hyperactive groups were currently (in last 3 months) using nonmedical drugs. For the vast majority in both groups this is marijuana and hashish, and most subjects use it to a mild degree, with none falling into the abuse category. The findings are similar when marijuana/hashish use in the last 12 months is examined. A very distant second is cocaine, with 6 subjects in each group using this drug. Again the extent of use is mild for most of the subjects, with 1 hyperactive falling into the abuse categories. Only 1 or 2 subjects were using stimulants or hallucinogens, and no subjects are involved with heroin or barbiturates. These findings are similar for the hyperactive and control groups.

In assessing the use of nonmedical drugs in the last 3 years (Table 8-6), the picture is similar. Most subjects in both groups have used some nonmedical drug, and for the majority this was marijuana/hashish, with cocaine a distant second. Few subjects in either group had had any history of drug abuse in the last 3 years. There was a trend (p < .09) for more hyperactives to have tried heroin (4 vs. 0) compared

TABLE 8-5. Current (Last 3 months) Nonmedical Drug Use at 15-Year Follow-Up

	Controls (n = 41)	Hyperactives (n = 61)
Used any nonmedical drugs	19	35
Hashish/marijuana (extent and frequency)	19	35
Mild	16	29
Moderate	3	6
Hallucinogens (extent)	0	2
Mild	0	2
Cocaine (extent)	6	6
Mild	5	5
Moderate	1	0
Abuse	0	1
Stimulants (extent)		
Mild	1	1
Heroin	0	0
Barbiturates	0	0

to controls. In looking at each year separately for each drug, no additional significant differences were found between the groups.

It is interesting to note that when subjects were asked if they had intentionally stopped using any or all drugs for at least 6 months in the past 3 years, significantly more hyperactives compared to controls had done so (19 vs. 5, $p < .02$). Reasons for stopping drug use were explored and generally fell into the following categories: impaired func-

TABLE 8-6. Nonmedical Drug Use (Last 3 years) at 15-Year Follow-Up

	Controls		Hyperactives		
	Any use	Abuse	Any use	Abuse	Significance
	(n = 39)		(n = 60)		
Any nonmedical drug	27	4	42	12	
Hashish/marijuana	28		41		
Hallucinogens	4		10		
Cocaine	13		15		
Stimulants	3		5		
Heroin	0		4		$p < .09$
	(n = 28)		(n = 41)		
Stopped drug use (for 6 months in last 3 years)	5		19		$p < .02$

Note. In looking at each year separately for each drug, no added significant differences were found between the groups.

tioning, health worries, lack of funds, legal–social consequences, shift in life-style. Generally no particular reason was cited more frequently than any other, nor were there any particular reasons associated with particular drugs. These findings were similar for hyperactives and controls.

DRUG SELLING (Table 8-7)

There was a trend for more hyperactives to be involved in selling nonmedical drugs when compared to controls (13 vs. 3, $p < .09$). Most subjects sold marijuana, either for profit or to pay for their own drug use. However, it was the major source of income for only 1 hyperactive.

SADS DRUG AND ALCOHOL USE (Table 8-8)

It should be stressed that only a subgroup (37 controls, 51 hyperactives) agreed to do the SADS. We modified the test to focus on the last 5 years versus lifetime history, thus preserving the blindness of the interviewer. Findings on the SADS generally support and confirm the findings obtained on our scales from subject interviews. There were no significant differences between hyperactives and controls on alcohol or drug use. Alcohol use was greater than drug use in both groups. Most subjects in both groups showed no or clinically insignificant effects on their functioning from their drug use. Only 4 hyperactives, and no controls, showed important modification or major disruption in their functioning due to drug use in the last 5 years.

TABLE 8-7. Selling Nonmedical Drugs

	Controls ($n = 41$)	Hyperactives ($n = 60$)	Significance
Sold drugs last 3 years	3	13	$p < .09$
Sold for			
Major income		1	
Profit		7	
Own drug use	3	6	
Sold mostly			
Marijuana	2	10	
Hallucinogens			
Stimulants		1	
Cocaine	2	2	
Heroin			
Barbiturates		1	

TABLE 8-8. Drug or Alcohol Use on Modified SADS

	Controls (n = 37)	Hyperactives (n = 51)
Was there period when drank too much	11	18
Others objected to drinking	8	15
Wanted to stop and couldn't	1	1
Drinking heavily for a month	7	12
Drug abuse or dependence		
Not at all	12	14
Clinically insignificant	22	22
Minor interference	2	1
Important modification	0	2
Major disruption	0	2

Discussion

Generally one has the impression that hyperactives and controls are comparable in their current drug and alcohol use. These findings are similar to our 10-year follow-up data[32] and to those of others who have followed hyperactives into adulthood.[24-27]

Even though no statistically significant differences were found between the hyperactive and control groups with regard to drug and alcohol use, some trends are worth mentioning. There was a trend ($p < .08$) for more hyperactives than controls to fall into the abuse category when the average use of alcohol in the last 12 months was assessed. In the last 3 years, more hyperactives than controls tried heroin ($p < .09$), and significantly more ($p < .02$) actively stopped using a drug for at least 6 months. All this suggests that there is slight but consistent increased use of drugs and possibly alcohol by the hyperactive group, though this does not reach statistical significance nor result in significant dysfunction. This slight increase was also noted by Loney et al.[27] in comparing hyperactives with the national survey sample, though not with their brothers. Feldman et al.[5] too, noted some slight increased alcohol use in their hyperactive adults, but their state norms were equally high. This persistent slight increase may have no significance; it may reflect a small poor-outcome group that will be heavily involved in alcohol or drugs; or it may be a trend that will increase and become significant as more pressures and responsibilities accumulate for the subjects. This latter possibility is unlikely in view of Borland's and Heckman's[25] study, which found no alcoholism in their 20 hyperactives at age 30. The existence of a small subgroup that is more heavily involved in drugs and alcohol is a possibility. What contributed to some individuals becoming part of this subgroup is probably not one factor but the cumulation of various aspects, such as IQ, socioeconomic status and family functioning, including parental alcoholism or drug abuse. (These factors will be dealt with at greater length in the predictive section.) Thus the link between childhood hyperactivity and adult drug and alcohol abuse is weak. In the few instances where it does exist, it is strengthened by the cumulative stress of having several concurrent problems rather than hyperactivity alone.

Stimulant treatment in childhood does not predispose these individuals to greater drug or alcohol use in adulthood.[5,11,24,26] In fact, some authors[27] have suggested that successful stimulant treatment decreases adult drug and alcohol use. Despite this optimistic picture, the challenge of identifying and treating the subgroup, with its multiple-risk factors and poorer outcome, remains.

WORK RECORD

Only through labour
Is one at home in the world.
—From "Das Landhaus am Rhein,"
by Berthold Auerbach, 1812–1882

Few retrospective or prospective follow-up studies exist whose aim it was to systematically evaluate the work record and work status of hyperactive adults. The retrospective study of Menkes and coworkers[1] published in 1967 (which was described in more detail in Chapter 5, p. 62–63) suggested that of 14 adults retrospectively diagnosed as having had hyperactivity and Minimal Brain Dysfunction (MBD) 25 years earlier, only 8 were currently self-supporting. However, these authors pointed out that of their 9 patients who had IQ's above 90, 7 were currently self-supporting. This suggests that the poor employment record and economic dependency of the remaining 6 subjects were related to low intelligence. Feldman and coworkers,[2] who studied 48 young adults who had been diagnosed earlier as MBD or Hyperkinetic Impulse Disorder found that 90% were currently employed or at school.

The first retrospective study which systematically assessed work record and work status was that of Borland and coworkers[3] in Allentown, Pennsylvania (described in detail in Chapter 5, p. 63). These investigators traced and interviewed 20 of 37 men who in their childhood (20–25 years earlier) had conformed to Mendelson et al.'s[4] diagnostic criteria for the hyperactive child syndrome. As a comparison group 19 brothers were also interviewed; mean ages of the two groups were 30.4 years and 28.1 years respectively. All men in the study (probands and their brothers) were currently working full time and were self-supporting, with the exception of 2 brothers who were attending college.

Results showed that the socioeconomic status of both probands and their brothers was significantly higher currently than it had been at age 20. While both groups were upwardly mobile and had reached middle-class status, the socioeconomic status of the brothers was higher both at age 20 and at the time of the study, although the gap between the two groups was narrowing over time.

The hyperactive men worked more hours than their brothers, had more part-time jobs (in addition to their full-time jobs), and changed jobs more frequently. The 4 men who were diagnosed "sociopathic" changed jobs more frequently than the other 16, but this difference was not statistically significant. The main reason given by the hyperactive men for their additional part-time jobs was the increased income. However, these jobs involved activities of personal interest, or work they had previously done as a hobby, and each of the probands described his extra work as a means of avoiding feelings of restlessness and nervousness in periods of inactivity. For many of the probands, but for few of the brothers, changing from one job to another was preceded by dissatisfaction with what they regarded as the uninteresting and repetitious nature of their work, and the lack or promotion they felt they had earned.

This study indicates that while the work status of hyperactive adults is somewhat inferior to that of normals, their rate of full-time employment and self-sufficiency is similar to that of controls. The study also suggests that the hyperactive adults changed jobs more frequently because they more easily became impatient with what they felt was the boredom of the job. In addition about half of the hyperactive adults in this study carried additional part-time jobs to make more money but also to avoid feelings of restlessness and nervousness in periods of inactivity. As a result they worked extremely hard.

Weiss and coworkers[5] sent questionnaires to current employers and to classroom teachers (of the last grade of high school completed) of both young hyperactive adults and matched controls whose mean age was 19 years. (The employers' questionnaire used is described later in this chapter on p. 145.) It was found that employers rated hyperactive adults no different from controls on any of the questions, whereas high school teachers rated hyperactives significantly inferior to controls on all 7 items of the questionnaire. It seemed that the many choices of types of work, as compared to the relative lack of choice of activities in the secondary-school setting, as well as the degree of physical activity permissible (or even desirable) on the job, might account for the discrepancy in how hyperactive adults are viewed by employers and by teachers. Successful school performance requires not only intelligence but a high level of prolonged listening ability, reflective cognitive style, organizational ability, neatness, and the ability to memorize rote material, traits which are particularly poorly developed in hyperactive subjects. It is possible that for successful achievement at work different traits are valued, that at work hyperactives may do as well as or better than normals in some aspects of their work record (e.g., amount of work done), as was shown by Borland and Heckman's study.

We evaluated the work record of hyperactive adults and matched controls at the conclusion of the 10-year follow-up evaluation when they were 21 years old, having been encouraged by the favorable reports by their employers as seen on the employers' questionnaire, 2 years earlier. We obtained detailed work records on 53 hyperactive adults and 38 controls, as part of our 10-year follow-up evaluation of 75 hyperactive subjects. (Eleven refused to be interviewed again so soon, 5 had moved out of Montreal, 4 did not keep appointments or did not finish the evaluation, and 2 subjects had died.)

The most significant findings were:

1. At a mean age of 21 years half of the subjects in the group of normal controls (53%) were continuing full-time education, whereas only a minority (20%) of hyperactives were continuing their education.

2. On the job, hyperactives were not found at this age to be inferior to normal controls. Such factors as being fired, laid off, quitting or changing jobs more frequently, being unemployed, doing nothing, and length of time spent in the longest job held did not differentiate the hyperactives from the normal controls.

3. On the last job held a detailed enquiry on the percentage of time in a typical workday during which the subject was required to be active (vs. sedentary) showed that the hyperactives eventually chose jobs at which more activity was required.

The findings of this study were not published (although they were presented at a meeting[6]), because it was clear to us that at age 21 final work status had not been reached, particularly by the control group, most of whom were continuing their education. For this reason work status on the Hollingshead Scale of Work Status was not calculated for the two groups, since it would have been applied to a nonrandom sample of the controls. We postulated that the controls, because so many of them were continuing their education, would eventually achieve a higher work status, and we waited until the 15-year follow-up study before evaluating this aspect.

FIFTEEN-YEAR FOLLOW-UP: WORK STATUS[7]

The methodology of this study was described in detail in Chapter 5 (pp. 66–68). As part of this study the same Employers' Rating Scale (see Table 9-1) used in the 10-year follow-up study was sent to all employers of hyperactive adults and controls who gave permission for this. It was interesting that 33 of 41 controls and only 37 of 62 hyperactives agreed to let us contact their employers, even though the letter to the employer stated, "Mr. _____ has agreed to take part in a study of normal young adults, and has given us permission to contact you in order to fill out the enclosed questionnaire." The reluctance of the hyperactive adults to give us permission was probably related to their fear of being identified as abnormal. And indeed, one employer replied, "If you are doing a study of *normal* young adults I do not think you should be including this employee."

Employers' Questionnaire

The questionnaire sent to 33 controls' and 37 hyperactives' employers contained seven questions, each to be rated on a scale of 1 to 5 (hardly ever, sometimes, usually, nearly always, always). Each question was analyzed separately by the chi-square method. All significant differences favor the control group.

As can be seen from Table 9-1, employers scored hyperactive subjects significantly worse than controls on four of the seven questions (fulfilling tasks adequately, working independently, completing tasks, getting along with supervisors), and there was a trend for employers not to wish to rehire hyperactives versus controls. No significant differences were reported by employers with respect to punctuality or getting along with coworkers. Reasons for the discrepancy between the employers' ratings at the 10-year and 15-year follow-ups will be discussed at the end of this chapter.

The hyperactive adults and control subjects were interviewed in order to obtain a detailed record of their work history in the past 3 years. During this interview subjects were asked about the number and types of jobs they had held, the number of jobs from which they had been fired or laid off or had quit, and reasons for difficulties and/or enjoyment of their work. We also probed whether subjects had had any difficulties with concentration while at work. In order to determine whether hyperactive adults looked for jobs which required more activ-

TABLE 9-1. Employers' Rating Scale

Question	Significance
Does he fulfill his work adequately?	$p < .03$
Does he work independently?	$p < .01$
Does he complete tasks?	$p < .02$
Does he get along well with his supervisors?	$p < .05$
Does he get along well with his coworkers?	
Is he punctual?	
Would you hire him again?	$p < .09$

ity, subjects were asked to estimate the amount of time during a typical workday when they were physically active versus sedentary.

Results, as seen from Table 9-2, indicate that hyperactives leave school to start work earlier (mean age 18 years vs. 19.9 years for the controls). Once working, as reported for their last 3 years of work, they both quit and are laid off more frequently than controls, but they are not fired more frequently. It is likely that bosses prefer to "lay off" rather than to fire, and the distinction between these two may not be valid. There is a trend which did not reach significance for hyperactives to spend longer out of work and not at school. Hyperactives had significantly more full-time jobs than controls, indicating that they change jobs more frequently.

Hyperactive adults, as compared to normal controls, have a significantly worse work status (judging from their last or current job held) on the Hollingshead Scale (Table 9-3). However, there is no difference with respect to their average annual income. When they were asked to state in detail their final goals with respect to work, their aspirations were significantly lower than those of normal controls.

All subjects were asked what they enjoyed most with respect to their work and what they found most difficult, including questions related to ability to concentrate on the job (Table 9-4). Significantly more hyperactive adults reported that some tasks at work were too difficult for them, but there was no indication that they had more difficulties than normal controls with respect to concentrating on their

TABLE 9-2. Work History during Past 3 Years

	Controls	Hyperactives	Significance
Age when first left school	19.9 years	18.0 years	$p < .003$
Number of full-time jobs (at least 2 months' duration)	1.3	1.9	$p < .007$
Number of full-time jobs lasting 1 week to 2 months	0.3	0.1	
Number of full-time jobs quit	0.3	0.6	$p < .07$
Number of full-time jobs (at least 2 months' duration) from which subject was fired	0.05	0.09	
Number of full-time jobs (at least 2 months' duration) from which subject was laid off	0.03	0.3	$p < .01$
Number of jobs left for school	0.08	0.01	
In the past 3 years number of weeks not working or at school	8	17	$p < .1$

TABLE 9-3. Current Work Status, Income, and Job Aspirations

	Controls	Hyperactives	Significance
Work status (Hollingshead Scale)			
Full-time job	2.8	4.3	$p < .001$
Annual income (Canadian $)	17,296	17,444	
Goals for final work status	2.5	3.8	$p < .0001$

work. There was a trend ($p < .06$) for hyperactives to enjoy a job most because of the social interaction it offered, whereas for normal controls there was a trend ($p < .06$) to enjoy the learning experience and challenge of a job the most. One can interpret this trend as indicating that normal adults enjoy challenge at work, whereas hyperactive adults may be more threatened by this. In addition, normal adults may not rely on social interaction at work as much as hyperactive adults, who are more socially isolated outside of work. Both hyperactives and controls preferred "active" versus "sedentary" jobs (80% of each group). No significant differences between hyperactive adults and controls were found regarding their reasons for choice of a job (e.g., active vs. sedentary easy vs. challenging, and so on).

In general the above results indicate that while hyperactive adults are no less self-supporting or fully employed than normal controls, several aspects of their work record are inferior. Employers rate them as inferior to controls on most questions related to their work performance, with the exception of punctuality and getting along with co-workers. With respect to the latter, it is possible that employers may not notice if a hyperactive adult is socially isolated at work, provided he is not in excessive open conflict with other employees.

The same Employers' Rating Scale sent to employers of both hyperactive and control subjects 5 years previously, when their mean

TABLE 9-4. Difficulties and Assets of Last Full-Time Job

	Controls	Hyperactives	Significance
Number of subjects reporting that tasks were too difficult for them	1	7	$p < .09$
Number of subjects reporting that they had difficulty concentrating on the job	10	21	
Number of subjects who chose a job because it was a good learning experience	15	13	$p < .06$
Number of subjects who chose a job because they liked the people working there	7	21	$p < .06$

age was 19 years, did not at that time differentiate the two groups. It could be that the reason for this discrepancy is that control subjects improved their performance at work during these years more than did hyperactives. It is also possible that 5 years previously employers did not know their employees (hyperactives and controls) as well as now, since both had had a shorter duration of work. The fact that hyperactives achieved less education supports the former.

Findings indicated that hyperactive adults were laid off and quit jobs more frequently than controls and reported more difficulties in carrying out some of the tasks required of them. They did not feel that this was due to any difficulties they had concentrating on the tasks at work.

The poorer work record of hyperactives than normals in our study may be due to all or any of the following. Firstly, they were handicapped by their lower educational status. Secondly, the fact that they complained (significantly more often than normals) that they had difficulties with some of the tasks required of them at work may be the result of previous learning disabilities which they did not overcome. Several subjects indicated to us that they were aware of learning disabilities affecting their work. For example, 1 hyperactive adult who worked as a shipper could not sort objects into boxes when style, color, and size had to be taken into account and speed was a factor. While hyperactive adults did not feel that concentration at work was a problem, it is possible that they were hindered by not paying attention without being aware of it. It is also possible that they gravitated into jobs where sustained attention was relatively less significant. It is likely that hyperactive adults were also hindered at work by impulsivity and by characterological difficulties and general malaise, which were present in hyperactive adults more frequently than in controls, as outlined in Chapter 5.

These results confirm several of the findings of Borland and co-workers,[3] with respect to hyperactive adults' lower work status and more frequent job changes. It seemed that in Borland's subjects the job changes were initiated by the subjects because they became bored with their jobs. This was also the case in our study, but in addition to this our hyperactive subjects were laid off more frequently. Both studies indicated that hyperactives were in general self-sufficient economically and fully employed. The worse job status of our hyperactive subjects could be partly explained by their lower educational level, whereas this was not the case for the hyperactive subjects of Borland's study.

It is of interest that in spite of quite thorough structured probing, the adults who had been hyperactive as children did not complain of difficulties related to attention or distractibility at work. The probed questions include the following:

- Was it ever difficult to concentrate at work?
- Was it ever difficult to concentrate at work, because of too much work?
  - because of too little work?
  - because the job was boring?
  - because of distractions around you at work?
  - Any other reasons?

The hyperactive and control groups were identical in their responses to the above. This could indicate any one or more of the following:

1. Most hyperactives have outgrown significant attention deficits.

2. Hyperactives select jobs in which they do not experience problems of concentration.

3. Hyperactives lack insight into the existence of their attentional deficits.

In the 15-year follow-up study we did not measure attention in a laboratory task, which might have given us a clearer answer. However, in the 10- to 12-year follow-up study we gave an auditory version of the Continuous Performance Test (CPT) to 20 hyperactive adults and 20 individually matched controls. The two groups were matched on age, Wechsler Adult Intelligence Scale IQ, education received, and socioeconomic status. The mean age of the group was 19 years.

Results indicated (unpublished manuscript) that the two groups did not differ from one another on errors of either commission or omission. We wondered if the version of the CPT given was somehow "too easy" to detect actual but small differences. But then one may well ask whether small remaining differences in sustained attention, if present, would be of practical significance for most jobs chosen by the hyperactive subjects. One may conclude that while hyperactives as adults generally become economically self-sufficient, they have a poorer work record than do controls. The reasons for this are probably multiple and interactive.

CHAPTER TEN

SELF-ESTEEM AND SOCIAL SKILLS

If you can trust yourself when all men doubt you. . . .
—From "If," by Rudyard Kipling, 1865–1936

It has long been assumed that self-esteem or self-concept is derived to a large extent from interactions with significant others: initially mother; later other family members; and finally peers, teachers, and others in one's expanded environment.

It is therefore reasonable to assume that hyperactive children who present behavior problems at home and at school and thus have difficulties in their relationships with family members, teachers, and peers should suffer from poor self-esteem. Poor performance at school and other activities such as sports may also contribute to poor self-concept. (These problems are presented in greater detail in Chapter 3.) Few follow-up studies have systematically looked at measures of self-esteem or social skills, though many have made clinical reference to the fact that hyperactive subjects appeared to have poor self-esteem and "social problems." In this chapter, we will briefly discuss some follow-up studies of hyperactive adolescents and adults that have touched on the question of self-esteem and social skills. We will also present the results of both our 10- and 15-year follow-up studies, which attempted to measure and compare self-esteem and social skills in the hyperactive young adults and their matched normal controls.

ADOLESCENT FOLLOW-UP STUDIES

Weiss and her associates,[1] in the prospective controlled follow-up study (described in greater detail in Chapter 4) of adolescent hyperactives, stated that it was apparent that the hyperactives were highly aware of their past and continuing failures and had a markedly low self-esteem. Many had very low expectations of any success in the future, thus lacking ambition, and this hopelessness often prevented them from making any real efforts. Socially almost 30% of the hyperactive adolescents were described by their mothers at follow-up as having no steady friends.

Hoy et al.[2] attempted to further clarify these clinical impressions by conducting more detailed tests pertaining to self-esteem, cognitive, social, and academic functioning, and career aspirations on a subgroup of 15 hyperactive adolescents and matched controls studied by Weiss. The two groups had a mean age of 14.7 years, a mean IQ of 108, and a mean social class (Hollingshead)[3] of 3.5 (middle class). Self-esteem was measured by the Davidson and Lang checklist[4] and a modified version of the Ziller[5] Self–Other Social Orientation Test. (These tests were also used in our 10- and 15-year follow-up studies and will be described in greater detail later in this chapter.) Social life, academic status, and career aspirations were measured by the Behavioral Information questionnaire, constructed by the authors specifically for that study. It examined activity and distractibility problems, social difficulties, academic status, and career aspirations. The authors found that results of all self-esteem measures were in the predicted directions, namely with the hyperactives showing lower self-esteem than controls. However, only two of these measures reached statistical significance (Ziller Self–Other total score and "pleased with self" item). Hyperactives indicated that they were less pleased with themselves and placed themselves closer to unsuccessful, unhappy, failing, and cruel people than did the controls. Hyperactives did not differ from controls in the total score of the Davidson and Lang checklist, nor on the "distance from the smartest person in your class" item. However 4 of the 36 items on the checklist yielded significant differences. Hyperactives rated themselves as more unkind, more noisy, and more of a nuisance, but also as more valuable, than controls. Generally the authors felt that the specific tests of self-esteem supported the clinical impression that hyperactives had a somewhat lower self-concept.

Socially the hyperactive adolescents reported spending more of their spare time alone or with younger children rather than with peers than did the controls. However there was no significant difference between the two groups in the reported number of friends. Career aspirations were also not significantly different for the two groups. These latter two findings are somewhat different from the clinical impressions of the Weiss[1] study. The difference may be due to the use of mothers' reports on the friends in the Weiss study versus subjects' own reports measured by Hoy. Ambition in the Weiss study may have referred to more current aspiration, as opposed to more distant future jobs explored by Hoy. Finally, Hoy's study looked at a subgroup of 15 hyperactives which may not have included some of the more isolated or hopeless subjects.

Mendelson et al.'s[6] retrospective follow-up study of 83 hyperactive adolescents was less well controlled (no control or comparison group) and specific (no direct measures of self-esteem or social functioning). However, mothers of the hyperactive adolescents reported that 54% of the subjects had low self-confidence, 42% felt that they were a failure in school, 57% felt that they were not liked, and 46% were described as loners with no friends; 51% were involved in frequent fighting. From these figures the authors concluded that the hyperactive adolescents had poor self-esteem and social problems.

Stewart et al.[7] conducted direct interviews with these hyperactive adolescents whose mothers had been seen by Mendelson. Two-thirds of the subjects reported that they were quick tempered or irritable and that they lied and fought often. Sixty-two percent said they were disgusted with themselves. The subjects' negative self-image is evident in these reports, and the authors concluded that 40–60% of the hyperactives had feelings of low self-esteem.

Ackerman and coworkers'[8] prospective study comparing hyperactive, normoactive, and hypoactive learning-disabled adolescents at age 14 with an age-matched normal control group was better controlled and more specific. The authors reported that all three learning-disabled groups rated low on self-confidence. More specifically, on the "self-confidence" cluster of the Minnesota Counseling Inventory (MCI), a Minnesota Multiphasic Personality Inventory type instrument for adolescents, both hyperactive and hypoactive learning-disabled groups had significantly worse scores than either normoactives or controls ($p < .02$). Thus it is not surprising that subjects with the dual handicap of hyper- or hypoactivity and learning disability do worse than those who have only the learning disability to contend with. The social consequences of the activity problems may be particularly influential in affecting these subjects' self-confidence.

Another study that followed subjects who were learning disabled and hyperactive was the longitudinal study on the island of Kauai.[9] The authors found that three-quarters of the children identified as learning disabled/hyperactive at age 10 had poorer outcomes at age 18 on measures of achievement, interpersonal relationships, and self-esteem when compared to normal controls.

Self-image problems were also noted by Feldman et al.,[10] who followed 81 adolescent hyperactives (mean age 15.5) and felt 16% required counseling particularly for this difficulty. Loney and her associates Langhorne and Paternite have suggested that factors other than hyperactivity (e.g., level of aggressivity and socioeconomic status) may have more of an influence on self-esteem of hyperactive adolescents than hyperactivity per se.[11,12] Thus Langhorne[11] found that it was the degree of aggression at referral, and not the degree of hyperactivity, which significantly predicted self-esteem deficits in adolescence. Paternite[12] showed that self-esteem deficits were greater in hyperactive subjects from low socioeconomic statuses than in those of higher socioeconomic status. However, the high- and low-socioeconomic-status groups of hyperactives also differed in the type of parenting they received as well as in level of aggressive interpersonal behavior and impulse-control deficit. It is therefore unclear which of the above factors most contributes to poor self-esteem. More likely all act together to result in the negative self-image many adolescent hyperactives possess.

On a more optimistic note, Satterfield and associates[13] in their 3-year follow-up of 100 hyperactive boys offered multimodal treatment and found that those subjects who had received more (2 years or more) treatment were further ahead academically, had less antisocial behavior, were more attentive, and had better school and home adjustment than a comparable group of hyperactives who had received less (less than 2 years) treatment. Specifically, after comprehensive assessments, children received (in addition to stimulant medication) any number of the following interventions: individual or group psychotherapy for the child, psychoptherapy for the parents including family therapy, and group or individual educational help for the child. At 3-year follow-up the hyperactive group that had received more treatment showed greater improvements in school adjustment, mood, self-concept, insight, social judgment, peer relations, and home relations, when compared to the less-treated group. One is tempted to conclude that appropriate, significant, long-standing intervention may prevent the negative self-esteem and social difficulties that many studies of hyperactive adolescents have reported.

ADULT FOLLOW-UP STUDIES

Few studies of adult hyperactives have addressed themselves specifically to self-esteem and social skills. Feldman et al.'s[10] was one such study, which specifically measured self-concept in 48 adult hyperactives (mean age 21) and compared these measures to those of their siblings (mean age 26) and comparable normative values. The authors used the Tennessee Self-Concept Scale and found that the hyperactive young adults fell within the normal range (i.e., 30th percentile). However, the siblings were significantly higher (i.e., at the 70th percentile), and so hyperactives scored significantly lower ($p < .01$) than their siblings on self-concept. It is interesting to note that most (81%) of these adult subjects received multiple therapies, including stimulant medication in childhood. The other therapies involved individual counseling, family therapy, visual–perceptual training, language therapy, and special education. Again the fairly positive outcome (including normal self-concept) of their adult hyperactives may in part, be a function of use of multiple therapies to deal with these subjects' various problems (educational, social, emotional).

Borland and Heckman's[14] study, though much more general and less specific, had similar findings. The 20 hyperactive subjects (mean age 30) and their 20 brothers (mean age 28) were thought to have comparable social functioning. For example, 14 of the probands and 15 of the brothers were married, and only 1 of the probands was separated from his wife. In addition, 8 probands lacked friends, as compared to 2 brothers. This difference was not significant. The authors concede that early social and academic difficulties of the hyperactive men in the study may have led to low self-esteem and reduced motivation for successful school performance. However they conclude that the effect of lowered self-esteem or motivation for educational attainment seems to have been limited, since the hyperactives' final level of education was comparable to that of their brothers.

Findings were somewhat different in Milman's[15] prospective study of 73 hyperactives (mean age 19.4 years). She found that 67% of her subjects had social problems and only 27% had achieved any degree of heterosexual maturity as reflected by dating and being engaged or married. The difference in Milman's results as compared to Feldman's or Borland's may be a function of age of the subjects (Milman's are considerably younger) and degree of organicity (62% of Milman's subjects were thought to have Organic Brain Syndrome).

We thus see that most adolescent follow-up studies strongly suggest that hyperactives have problems of self-esteem and socialization. Adult follow-up studies are few and generally have not addressed the issues of self-esteem and social skills directly. For this reason we undertook the portion of the 10-year follow-up study[16] (see Chapter 5) that dealt specifically with self-esteem and social skills.

TEN-YEAR FOLLOW-UP STUDY

In our study we showed that even though these subjects continued to have some difficulties, they did not load the psychiatric or antisocial populations, and only a small subgroup had serious problems in these areas. However, the psychiatric interview and the self-rating scales, such as the California Psychological Inventory (CPI), suggested that the hyperactive young adults nevertheless had more problems with socialization and self-esteem when compared to matched controls.[16,17] This part of the study was an attempt to clarify clinical impressions by trying to answer the following questions:

1. Do various self-esteem tests distinguish hyperactive young adults from matched controls and thus support the clinical findings of a lower self-esteem in these young people?

2. What aspects of social skills are deficient in the hyperactive group when compared to controls matched for age, sex, IQ, and socioeconomic status?

3. What is the correlation between social skills and self-esteem in this group of young adults?

Subjects

Subjects consisted of 18 matched pairs of hyperactive young male adults and normal controls selected randomly from the pool of hyperactives and controls seen in the 10-year follow-up study[16] and described in detail in Chapter 5. Pairs were matched within 12 months of age, 10 IQ points, and 1 year of education completed. No variability on sex and socioeconomic status existed. Thus, the means for the hyperactive versus the control group showed no significant differences on these parameters; for example, mean age of hyperactives was 22 years 2 months and mean age of controls was 21 years 10 months; mean IQ was 112 for both groups; education completed was 12.7 years for hyperactives and 13.0 years for controls; and socioeconomic status was 3.16 for both groups.

The matched-pair group of both hyperactives and controls was compared to the overall male group of hyperactives and controls. No significant differences were seen in age and socioeconomic status. However, the IQ's of both hyperactives and controls in the matched-pair group were significantly higher than in the overall group. The reason for this difference may be related to the fact that the education-completed requirement was relatively high (13 years), thereby inadvertently preselecting a higher IQ group.

The matched pairs of subjects came for three test sessions, each lasting about 2 hours, occurring about 1 week apart. During the first test session, subjects were given the first social-skills test, namely, the Situational Social Skills Inventory (SSSI; direct oral response).[18] The second test situation included the Means–End Problem Solving Procedure (MEPS) test of social skills.[19] The third session consisted of the written SSSI[18] and three self-esteem tests. All these tests were used because they have an established validity for the age group in question.

Social-Skills Tests

A total of three tests were given. Two of them [18] dealt with three distinct areas: job interviews, heterosocial interactions, and assertion situations. All three areas were investigated in two different ways. The first form of testing was via direct response, that is, a prerecorded situation was described to the subject, then the response the subject thought he would actually make in that situation was taped and later scored. The second form of testing was a paper-and-pencil task where subjects chose the best response from five possible available responses. The third social-skills test was also a paper-and-pencil task. This was the MEPS,[19] wherein the beginning and end of a situation are described and the subjects have to supply the intervening steps. The purpose of this test is to evaluate whether the subjects have a good grasp of social sequencing.

Self-Esteem Tests

Three different self-esteem tests were administered. The first—the Davidson and Lang checklist[4]—is a test where the subject indicates how he sees himself on a 5-point scale ranging from "some of the time" to "almost never" on a series of polarized adjectives such as "intelligent" versus "unintelligent." The second test—the Ziller Self-Other[5]—involves the subject placing himself and five other people in a series of circles that are linearly arranged. The score for self-esteem is the number of circles between the subject and the negative person—for example, someone who is cruel, unsuccessful, or failing. The third self-esteem test—the Area Test developed by Elizabeth Hoy[2]—required the subjects to score themselves in comparison to their peers (same, better, worse, on a 5-point scale) on various parameters, for example, physical appearance, health, creative ability.

Results

SOCIAL SKILLS

Of the three types of social-skills test (i.e., the SSSI oral response, the SSSI written response, and the MEPS), only the oral-response test significantly differentiated the hyperactive and control subjects. Hyperactives had significantly more difficulties with responses in hetero-social situations ($p < .02$) and tended to have more difficulties in asser-tion situations ($p < .09$) when compared to matched controls. No differences were seen in their responses dealing with job interviews.

The written form of the SSSI showed no differences between hyperactives and controls. The MEPS also failed to differentiate the two groups.

SELF-ESTEEM

DAVIDSON AND LANG CHECKLIST. This test found the hyper-actives rating themselves significantly worse on 8 of the 30 adjectives. These were: obedient–disobedient ($p < .03$); strong–weak ($p < .01$); calm–nervous ($p < .001$); nice–awful ($p < .017$); careless–careful ($p < .02$); attentive–inattentive ($p < .02$); disorderly–orderly ($p < .028$); ungrateful–grateful ($p < .027$). The hyperactive subjects scored them-selves better than controls on only one item, sad–happy ($p < .05$). The other 21 items did not significantly differentiate the two groups.

AREA TEST. The Area self-rating test assessing how subjects compare themselves to peers on 11 different parameters (e.g., health, intelligence) also failed to differentiate the two groups.

ZILLER SELF–OTHER TEST. This test did show significant differ-ences between hyperactives and controls. Hyperactives placed them-selves significantly more closely to someone who was cruel ($p < .03$) and tended to place themselves near someone who was unhappy ($p < .08$). No differences were seen for the other two types of people, that is, "someone who is flunking" and "someone who is unsuccessful."

CORRELATION OF SELF-ESTEEM AND SOCIAL-SKILLS TESTS

There were no significant correlations between the various social-skills tests and the self-esteem tests.

Discussion

Our findings suggested that the social-skills deficit in hyperactive young adults appeared to be behavioral rather than cognitive. When hyperactive subjects were asked to orally respond to heterosocial situa-tions requiring appropriate responses and, to a lesser extent, situations requiring personal assertion, they did less well than their nonhyperac-tive peers. This may imply that the hyperactives know what ought to be done in these situations, as witnessed by their competence on the written parts of the social-skills test, but have problems actually doing it. Whether this inability is due to a lack of practice or a hesitancy stemming from many years of social ostracism is unclear. It should also be a reflection of the persisting impulsivity these young adults show in many life situations[15] but may well be due to a combination of all these factors.

As expected, hyperactives scored themselves worse on some items of self-esteem when compared to matched controls. This was particularly true of the Davidson and Lang test and the Ziller Self–Other test, but not of the Area Test. On only one item did hyperactives score themselves better than controls (sad–happy, $p < .05$).

Some of the items differentiating the two groups seemed to have an intrinsic validity. For example, hyperactives saw themselves as more disobedient, nervous, careless, inattentive, and ungrateful, all areas in which these children traditionally have difficulties. On the other hand, these young men perceived themselves as equally fair, friendly, reliable, popular, and mature as their control peers. This again confirms that although these youngsters continue to have some problems, they do not constitute a markedly pathological population as was once assumed. This supports the clinical impressions of the psychiatric assessment and the self-rating on the CPI done at 10-year follow-up.

It was somehwat disappointing that no significant correlations were found between the social-skills-tests results and those of self-esteem. This may be a function of the number of subjects (small) or the number of items looked at (large). It may also be that these particular tests or items do not correlate highly. Whatever the reason, it is clear that self-esteem is a complex, multifaceted parameter of which social skill is but a part.

FIFTEEN-YEAR PROSPECTIVE FOLLOW-UP

The decision to repeat self-esteem and social-skills measures at 15-year follow-up was prompted by two factors. First, the 18 hyperactives selected for the matched pairs were only 23% of the overall 10-year follow-up sample and may have been not wholly representative of the overall group, in that they had significantly higher IQ's. Secondly, the 15-year follow-up results[20,21] suggested (see Chapters 5, 6, and 8) that at this time hyperactives were encountering slightly more difficulties than they did at 10-year follow-up. It therefore became important to evaluate self-esteem and social-skills measures for the entire 15-year follow-up group and assess whether these measures had also changed.

Subjects included 39 of 41 controls and 58 of 61 hyperactives matched for age (mean age 25 years), sex, and socioeconomic status followed in the 15-year follow-up study and described in detail in Chapter 5. The social-skills tests included the SSSI[18] (direct oral and written forms) described earlier in this chapter. The self-esteem tests included the Davidson and Lang test,[4] the Ziller Self–Other test,[5] and the Area Test,[2] also described earlier.

Results

SOCIAL SKILLS (Table 10-1)

It is striking that all hyperactive adults were significantly worse on all aspects of the social-skills tests when compared to their matched controls. Thus, on the behavioral or direct-oral-response test, hyperactives were significantly worse in situations involving job interviews ($p < .02$), heterosocial interactions ($p < .01$), and assertion ($p < .009$). In addition, on the questionnaire test, hyperactives again were significantly worse than controls in situations involving job interviews ($p < .008$), heterosocial interactions ($p < .002$), and assertion ($p < .02$).

This finding is significantly worse than the 10-year follow-up results, which showed hyperactives having more difficulties only in the direct oral response in situations involving heterosocial relations and assertion. Hyperactives may have experienced more social difficulties in the intervening years, accounting for the worsening scores. However, it is more likely that the 18 hyperactives in the matched pairs at 10-year follow-up were not truly reflective of the whole group's functioning in this regard, and the 58 subjects now evaluated give a more representative picture.

TABLE 10-1. Social Skills at 15-Year Follow-Up

	Controls	Hyperactives	Significance
Behavioral			
Job interview	17.4	15.3	$p < .02$
Heterosocial interactions	20.95	18.39	$p < .01$
Assertion	20.36	17.95	$p < .009$
Total	58.69	51.59	$p < .002$
Questionnaire			
Job interview	45.85	44.02	$p < .008$
Heterosocial interactions	42.38	39.74	$p < .002$
Assertion	43.08	41.13	$p < .02$
Total	131.31	124.89	$p < .001$

SELF-ESTEEM (Table 10-2)

Two of the self-esteem tests (Davidson and Lang and Area) showed hyperactives to have significantly worse ($p < .04$, $p < .02$ respectively) self-esteem than their matched normal controls. The third test, Ziller Self–Other, showed no significant differences between the two groups. These results are generally similar to our 10-year follow-up findings, where hyperactives were significantly worse than controls on two of the three self-esteem tests. However, at 10-year follow-up the differences were on the Davidson and Lang and Ziller Self–Other tests but not on the Area Test. In an effort to clarify why different tests distinguish the groups at one point in time and not at another, we compared our 10- and 15-year follow-up findings with those of Hoy et al.,[2] who used two of the same tests on a subgroup of our subjects at 5-year follow-up in adolescents. We thus see that the Davidson and Lang test was not significantly different at 5-year follow-up but was significantly different at 10- and 15-year follow-up.

The Ziller Self–Other was significant at 5- and 10-year follow-up but not at 15-year follow-up. The Area Test was not used at 5-year follow-up, was not significant at 10-year follow-up, and was significant in the 15-year study. It may well be that some of these self-esteem tests are better suited for one age group versus another. Thus, the Davidson and Lang, with its polarized adjectives, may be better suited to the older age group, while the Ziller Self–Other test, which requires subjects to place themselves and other people in circles, is better suited to a younger age group. There is also some suggestion that the Area Test, which looks at subjects' comparison of themselves to peers, is better suited to the older age group. It is therefore most important to use several measures and to try to use tests best suited to the particular age group. There is also some evidence that the subjects' perceptions and preoccupations about themselves shift with time. For example, in the Ziller Self–Other test at 5-year follow-up, hyperactives rated themselves as more unsuccessful, unhappy, failing, and cruel. At 10-year follow-up, hyperactives rated themselves as more unhappy and cruel but not more unsuccessful or failing. Being out of school may be one of

TABLE 10-2. Self-Esteem at 15-Year Follow-Up

	Controls ($n = 39$)	Hyperactives ($n = 58$)	Significance
Davidson and Lang total	123.87	117.90	$p < .04$
Ziller Self–Other total	7.87	7.29	
Area Test total	39.12	37.07	$p < .02$

the reasons for this. Similarly on the Davidson and Lang test at 5-year follow-up, hyperactives rated themselves as more unkind and noisy and more of a nuisance when compared to controls. At 10-year follow-up they rated themselves as more disobedient, weaker, more nervous, less nice, more careless, more inattentive, more disorderly, and more ungrateful when compared to the matched controls. At 15-year follow-up, hyperactives still rated themselves more nervous and less nice, but also as less honest, more foolish, and more indifferent when compared to the control group. It is striking that hyperactives rarely rate themselves better than controls.

In summary, one can say that the social-skills and self-esteem deficits suspected clinically were substantiated by the specific tests used to measure these entities. These measures at 15-year follow-up are worse for the hyperactives when compared to controls than they were at 10-year follow-up. This may be a function of the use of a subgroup of 18 subjects at 10-year follow-up versus most of the group (58 subjects) at 15-year follow-up.

It may be that with the changing age of the subjects, some tests become more sensitive, giving more clear-cut results. However, it may also be that as the subjects get older they see more clearly the growing gap between their hopes and aspirations and their achievements. Hyperactives may also be more aware of where they are in various areas of functioning compared to their peers. The greater awareness of these gaps with increasing maturity may affect their self-esteem and result in more negative self-ratings. There is some evidence that early, prolonged multiple intervention[10,13] may prevent the negative self-esteem so often seen in these hyperactives. The need to recognize and address the problems of social skills and self-esteem in hyperactive children and adults seems clear.

CHAPTER ELEVEN

PHYSIOLOGICAL MEASURES

Men ought to know that from nothing else but the brain come joys, delights, laughter and sports, and sorrows, griefs, despondency and lamentations—All these things we endure from the brain when it is not healthy, but is more hot, more cold, more moist, or more dry than natural.—From "The Sacred Disease," by Hippocrates, 460–377 B.C.

Interest in various physiological measures and their relationship to hyperactivity or Attention Deficit Disorder has three main, though overlapping, purposes. The first is to explore possible biological under-pinnings for the condition, and in so doing to clarify possible etiology and pathogenesis, as well as effectiveness of various treatments. Thus, height, weight, and various neurological and autonomic measures have been used to support or negate the hypothesis of immature biological development in these children. Furthermore, cardiovascular–pulmo-nary measures (e.g., heart rate, blood pressure, pulse, respiration, oxygen utilization), electroencephalograms (EEG's), and measures of skin resistance have all been used to support or negate the hypothesis that these children have increased or decreased basal (tonic) arousal or some abnormality in responsivity (or phasic arousal).

The second purpose for the interest in physiological measures pertains to how stimulant medication affects these measures. The aim is to continue to clarify the underlying problem in the condition and to delineate possible mechanism of action and possible side effects of the drug. The third purpose relates to long-term outcome. Namely, what is the natural course into adulthood of this condition for the various physiological measures? And finally, what is the impact of stimulant medication on the natural course of these physiological variables into adulthood?

This chapter will briefly summarize studies dealing with the first two issues, namely, possible physiological differences in hyperactive children and the effects of stimulant medication on these physiological measures; then it will present our findings in greater detail on the third question, namely, the long-term outcome of these physiological measures in adult hyperactives who received and did not receive stimulant treatment in childhood.

PHYSIOLOGICAL DIFFERENCES IN HYPERACTIVE CHILDREN

There has been considerable controversy as to whether or not hyperactive children differ physiologically (i.e., with regard to cardiovascular-pulmonary measures, skin conduction/resistance, electroencephalographic recordings, stature) when compared to nonhyperactive children.

Autonomic Measures

Many studies have focused on "autonomic" measures to support or negate the hypothesis that these children suffer from overarousal, underinhibition, or underarousal. Studies suggesting that hyperactive children suffer from overarousal due to excessive excitatory processes and reflected in increased autonomic activity are relatively few and include Laufer et al.,[1] Freibergs and Douglas,[2] and Buckley.[3] Also supporting the overarousal hypothesis but due to underactive inhibiting processes are Wender[4] and Dykman et al.[5]

Other authors [6-9] have suggested that hyperactives are underaroused in central nervous system (CNS) functioning, thereby accounting for their positive response to stimulant medication. In an extensive review Rapoport and Ferguson[10] suggested that data support the hypothesis of CNS underarousal for at least a subgroup of hyperactive children. However, most studies have found no differences between hyperactive and normal children in resting levels of autonomic activity.[11-17] Thus, generally results from cardiac and electrodermal variables indicate that basal (or tonic) arousal levels appear to be normal. However, there has been some suggestion that hyperactives are less "arousable" in their psychophysiological responses to environmental stimuli. Barkley et al.[17] have proposed that the CNS functioning of some of these children might be slower in responding to environmental stimuli and may show less than normal levels of responding once stimulated. Such findings were seen with regard to galvanic skin response by Satterfield and Dawsons,[7] Spring et al.,[13] and Zahn et al.,[15] and with regard to cardiac measures by Porges et al.[18] It is important to note that other studies [16,17] did not find such differences.

The complexity of this issue has been further addressed by Douglas, [19] who stressed the importance and influence of the nature of the task and the incentive value of reinforcers on measures of arousal, inhibition, attention, impulsivity, and performance. Douglas has stressed that hyperactive children may show both under- and overarousal depending on a variety of circumstances, and therefore the underlying problem was one of regulation of arousal.

Studies on the effect of stimulant medication on these autonomic measures are inconsistent. Some studies suggest that stimulant medication decreases arousal. For example, Montagu[14] showed decreased ectodermal measures, while Zahn et al.,[15] Porges et al.,[18,21] and Sroufe et al.[20] showed increased cardiac deceleration on stimulant medication. Other studies found evidence of increased arousal in hyperactive children on medication.[15,22] Ballard,[22] for example, showed heart rate and blood pressure both increased with increases in dosages of methylphenidate medication. Still others found no change in these measures with stimulants.[13,16,17] Some of the inconsistencies stem from the fact that certain studies measured autonomic responses during rest, while others took the measurements during required task performances. A second factor which confuses the results is that some aspect of a measure may increase (e.g., amplitude of nonspecific responses) while another may show no change (e.g., resting conductance or amplitude of specific response[7]).

A number of authors have suggested that efficacy of stimulant medication may be predicted by these autonomic measures.[12,15,18] Thus good responders are said to have lower heart rates and skin conductance when compared to poor responders. However, Ferguson et al.[16] and Barkley et al.[17] have not found such distinctions in good responders.

Even though it is attractive to think that hyperactives have an abnormality in their arousal system which can be documented by a variety of autonomic measures and that this deviation can be normalized by stimulant medication, various studies to date have given inconsistent and contradictory results, and the question must await further research.

Electroencephalographic Measures

There is some controversy regarding the significance and value of electroencephalographic measures in hyperactive children. The controversy is fueled by four factors. First, a certain proportion (10–15%) of normal children have abnormal EEG's, so that the significance of abnormal EEG's in hyperactive children is decreased. Even though there is general agreement that hyperactive children have an increased frequency of abnormal EEG's when compared to normal controls, [23-25] there are some studies[26,27] that have shown no greater EEG abnormality in hyperactives when compared to matched normal controls or nonhyperactive emotionally disturbed children. Secondly, some hyperactives have abnormal EEG's (35–50%)[28], while others do not. Thirdly, studies have varied in the type of abnormality they have pinpointed in hyperactive children; and finally, the effects of stimulant medication on EEG abnormalities of hyperactive children have also varied.

Despite these difficulties many studies have noted a high incidence of diffuse nonspecific changes and of extensive slow EEG activity in hyperactive children.[12,23,29–31] Shetty[32] indicated that in his series of 75 hyperactive subjects the most consistent abnormality was the absence of an appropriate amount of well-organized alpha waves for age.

In addition to this increase in slow-diffuse-wave activities, it has been suggested that hyperactives have EEG abnormalities associated with their evoked potential. Thus, Satterfield[33] reported that auditory evoked potentials in hyperactives had longer latencies and lower amplitudes when compared to those of age-matched controls. Buchsbaum and Wender[34] studied visual and auditory average evoked responses and again found that hyperactives showed increases in amplitude and latency with increases in intensity of the visual stimuli, while age- and sex-matched controls showed lesser increases in amplitude and decreases in latency. On the other hand, Hall et al.[35] recorded evoked potentials in response to four stimulus intensities under conditions of attention and inattention. They found no differences in stability, amplitude, or latency between hyperactive and control children.

The third type of EEG abnormality described in hyperactive children involves difficulties with attenuation of alpha waves, which presumably reflect the decreased capacity of hyperactive children to disattend to redundant events. This has been reported by Milstein et al.[36] and Fuller.[37] All of the above abnormalities have been described as immature patterns and interpreted as representing delayed maturation of the CNS in hyperactive children. This hypothesis is supported by the increased normalization of EEG's of hyperactives with increasing age, particularly in late adolescence. Details of this normalization process and EEG findings for the adult hyperactive will be presented later in this chapter.

The question as to whether hyperactives with abnormal EEG's differ from those with normal ones is of some clinical as well as theoretical interest. Indeed Satterfield et al.[30] and Quinn and Rapoport[38] showed that hyperactives with abnormal EEG's had greater anxiety at home and at school, more motor restlessness in the classroom, higher Wechsler Intelligence Scale for Children Full Scale and Performance IQ's, lower Bender performance scores, and were more likely to respond to stimulant medication.

It has further been suggested that "good" (clinical) stimulant treatment response is accompanied by normalization of the EEG on the medication while "poor" stimulant treatment response is not. Thus, Shetty[39] found that good responders showed increased EEG alpha activity, while poor responders did not. Knights and Hinton[29] showed that abnormal EEG records (mostly increased slow-wave activity) were reduced by 30% on methylphenidate, while Satterfield et al.[12] reported that poor responders to methylphenidate showed increased slow-wave activity and good responders showed no change. Furthermore, good responders in the Satterfield study showed decreases in amplitude of auditory evoked potential. Recent sleep studies by Greenhill et al.[40] and Nahas and Krynicki[41] have shown that hyperactives on stimulant medication show no differences in any of the sleep measures (e.g., total sleep time, rapid-eye-movement [REM] latency movement time, or any of the stages of sleep).

It is thus tempting to tentatively conclude that some hyperactives have certain types of EEG abnormalities, that these abnormalities are suggestive of maturational delays and that stimulant treatment normalizes some of these abnormalities.

Growth Measures (Height and Weight)

Oettinger et al.[42] lent support to the concept of an underlying physiological immaturity in hyperactive children by showing, via single anterior–posterior x-rays of the left wrist, that two-thirds of 53 children diagnosed as having Minimal Brain Dysfuction (MBD) had lower bone age than chronological age. Ten of these children had bone age which was two standard deviations below the norm, while one had a significant increase in bone age. However, in an extensive review on the subject, Roche et al.[43] tentatively concluded that untreated hyperkinetic children are near normal in stature, weight, and skeletal maturity. They cautioned, however, that in untreated hyperkinetic children the condition may be less severe than in those who are treated.

The major interest in height and weight of hyperactive children has centered around how these measures are affected by stimulant medication in the short and long term. Safer and colleagues[44,45] reported depression of growth in hyperactive children taking stimulant drugs and rebound of growth after termination of such therapy.[46] Similar concerns were expressed by Weiss et al.,[47] who found that 8 of 12 children treated with methylphenidate for 3 to 5 years might not have grown at expected rates. Quinn and Rapoport[48] also showed mean gains in stature and weight during 1 year of treatment that were slightly less than expected. Other authors expressing conerns over growth suppression included Puig-Antich et al.,[49] who showed growth retardation in their index group treated with d-amphetamine for 1 year; and Mattes and Gittelman,[50] who studied the height and weight of 86 hyperactive children on methylphenidate (40 mg/day) for up to 4 years. They found that significant decreases in height percentiles were apparent after 2, 3, and 4 years of treatment, but not after 1 year.

On the other hand, some authors have reported no growth suppression in hyperactive children treated with stimulants. McNutt and associates[51] compared growth and body composition in nonmedicated hyperactives, hyperactives medicated (10–40 mg/day) for 1 and 2 years, and normal controls. They found no significant differences in these measures in any of these groups and thus concluded no growth suppression had taken place. Similarly, Knights and Hinton,[29] in a 6-month study, found a mean weight loss of 0.9 kg, but no difference in rate of growth in stature when compared to untreated hyperactive children. Eisenberg[52] also reported no evidence of growth suppression in 83 hyperactive children treated from 1 to 11 years with stimulants.

Between these two divergent and contradictory positions is a group of authors who have suggested that the growth retardation is temporary, usually in the first year or so, and that even with the continuation of stimulant treatment hyperactive children catch up, and their stature and weight are not significantly affected. Thus, Gross[53] showed that initial stature and weight gains which were less than expected were compensated for later by greater than expected gains. This compensation occurred while the patient was still on medication and after it had been discontinued. He thus concluded that long-term use of methylphenidate, dextroamphetamine, or imipramine did not retard growth in the long term. These findings are in general agreement with those of Millichap and Millichap.[54]

Similarly, Satterfield et al.,[55] who studied the height and weight of 72 hyperactive boys treated continuously with methylphenidate, found that adverse effects on growth in the first year were offset in the second year by greater than expected growth rate. The pattern of initial deficit in height and weight (in the first 18 months), followed by no significant differences in these measures when compared to controls, was also reported by Friedmann et al.[56] for pemoline-treated hyperactives. Attention thus shifts to the long-term rather than short-term outcome of these measures in hyperactive children who received stimulant treatment in childhood.

Two studies which particularly looked at the adolescent age group were Beck et al.[57] and Loney et al.[58] Beck et al. found no differences in the mean heights in the hyperactive group aged 14–19 compared to a matched control group. The subjects in the hyperactive group had a minimum of 6 months stimulant therapy in childhood. Loney et al., on the other hand, used stepwise regression analysis in determining what factors affected the adolescent height and weight of their subjects, now

12–18 years of age, who had received 5 years of stimulant treatment. Loney concluded that some hyperactives were at risk for growth suppression. This risk was associated with factors such as dose and duration of medication treatment and the prevalence of side effects (e.g., early weight, appetite suppression, nausea, vomiting).

Other authors have also stressed the importance of dosage[44,45,50] in growth suppression. For example, Safer[45] pointed out that growth suppression was more likely to occur if methylphenidate dosages exceeded 20 mg/day. These authors also suggested that amphetamines seem to have greater growth-suppression effects than methylphenidate.

Another factor given imprtance is the presence of drug holidays— for example, 2 months in the summer—which are thought to allow for rebound growth and some, though incomplete, catch-up.[46] Satterfield et al.[55], however, felt that deficits in height were not related to total dosage or summer drug holidays, but wieght deficits might be. Nonetheless, in their review of the literature, Roche et al.[43] felt that growth suppression, though temporary, was influenced by dosages and drug holidays. Few studies have treated adolescents during their growth spurt, and this may have a more lasting adult effect. We will report the height and weight status of the stimulant-treated and untreated adult hyperactives and how they compare to matched controls later in this chapter.

However, the interest in stimulant effects on growth has given rise to a large number of studies that have sought to clarify possible mechanisms by which stimulants affect height and weight. Many of these studies are neuroendocrine in nature and seek to measure the effects of stimulants on growth-hormone secretion and/or prolactin levels. Several studies have shown an increase of growth-hormone levels in respose to stimulant medication. Shaywitz et al.[59] compared methylphenidate effect on growth-hormone and prolactin level in hyperactive boys 7–12 years of age. He found that methylphenidate increased levels of growth hormone and decreased prolactin levels, and this was similar for those receiving acute and chronic methylphenidate treatment. Aarskog et al.[60] compared the acute effect of L-dopa, dextroamphetamine, and methylphenidate on growth-hormone secretion in 20 hyperactive children. All three stimulants resulted in peak growth-hormone concentration in serum within 60 minutes. Seven of the children were retested after 6–8 months of methylphenidate treatment. After this "chronic" treatment, there was a higher zero-time level of growth hormone and a delay in dextroamphetamine stimulation of growth-hormone secretion. The author thus concluded that there are acute and probably long-term effects of dextroamphetamine and methylphenidate on the homeostasis of growth hormone. In contrast, Puig-Antich et al.[49] did not find any changes in growth hormone of 7 boys who had amphetamine treatment for 1 year, though significant decrease in prolactin levels was seen. Even though the number of subjects was small, the correlation between decreased prolactin levels and growth suppression was extremely high. The mechanism by which prolactin may affect growth is unclear, as is the process by which stimulant medication modifies growth-hormone and prolactin secretion. These are, however, interesting and important areas for future research.

PHYSIOLOGICAL MEASURES IN ADULTHOOD

As stated earlier, the interest in physiological measures in adults who were hyperactive as children is twofold. First, what is the natural history of these measures? Does the "maturational lag" disappear with time, or do differences seen in childhood persist in adulthood? Secondly, what is the long-term effect of stimulant medication taken in childhood? Does it affect adult physiological measures? Our follow-up study addressed both these questions.

Natural History

Hyperactive subjects who had not received any ongoing stimulant medication during childhood and their matched normal controls were evaluated with respect to height, weight, blood pressure, and pulse to determine the fate of these measures in adulthood in a relatively untreated hyperactive population (see Chapter 5). We thus obtained some view of the natural history of these measures.[61]

Subjects included 65 young adults (aged 17–24 years) who had been judged hyperactive 10 years before and were participating in an ongoing follow-up study and 39 "normal" individuals matched for age, sex, IQ, and socioeconomic status. Height and weight were measured on a standard upright scale, with the subjects dressed in casual indoor clothing without shoes. The pulse rate was measured over a 1-minute period after the subject had been seated for about 1 hour discussing general information, this part of the psychiatric interview being considered by us to be the least likely to evoke emotional reactions. Blood pressure was measured at the same time as the pulse rate, with the subject seated. The height and weight of a subgroup of subjects (24 hyperactive and 24 matched control subjects) were measured again under similar conditions approximately 2 years later to determine whether the measurements obtained at the 10-year follow-up assessment reflected final adult values. All measurements were obtained by the same two examiners (L. H. and G. W.), whose findings correlated highly, and all findings were studied by analysis of variance.

At the 10-year follow-up assessment there were no significant differences between the 65 hyperactive individuals and the 39 matched control subjects in height, weight, pulse rate, or blood pressure (Table 11-1). Similarly, at the 12-year follow-up assessment there were no significant differences between the 24 hyperactive and 24 matched control subjects for any of these physiologic measures (Table 11-2). The mean heights and weights of the hyperactive and control subjects were not significantly different at the two follow-up assessments (Table 11-3), which suggests that a growth plateau had been reached by both groups at the time of the 10-year follow-up assessment. The correlations between the mean heights at the 10-year and 12-year follow-up assessments were very high—0.981 for the hyperactive individuals and 0.968 for the controls—which indicates that our findings were not subject to significant measurement error.

Our findings indicate that hyperactive individuals 17–24 years of age who have never taken stimulant medication show no differences in height, weight, pulse rate, or blood pressure from matched control subjects. This suggests that whatever the problems of physiologic maturation of hyperactive individuals referred to by Beck[57] and Oettinger[42] and their colleagues may be, they do not significantly influence adult height and weight or cardiovascular measures; hence hyperactivity itself does not significantly affect final growth measures. One cannot say on the basis of our data that the hyperactive and control subjects reached their growth plateau at the same time. Only sequential measurements during adolescence would reveal the plateau for

TABLE 11-1. Physiological Measures (Means) at 10-Year Follow-Up Assessment of Hyperactive and Control Subjects Aged 17 to 24 Years

Measure	Hyperactives ($n = 65$)	Controls ($n = 39$)
Height (cm)	173.38	172.98
Weight (kg)	71.25	71.18
Pulse rate (beats/minute)	75.98	77.68
Blood pressure (mm Hg)		
Systolic	120.30	123.45
Diastolic	77.36	80.02

Note. No significant differences were found between the groups for any measure.

TABLE 11-2. Physiological Measures (Means) at 12-Year Follow-Up Assessment of Subgroup of Hyperactive and Control Subjects

Measure	Hyperactives ($n = 24$)	Controls ($n = 24$)
Age at 12-year follow-up assessment (years)	22 1/12	21 5/12
Interval between assessments (years)	2 5/12	2 1/12
Height (cm)	172.10	173.20
Weight (kg)	74.87	75.25

Note. No significant differences were found between the groups for any measure.

each group. However, one can assume that the plateau for both groups was reached sometime between 17 and 24 years of age.

Our data also provide a baseline against which the height, weight, pulse rate, and blood pressure of hyperactive individuals who have taken stimulant medication at various ages, for various durations, and in various dosages can be compared.

Physiological Measures of Adult Hyperactives Who Received Stimulant Treatment in Childhood

We also followed a group (25 subjects) of hyperactives who had received at least 3 years of sustained stimulant medication (20–50 mg/day) between 6 and 12 years of age. These hyperactives were reassessed in adolescence in a 5-year follow-up study,[47] where there were some concerns regarding growth suppression due to medication treatment. More recently[62] 20 of these subjects and 20 matched normal

TABLE 11-3. Physiological Measures (Means) at the Two Follow-Up Assessments

Measure and subjects	10-year ($n = 24$)	12-year ($n = 24$)
Height (cm)		
Hyperactives	172.35	172.10
Controls	172.37	173.20
Weight (kg)		
Hyperactives	70.12	74.87
Controls	71.95	75.25

Note. No significant differences were found between 10-year and 12-year values; correlation of heights was 0.981 for hyperactive subjects and 0.968 for control subjects.

controls were seen in a 10 to 12-year follow-up study. The inclusion criteria for both the hyperactive and control groups were similar to those used for the untreated hyperactive follow-up group (see Chapter 5). The physiological measures of height, weight, blood pressure, and pulse were obtained in the same manner and sequence as with the untreated hyperactive group described previously.[61] In addition, heights and weights of both parents were obtained whenever possible to determine if the subjects deviated significantly from their parents in these measures.

Comparison of the three groups—namely, stimulant-treated hyperactives, their control group, and untreated hyperactives—revealed that the three groups matched on socioeconomic status. The stimulant-treated hyperactive group and their control group matched in age (mean age 21 years) but were slightly older than the untreated hyperactive group when the physiological measures were taken (mean age 19.6 years). Finally, the two hyperactive groups were matched on IQ but the control group had slightly higher IQ, 115 compared to 107. As Table 11-4 shows, no significant differences with regard to weight, height, pulse, or blood pressure were seen in the three groups. Measures of parental heights and weights were similar for the stimulant-treated and control groups. Offspring did not deviate significantly from parental measures. These findings suggest that the amount, duration, and time of administration of the stimulants for this group of hyperactives did not significantly affect their growth or cardiovascular status.

However, even though group means showed no differences on these measures, it should be pointed out that some (3 or 4) of our subjects appeared particularly short. It was unclear whether the short stature was due to familial factors (some of the families of these subjects were also short), metabolic factors (some of these subjects had metabolic problems), or long-term medication side effects. It may well be that subjects already vulnerable to short stature because of genetic or metabolic factors are more affected by stimulant medication, since this may further decrease their eventual height, which is already somewhat compromised.

Electroencephalographic Measures in Adult Hyperactives

To test the hypothesis outlined earlier, that EEG abnormalities in hyperactive children reflect immature patterns which will normalize with age, we compared the EEG's of hyperactive young adults who had received no sustained stimulant treatment with EEG's of matched normal controls.[63] We also examined the EEG's of the hyperactive subjects longitudinally (i.e., initially, at the 5-year follow-up assess-

TABLE 11-4. Physiological Variables

	Hyperactives		Controls
Measure	Ritalin	Non-Ritalin	Ritalin
	($n = 17$)	($n = 60$–62)	($n = 17$–19)
Weight (kg)	70	71	79
Height (cm)	170	173	158
Pulse	73	76	74
Blood pressure			
Systolic	118	120	116
Diastolic	79	77	78
	($n = 15$)		($n = 17$–18)
Father's weight (kg)	78		78
Father's height (cm)	174		174
Mother's weight (kg)	57		62
Mother's height (cm)	163		162

Note. The Ritalin hyperactive group was comprised of subjects who had had 3–5 years of stimulant therapy in childhood. Control subjects were normals who were matched and compared only to the Ritalin group.

No significant differences were found between the groups for any measure.

ment, and currently, at the 10-year follow-up assessment) to see how they changed with time.

The relation of behavioral and functional measures to EEG findings is also unclear and controversial. Satterfield and colleagues[30] found no difference in intelligence, school achievement, or behavior problems at school or at home between hyperactive children with normal EEG findings and those with abnormal EEG findings. Others (e.g., Stevens *et al.*[64]) have postulated a close correlation between EEG and behavioral abnormalities. To clarify this issue we looked at global outcome measures in hyperactive individuals at the 10-year follow-up assessment and compared them with EEG findings at the initial assessment and after 5 and 10 years.

Methods

Subjects were part of the 10-year prospective follow-up study described in detail in Chapter 5. They consisted of 37 of 75 hyperactive individuals (49%) and 27 or 44 controls (61%) matched for age (mean ages 19.17 and 19.59 years respectively) and sex. Though most of the

75 hyperactive and 44 control subjects agreed to have EEG's recorded, few completed the examinations.

The EEG's were recorded in a regular adult EEG laboratory under standard conditions of rest, hyperventilation, and photic stimulation, but not during sleep. All EEG's were interpreted by the same trained neurologist and encephalographer (F. A. Andermann), who was uninformed as to the research design and did not know that any of the subjects were normal controls, but assumed them all to be hyperactive. The interpreted EEG's were then scored by another trained encephalographer (K. M.), who had read and scored the EEG's of these subjects at the initial assessment and at the 5-year follow-up assessment. Each EEG was scored according to the items in Table 11-5. Initial, 5-year

TABLE 11-5. Comparison of Findings in EEG's of Hyperactive and Control Subjects (Young Adults) at 10-Year Follow-Up Assessment

EEG findings	Hyperactives ($n = 37$)	Controls ($n = 27$)
Normal	26	18
Abnormal		
Diffuse	6	5
Focal	0	0
Paroxysmal	5	4
Severity		
Mild	9	9
Moderate	2	0
Severe	0	0
Epileptic discharges		
None	30	20
Spikes	0	0
Spindle-wave complex	1	0
Sharp waves	3	0
Other	0	0
Abnormality occurs during		
Rest	6	5
Hyperventilation	5	7
Sleep	0	0
Photic stimulation	2	0
Drowsiness	0	0
Abnormal activity		
Slow	8	9
Fast	1	0
Sharp	1	0
Mixed	0	0

Note. There were no significant differences between the two groups.

follow-up, and 10-year follow-up EEG's were compared in more general terms and categorized as follows:

- Normal
- Minimal abnormality
- Moderate abnormality
  1. not epileptiform
  2. epileptiform
- Severe abnormality
  1. not epileptiform
  2. epileptiform

At the initial EEG assessment the 59 hyperactive subjects were 6–13 years of age (mean $\pm SD$ = 8.33 $\pm$ 1.47 years). At the 5-year follow-up the remaining 25 hyperactive subjects were 10–16 years of age (mean $\pm$ SD = 13.12 $\pm$ 1.62 years). Only 12 hyperactive subjects underwent assessment at all three specified times. Sequential EEG's were not available for the control subjects, since most of this group joined the study at the time of the 5-year follow-up assessment, but did not receive EEG's at that time.

EEG differences between hyperactive and control subjects and for hyperactive subjects at various stages were analyzed by the chi-square test. Global outcome measures included work or school record, quality of emotional adjustment and interpersonal relations, and record of persistent antisocial behavior or extensive nonmedical use of drugs. Subjects were divided into groups of good, medium, or poor outcome on the basis of these measures by two psychiatrists (L. H. and G. W.), who correlated highly in the scoring. Comparison was then made between these outcome measures and the EEG findings at the three assessments.

Results

EEG'S OF HYPERACTIVE VERSUS CONTROL SUBJECTS AT 10-YEAR FOLLOW-UP ASSESSMENT (Table 11-5)

Comparison of EEG's of hyperactive and control subjects at the 10-year follow-up assessment showed no significant differences between the two groups. Most of the EEG's in both groups were thought to be normal (26 of 37 in the hyperactive group and 18 of 27 in the control group). Most of the abnormalities that did occur were assessed to be mild (9 of 11 in the hyperactive group and all 9 in the control group), and most in both groups occurred during rest or hyperventilation and were mainly characterized by slow-wave activity.

SEQUENTIAL EEG'S OF HYPERACTIVE SUBJECTS

At the initial and 5-year follow-up assessments about 50% of the EEG's of different groups of hyperactive subjects were abnormal, but at the 10-year follow-up assessment only about 30% were abnormal (Table 11-6). Statistical analysis could not be performed because the EEG's of some subjects appeared in more than one time grouping and hence did not represent independent measures. Unfortunately, few hyperactive subjects had EEG's recorded at all three assessments. No significant changes were seen in the EEG's from one assessment to the next (Table 11-6), but this may have been due to the small numbers included in this analysis. At all three times 69–88% of the abnormalities were mild.

CHANGES IN EEG'S OF HYPERACTIVE SUBJECTS WITH PARTICULAR TIME INTERVALS (Table 11-7)

Of the 14 subjects with initially abnormal EEG's, 11 had improved tracings at the 10-year follow-up assessment, and in only 5 of the 15 with initially normal EEG's were the tracings worse. These changes were significant ($p < .01$), thus indicating that the EEG abnormalities tend to lessen with time. Further, this improvement did not take place between the times of the initial assessment and the 5-year follow-up assessment: of the 10 subjects with initially abnormal EEG's, 7 still showed abnormalities at the 5-year follow-up assessment, and there were no significant changes during this period. The changes seemed to

TABLE 11-6. Comparison of Findings in Sequential EEG's of Hyperactive Subjects

Subjects and EEG findings	Time of assessment		
	Initial	5-year follow-up	10-year follow-up
Mean age (years)	8.3	13	19
Different groups			
Normal	30	13	26
Abnormal	29	12	11
Total	59	25	37
Same group			
Normal	6	5	6
Abnormal	6	7	6
Total	12	12	12

Note. Statistical analysis could not be performed between the different groups because the EEG's of some subjects appeared in more than one time grouping and hence did not represent independent measures. For the same groups the differences in findings at the three times were not significant; $\chi^2 = 1.09$, 0, and 0.01 for initial versus 5-year, initial versus 10-year, and 5-year versus 10-year results respectively.

TABLE 11-7. Changes in EEG's of Hyperactive Subjects with Particular Time Intervals

Time of assessment and EEG findings		Change in EEG findings		
		Better	Worse	Same
		At 10-year follow-up[a]		
Initial				
Normal	15	0	5	10
Minimally abnormal	12	9	0	3
Moderately abnormal	2	2	0	0
Total	29	11	5	13
		At 5-year follow-up[b]		
Initial				
Normal	11	0	2	9
Minimally abnormal	9	2	1	6
Moderately abnormal	1	0	0	1
Total	21	2	3	16
		At 10-year follow-up[c]		
5-year follow-up				
Normal	7	0	2	5
Minimally abnormal	6	3	0	3
Moderately abnormal	2	2	0	0
Total	15	5	2	0

[a]Changes significant; $p < .01$, $\chi^2 = 20.279$.
[b]Changes not significant; $\chi^2 = 3.217$.
[c]Changes significant; $p < .05$, $\chi^2 = 9.294$.

occur during the last 5 years—that is, between the 5-year and the 10-year follow-up assessments: the 8 subjects with abnormal EEG's at the 5-year follow-up had improved tracings at the 10-year follow-up. This finding was significant ($p < .05$).

OUTCOME MEASURES AND EEG'S (Table 11-8)

The EEG findings at the 10-year follow-up assessment did not differ between the groups of hyperactive subjects classified according to outcome. In each outcome group most of the EEG's were normal, so the correlation between current EEG findings and current functioning was not significant. As for the predictive value of initial or 5-year follow-up EEG assessment and global outcome measures at 10-year follow-up assessment, there was no significant difference in initial and 5-year follow-up EEG findings between any of the outcome groups.

TABLE 11-8. Comparison of Findings in Sequential EEG's of Hyperactive Subjects with Current Outcome Measures

Time of assessment and EEG findings	Outcome		
	Good	Medium	Poor
10-year follow-up[a]			
Normal	11	9	6
Minimally abnormal	2	5	2
Moderately abnormal	0	2	0
Total	13	16	8
No EEG's recorded[b]	10	18	10
5-year follow-up[c]			
Normal	5	5	3
Minimally abnormal	4	3	1
Moderately abnormal	0	2	2
Total	9	10	6
Initial[d]			
Normal	12	11	6
Minimally abnormal	5	14	4
Moderately abnormal	1	5	0
Total	18	30	10

[a]Correlation not significant; $\chi^2 = 4.223$.
[b]Distribution of these subjects was not significantly different from that of subjects with EEG's recorded; $\chi^2 = 0.7179$.
[c]Correlation not significant; $\chi^2 = 3.590$.
[d]Correlation not significant; $\chi^2 = 5.872$.

Unfortunately only 37 of 75 hyperactive and 27 of 44 control subjects had EEGs recorded. To determine whether this constituted a positive or negative bias we assessed the global outcome of the hyperactive subjects who did not have EEG's recorded. Since, as Table 11-8 shows, they did not fall predominantly into the good or the poor outcome group, it is unlikely that a positive or a negative bias existed.

Discussion

Our finding that at the 10-year follow-up assessment there were no significant differences in the EEG's of hyperactive and matched-control subjects supports the hypothesis that EEG's of hyperactive individuals normalize with age and that the mild diffuse slowing seen earlier in life and reported by others[33] reflects an immature pattern which disappears with age. Our sequential data suggest that this normalization is most significant toward the end of adolescence, in that a much larger proportion of the hyperactive subjects' EEG's were normal at the time of the 10-year follow-up assessment. Unfortunately, since we did not have EEG's recorded at all stages for all hyperactive subjects, some sequential comparisons could not be made. However, from the data available it seems that most of the improvement occurs between the times of the 5-year and 10-year follow-up assessment—that is, between 13 and 19 years of age.

Correlations of EEG findings at the three times of assessment with global outcome measures at the 10-year follow-up assessment were not significant. This supports the findings by Satterfield and colleagues[30] and by Hughes[65] of either no correlation or an inverse one between EEG abnormalities and learning or behavioral difficulties. We also see that the initial EEG is not a good prognostic indicator for long-term global outcome. Prediction of the latter by means of particular outcome measures, such as education completed and work status, is dealt with in Chapter 14.

In summary one can say that some hyperactives have physiological abnormalities. Often these abnormalities can be interpreted to reflect persistance of immature patterns. Stimulant medication seems to have a normalizing effect on some of these measures, though it also raises concerns regarding long-term side effects. Our findings in adults suggest that physiological abnormalities normally do not persist into adulthood but normalize with age and that stimulant treatment in childhood, in the amount, duration, and time of administration experienced by the hyperactive subjects we studied, did not have any long-term residual effect on the particular physiological measures studied—that is, height, weight, blood pressure, and pulse.

CHAPTER TWELVE

FAMILIES OF HYPERACTIVES

> Thus the story of Exodus
> Was told and retold from generation to generation
> Our Rabbis discovered centuries ago
> That there are four types of children
> Each one quite different from the rest;
> Each needs to be told the story
> . . . in a different way.
> —*The Haggadah*

Studies involving families of hyperactives generally fall into two large groups. One group focuses on siblings, either as a comparison group for the hyperactives or as a genetic cohort to see if there is an increased incidence of disorder in the siblings. The other group of studies addresses parents, again in an attempt to elucidate genetic factors—either in etiology or in order to postulate long-term outcome—or to evaluate the nature of interactions between hyperactive youngsters and their parents. Our own study, which will be described at the end of this chapter assesses how the family fares over time as the hyperactive child grows up and also after he or she leaves home.

SIBLING STUDIES

Most studies involving siblings of hyperactive subjects have used the siblings as a control or comparison group. In such studies hyperactives usually functioned worse than their siblings. Thus Borland and Heckman,[1] in a 20- to 25-year retrospective study, interviewed 20 men (mean age 30) who, from childhood medical records, conformed to the diagnostic criteria for hyperactive child syndrome. The authors compared this group with their brothers (mean age 28). Generally, they found that neither the hyperactives nor their brothers experienced serious social or psychiatric problems as adults. However, the hyperactive subjects had more emotional and work difficulties and lower socioeconomic status.

Feldman *et al.*[2] also carried out a 10- to 12-year retrospective follow-up study on 48 young adults (mean age 21) previously diagnosed as hyperactive and compared them to their siblings. Even though 91% of the hyperactives at age 21 were either in school or working, when compared to their siblings they had lower educational achievement and lower self-esteem. Some 10% of the hyperactives seemed to have significant problems with respect to drug use, inactivity, and Schizoid Personality Disorders. In addition, 10% drank alcohol before work or school, compared to none of the sibling controls. Again one gets the picture that siblings of hyperactives are functioning fairly well and better than the hyperactives.

Potentially the largest sibling study is now being carried out by Loney *et al.*,[3] with 200 hyperactives and 100 of their full brothers being followed up at 21–23 years of age. The data on 22 proband–brother pairs have been analyzed thus far. Again, there is a clear pattern that hyperactives do worse than their siblings in a variety of areas; for example, more hyperactives have significant unemployment, impaired interpersonal relationships, and lack permanent residence when compared to their brothers. Thus 45% of the hyperactives meet antisocial outcomes criteria (modified by excluding Impaired Interpersonal Relationships) compared to 18% of the brothers and only 6% of the normal control subjects in the extensive depression study. Even though there is no significant difference in the number of hyperactives and their brothers who were diagnosed as definitely and probably alcoholic— 27% and 23% respectively—this figure is greater than in the depression study, where only about 9% of the controls met alcoholic criteria.

There was also no significant difference with regard to nonmedical drug use between hyperactives and their brothers, but both groups differed from National Survey on Drug Abuse norms.[4] This difference was greater for the hyperactives who used more inhalants (glue, cocaine, sedatives, and stimulants) than was the norm in the national survey. There was a trend for the sibling group to use more stimulants than the national survey group. Hyperactives were more involved in crimes against persons, and this involvement tended to be more severe when compared to that of their brothers. Consequently, the hyperactives had more serious police involvement, with 41% having been convicted or having spent time in jail compared to 5% of their brothers. We thus see that though the hyperactives are not functioning as well as their brothers, the brothers in turn are not functioning as well as a normal control group; they have more Antisocial Personality Disorder and more alcoholism.

The differences between Loney *et al.*'s[3] siblings and those of Borland and Heckman[1] and Feldman *et al.*[2] may be a function of time seen

(Loney's are being seen in the 1980s; Borland's were seen in the early to mid-1970s), location, familial factors, and socioeconomic status. These discrepancies underline the importance of a matched control group to which siblings can be compared. A study comparing siblings of hyperactives with siblings of matched controls was carried out by Welner and colleagues.[5] They matched a group of hyperactives and a group of control subjects on sex (all males), race (all white), age (mean age 11 years), and roughly on socioeconomic status (roughly middle class). All had IQ's of 79 or above, were free of significant neurological abnormalities and psychosis, and were living with their mother. The workers' then compared all the siblings age 6 and older. They found that 26% of the brothers of hyperactives, but only 9% of brothers of controls ($p < .054$), met their diagnostic criteria for hyperactivity. However, no differences were found in the rate of hyperactivity in the sisters of hyperactives and controls. With regard to depression and anxiety symptoms, again 26% of brothers of hyperactives and only 6% of brothers of controls ($p < .02$) had three or more depression–anxiety symptoms. Again, no differences were found in the sisters. Interestingly, no differences were found in antisocial behavior in the brothers and sisters of hyperactives and controls, though hyperactives themselves showed more antisocial behavior. And finally, though control siblings had slightly higher IQ's than hyperactive siblings, the latter had somewhat higher achievements—a finding the authors had difficulty explaining.

In summary, siblings (particularly brothers) of hyperactive subjects function better than the hyperactives but seem to have more problems than siblings of controls (e.g., higher rates of hyperactivity and more depression–anxiety symptoms), although not more antisocial behavior. It remains unclear if these difficulties reflect familial patterns, genetic influence, or merely the stress of having a same-sex hyperactive sibling.

Studies of siblings which have tried to focus on genetic aspects have been few, with small samples and therefore inconclusive. For example, Lopez,[6] in a twin study, showed that 3 pairs of male monozygotic twins were all concordant for hyperactivity, while of 6 pairs of dyzygotic twins 5 were discordant. However, 4 of these discordant sets of twins were also discordant with regard to sex. In 3 of these pairs the male was hyperactive, while the female was not. This merely reflects the known fact that hyperactivity appears to be much more common in males compared to females and thus was not a function of zygocity.

In another study, Safer[7] looked at 19 sibs and 22 half sibs of 17 hyperactive probands who lived in foster homes. He found significantly greater occurrence of Minimal Brain Dysfunction (MBD) in full sibs when compared to half sibs. However, these families also had severe disorders, congenital anomalies, and low intelligence levels, and therefore would not today be included in most studies of hyperactive child syndrome.

PARENTAL STUDIES: INTERACTIONAL ASPECTS

Family studies have concerned themselves with interactional aspects as well as genetic possibilities. Many of the interactional studies were described in Chapter 3.

To summarize, Battle and Lacey[8] showed that mothers of highly active males were critical, disapproving, unaffectionate, and severe in their punishment. This was particularly true in the middle-childhood years. None of these maternal behaviors was associated with high activity levels in females. Some authors[9] have suggested that this type of maternal style was a primary etiological factor in the child's hyperactivity. Others[10] felt strongly that maternal behavior was simply a response to the child's behavior and not a cause of it.

There have been several studies which have supported this view that mothers of hyperactive children are merely responding to the type of behavior and difficulties that their children present and do not cause these problems. Campbell[11] compared observational data of three groups of mothers and children while performing easy and difficult tasks. The three groups represented reflective, impulsive, and hyperactive children. The authors found no differences in the mother–child interactions among the groups during the easy task. However, during the difficult task, mothers of hyperactives made more encouraging comments and provided more suggestions concerning impulse control. There was a trend for mothers of the hyperactives to be more disapproving, but this was not significant. Generally mothers of hyperactives were seen as supportive and not punitive. As no differences in mother–child interactions existed between the groups during the easy task, but only during the difficult task, the authors concluded that the mothers of hyperactives were responding to the child and adopting a more controlling style as the child experienced more difficulty. In a subsequent study,[12] which compared the interactions of hyperactive, learning-disabled, and matched normal boys and their mothers on the same easy and difficult tasks, the results were similar. Mothers of hyperactives provided more encouragement, impulse-control directions, and disapproval when compared to the other two groups. Again the authors concluded that mothers were responding to the child's behavior.

Humphries et al.[13] hypothesized that if stimulant medication modified children's behavior, and that if, under these circumstances, mothers in turn changed their interactions with their children—that is, became more positive and less controlling—this would support the idea that mothers were just responding to children's hyperactivity. The authors gave hyperactive children and their mothers a highly structured task to perform together under both drug and placebo conditions. Unlike Campbell's[11,12] studies where the mother's participation was optional, here it was required. While on medication, hyperactives and their mothers made fewer errors, praised each other more, and criticized each other less, and mothers gave fewer directions. This change in the nature of the mother–child interaction while the child was on stimulants led the authors to conclude that mother's intrusive, controlling, disapproving pattern was a response to the child's disordered behavior and not a cause of it, since it modified with changes in the child's behavior. However, Humphries did not have a control group with which the hyperactive mother–child dyad could be compared, so the degree of normalization achieved by stimulant medication could not be assessed. In addition, the authors used a very structured laboratory test which may not be relevant to real-life situations.

Both these shortcomings were addressed and controlled for by Cunningham and Barkley.[14] They compared the interactions of hyperactive (off medication) and normal boys and their mothers in both free-play and task settings. The authors found that during the free play, mothers of hyperactives interacted less with their children. They initiated fewer contacts, responded less, and encouraged play less. However, when they did interact they tended to be more controlling, but the hyperactives also complied less. In the task setting, again mothers of hyperactives initiated fewer contacts and responded less than mothers of controls. Mothers of hyperactives were more controlling, giving more commands, but even though the hyperactives complied less, their mothers rewarded compliance less and tended to be inconsistent in rewarding desired behaviors. The authors concluded that the intrusive, controlling style of the mothers of hyperactive boys, while initially a response to the child's overactive, impulsive, inattentive style, may further contribute to the child's behavioral difficulties.

These findings were almost identical to those of Mash and Johnston,[15] who also compared mother–child interactions in younger and older hyperactives (off medication) and an age-matched control group in structured-task and free-play situations. The mothers of hyperactives were more directive and negative and less responsive and approving. This was particularly true for the mothers of the younger hyperactives in the structured-task situation.

In a subsequent study, Barkley and Cunningham[16] compared mother–child interactions of hyperactive children in both drug and placebo states. When the hyperactives were on drugs they increased their compliance, and their mothers reduced their commands and increased their responsiveness. However, the level of responsiveness and interaction between the mothers of hyperactives and their sons did not equal that of the normal controls.

The fact that mothers of hyperactive children may get locked into a negative parenting pattern which extends to nonhyperactive siblings was pointed out by Mash and Johnston.[17] The authors compared interactions of hyperactives, their siblings, and their mothers with those of age-matched normal controls. Results showed that hyperactives and their siblings had more social conflict and high rates of negative behavior during play. The conflicts decreased during the mother-supervised situations. Mothers of hyperactives were less responsive, interactive, and rewarding and more negative than mothers of nonhyperactive children. This was true of their interactions with the siblings as well as the hyperactive children.

Few studies have looked at the parenting style of fathers of hyperactive children. Tallmadge and Barkley[18] found that fathers of hyperactives, like mothers, were more directive than fathers of controls. However, the hyperactive children were more likely to comply with fathers' than with mothers' commands.

It is thus not surprising that Mash and Johnston[19] found that parents of hyperactives reported less confidence in their parenting knowledge when compared to controls. In addition, mothers of hyperactives reported more stress, social isolation, self-blame, and depression.

In summary, one can conclude that the controlling, less responsive, and more negative parenting style of mothers of hyperactive children reported in several studies[8,12-15] is most probably a consequence and not a cause of the child's behavior. It is thus also not an intrinsic, predetermined aspect of the mother's personality. The evidence that the parenting style became markedly more positive (less controlling and intrusive and more rewarding) when the child's behavior improved on stimulant medication[13,16] shows that it is the child's behavior which initially influences the mother's behavior. However, even with stimulant medication, the mother–child interaction of hyperactives, though much improved, does not equal that of normal controls. It seems that old habits and patterns, once established, are modifiable but difficult to alter entirely. Therefore, even if the negative mother-child interaction seen in hyperactives is initially a response to the child's overactive, impulsive, inattentive style, it may affect the child's future development in terms of self-esteem and social competence and thus exacerbate his or her handicaps and symptomatology. Interventions (parental counseling, parent-training groups) which would foster appropriate parenting skills in parents of hyperactive children are therefore crucial.

PARENTAL STUDIES: GENETIC ASPECTS

In recent years, several studies have addressed themselves to the problem of psychiatric illness in families of hyperactive children. Morrison and Stewart[20] interviewed parents of 59 hyperactives and 41 control children and showed a high prevalence of alcoholism, sociopathy, and hysteria in fathers and mothers of hyperactive children. They also found that significantly more parents of hyperactive than of control children had probably been hyperactive as children themselves. This suggested associations of adult and childhood psychiatric disorders, and they questioned whether childhood hyperactivity might be related to alcoholism, hysteria, and sociopathy and whether the hyperactive child syndrome was transmitted genetically or socially from parent to child.

Cantwell's[21] findings were similar. He gave a systematic psychiatric examination to parents of 50 hyperactive children and 50 matched controls. Increased prevalence rates for alcoholism, sociopathy, and hysteria, but not affective disorders, were found in parents of hyperactive children. Ten percent of the parents of hyperactive children were thought to have been hyperactive as children themselves; and of this 10%, all were psychiatrically ill with alcoholism, sociopathy, or hysteria. Cantwell felt that the hyperactive child syndrome is passed from generation to generation and may be a precursor for certain adult psychiatric illnesses. Whether this transmission was environmental or genetic remained unclear.

In a later study, Cantwell[22] discussed the evidence of a genetic component in the hyperactive child syndrome and concluded that further family studies including twins and adoptees are needed. One such study, involving a comparison of adoptive and biological parents of hyperactive children, was carried out by Morrison and Stewart.[23] They interviewed the legal parents of 35 adopted hyperactive children. These children had had almost no contact with their biological parents, having been cared for by hospital nurseries, adoption agencies, or foster homes prior to placement at an average age of 15.7 weeks. The high prevalence of hysteria, sociopathy, and alcoholism found in biological parents of hyperactive children was not found in adopting parents.

Also, adopting parents were not as likely to have been hyperactive themselves. The authors concluded that this supported a genetic transmission. In two subsequent papers,[24,25] they tried to make a case for a polygenic mode of inheritance.

In another study involving adoptees, Goodwin et al.[26] connected alcoholism with the hyperactive child syndrome by showing that alcoholics as children were more often hyperactive, truant, antisocial, shy, aggressive, disobedient, and friendless. In addition they found alcoholism in 18.2% of adopted-away offspring of alcoholic fathers compared with 5.1% in adopted-away offspring of nonalcoholic fathers. The authors acknowledged the limitation of the retrospective approach to the problem, but cited literature suggesting the relationship between the hyperactive child syndrome and subsequent alcoholism, as well as a possible relationship between these disorders and antisocial behavior.

Thus, although several studies[20,21] have linked the hyperactive child syndrome with the prevalence of alcoholism, sociopathy, and hysteria in biological parents, the association with affective disorders is less pronounced. Stewart and Morrison[27] determined the incidence of Bipolar and Unipolar Affective Disorder among natural relatives of 59 hyperactive children, legal relatives of 35 adopted hyperactive children, and relatives of 41 control children. There were no significant differences in the incidence of the two conditions between the groups of relatives, except for a greater incidence of Unipolar Affective Disorder in the combined second-degree blood relatives of hyperactive children compared to relatives of controls. Moreover, the incidence of Bipolar Affective Disorder in natural parents of hyperactive children was much lower than figures reported for parents of patients with this type of affective disorder. Therefore, the data did not support a connection between hyperactivity in childhood and adult Manic Depressive Affective Disorder.

In a subsequent paper, Stewart et al.[28] have pointed out that earlier family studies[20,21] have suffered from three limitations. Firstly, investigators used normal children as controls rather than children attending a psychiatric clinic for reasons other than hyperactivity. Thus, the increased psychopathology seen in relatives of hyperactive children may be seen in all families who bring their children to child psychiatric clinics for emotional problems and may not be particularly related to hyperactivity. Secondly, hyperactivity is generally very broadly defined. Other behaviors—for example, resistance to discipline, aggression, and specific antisocial behaviors—have been included in the criteria for diagnosing this syndrome. The adult disorders found associated with hyperactivity in children may actually be related to some other dimension of the children's behavior—for example, aggressiveness or antisocial behavior. Finally, many of the studies were not done "blind." Interviewers were aware that the parents were relatives of a hyperactive or a control child, and this may have affected their ratings.

Stewart and his group have sought to show that when the above limitations are corrected, different results are obtained regarding psychiatric illness in parents of hyperactive children. The group has focused on the "unsocialized–aggressive" boy, and has found[29] that relatives of these boys (e.g., fathers, uncles, siblings) had a higher incidence of Antisocial Personality Disorders than a matched control group of boys coming for psychiatric help for other problems. Unfortunately, 14 of 17 boys in the unsocialized–aggressive group were also diagnosed as being hyperkinetic. It is thus unclear if the results reflect a connection with unsocialized aggression of the boys or a combination of hyperactivity and unsocialized aggression. Stewart et al.[30] distinguished between the two groups in the following way:

To qualify as hyperactive, a boy had to be described as being unusually active, energetic, and having difficulties concentrating or finishing tasks, both to a marked degree and persisting over at least the past year. To qualify as unsocialized aggressive, a boy had to have the following items: aggressiveness (shown by fighting, extreme competitiveness, attacks on adults or verbally abusing adults), resistance to discipline (not following directions, impossible to control, out late at night, or doing the opposite of what parents want), and either destructiveness (fire setting, destroying private property or destroying public property), or meanness (frequent quarrels, taking revenge or bullying). Again, these symptoms had to have been present to a marked degree for longer than a year.

Stewart et al.[30] reexamined the prevalence of alcoholism and antisocial disorders in parents of hyperactive and unsocialized–aggressive boys. Their finding that Antisocial Personality Disorder and alcoholism occur more frequently in the fathers of unsocialized–aggressive boys is not surprising. However, 27 of the 38 subjects classified as unsocialized–aggressive were also hyperactive—so again, it may well be this combination which is significant.

In a later study Morrison[31] sought to address the criticism that a comparison group of parents of psychiatrically ill children who were *not* hyperactive was lacking. He thus compared family histories of 140 children and adolescents with hyperactive child syndrome with family histories of 91 psychiatrically ill children matched for age and sex but who were not attention-deficit disordered. He found that parents of hyperactives were more likely to have Antisocial Personality Disorder and Briquet's syndrome (hysteria) than parents of nonhyperactive children. Approximately 11% of the hyperactive children had a parent with such a diagnosis. Parents of nonhyperactive children had more affective and psychotic disorders. Unlike previous studies by Morrison *et al.*[20,23] and Cantwell,[21,22] in this study the diagnosis of alcoholism was *not* significantly greater in the parents of the hyperactive children. The incidence in both groups of parents was fairly high, casting doubt on the specific link between alcoholism and hyperactivity.

We thus see that earlier studies (Cantwell[22,22] and Morrison *et al.*,[20,23] whose methodological limitations were eloquently pointed out by McMahon[32]) have suggested a strong relationship between childhood hyperactivity and parental problems with alcholism, antisocial disorders, and hysteria. More recent work,[28–30] which is somewhat better controlled, has questioned the relative significance of hyperactivity in children versus unsocialized aggression in connection with this adult psychopathology. However, the very significant overlap, with many children showing both these symptoms, leaves the issue unclear.

Morrison's[31] more recent family study with another psychiatrically ill comparison group supports the antisocial and hysterical findings but not the alcoholism. Furthermore, the hyperactive children whose parents had Antisocial Personality Disorder were not diagnosed as having conduct disorders in accordance with DSM-III criteria. This is contrary to Stewart's findings of a strong link between unsocialized aggression in boys and alcoholism and antisocial disorders in the parents. Obviously more comprehensive, well-controlled family studies are required to clarify some of these divergent and unclear findings. A description of our own long-term follow-up of families of hyperactive children[33] follows.

LONG-TERM FOLLOW-UP OF FAMILIES OF HYPERACTIVE CHILDREN

Preliminary findings of our 10-year prospective follow-up study of hyperactives as young adults[34] indicated that although these subjects continued to have problems in a number of areas (e.g., restlessness, cognitive style, social skills, and emotional well-being), they do not load the psychiatric or antisocial population, as reported by others.[35] It thus became important to assess if the families of our group of hyperactive subjects were also functioning differently (better) than has generally been reported by Cantwell[21] and others.[20]

The first part of our study, therefore, consisted of a comparison of 65 families of hyperactive young-adult subjects and 43 families of control subjects matched for socioeconomic status. In addition to the socioeconomic factors, areas such as child-rearing practices, physical and mental health of family members, and family relationships were assessed. The families of our hyperactive subjects had had similar assessments initially and at 5-year follow-up. We thus had an opportunity to evaluate if and how families had changed in these areas with time, and whether these changes had any relationship to the hyperactives' functioning. This sequential evaluation of families of hyperactives constituted a second part of our study.

The preliminary report on hyperactives as young adults[34] indicated that their functioning had improved when compared to the 5-year follow-up study during adolescence. We were also surprised to see many of the subjects still living at home in spite of previous marked conflicts with families. It thus became important to assess the families' view of the subjects' current functioning. Did the families also perceive their children's improvement? Had past conflicts between the hyperactives and families subsided, or had the past negative experiences and expectations of the families made it difficult for improvements to register with them? Thus, the families' view of the subjects' current functioning constitutes the third part of the study.

Finally, we compared the parents' view of their children's functioning at different ages in their development. What improvements or difficulties did they perceive at these various stages? This was the fourth and final part of the study.

Subjects

Sixty-five families of hyperactives being assessed in a 10- year follow-up study (detailed in Chapter 5) were compared with 43 families of normal control subjects matched with the hyperactives for age (range 17–24 years), sex, IQ (all above 85), and socioeconomic status (each group having equal representation from each status).

Family Interview

One of the parents, usually the mother (but occasionally the father or both parents), was interviewed in a well-outlined though open-ended interview by a psychologist or social worker. During the early part of the training of a new interviewer, two interviewers saw a family together, with one doing the interview and the other sitting in. The roles of the two interviewers were reversed for the next family. After the interview was completed, each interviewer independently scored all relevant variables in the family interview. The training process ended when the agreement on scores was high and the interviewing style was similar. At the beginning of the interview, examiners were blind as to whether this was the family of a hyperactive or control subject. Families were thus assessed on sociocultural factors, child-rearing practices, physical and mental health of family members, and family relationships. The same questionnaire was used to assess families of hyperactives initially, at 5-year follow-up, and at 10-year follow-up. Scores on various items were compared at each of these three stages.

Following the interview, families were asked to complete a number of forms which dealt with their view of their children's functioning, past and present.

These forms included the following.

FAMILY'S CURRENT ASSESSMENT OF YOUNG ADULT'S FUNCTIONING

This was determined by (1) the Katz family rating of subject's psychopathology (Katz Scale of Psychopathology[36]), which measured the family's impressions of its child on various psychopathological parameters, on a 4-point scale; and (2) a form outlining the family's current view of the child's functioning vis-à-vis plans, work, school, friends, money, drugs, etc.; possible areas of conflict were also noted.

FAMILY'S VIEW OF CHILD'S FUNCTIONING AT VARIOUS STAGES OF DEVELOPMENT

Three questionnaires—one for the preschool, one for the elementary-school, and one for the high-school period—were designed to tap social, academic, and hyperkinetic parameters. Parents were asked to complete these questionnaires, which required most items to be scored on a 5-point scale (1, hardly ever; 2, sometimes; 3, usually; 4, nearly always; 5, always). Data which included the assessment of families of hyperactive and control subjects and their responses on the various questionnaires outlined above were analyzed via chi-squares or analysis of variance, whichever was most appropriate.

Results

CURRENT ASSESSMENT OF FAMILIES OF HYPERACTIVE AND CONTROL SUBJECTS AT TEN-YEAR FOLLOW-UP (Table 12-1)

SOCIOCULTURAL FACTORS. In view of the fact that both groups were matched for socioeconomic status (each group having an equal representation from each status), most of the sociocultural factors reflecting socioeconomic status were, as expected, not significantly different for the families of hyperactives and controls. No significant differences were seen either in other social factors such as family size and whether the subject was adopted or an offspring of a previous

TABLE 12-1. Current Evaluation of Families of Controls versus Hyperactives: 10-Year Follow-Up

	Mean (hyperactives) (n = 61–65)	Mean (controls) (n = 41–43)	χ^2	df	Significance	Direction
Sociocultural parameters						
Mother's level of education	10.32	10.88				
Father's level of education	10.6	12.2				
Father's working status (Hollingshead)			4.8	6		
Mother's working status (Hollingshead)			5.82	6		
Mother working			.21	1		
Physical qualities of home			6.12	4		
Family size			4.2	5		
Child offspring of previous marriage			.57	1		
Child adopted			2.6	1		
Sibling order			12.19	4	$p = .01$	More hyperactives eldest
Child-rearing practices						
Continued presence of mother or stable substitute			3.36	4		
Inconsistent			6.7	4		
Lack controls			2.4	4		
Punitive-authoritative			8.4	4		
Overprotective			2.9	4	$p = .07$	Controls better
Health of family members						
Physical illness in family			.09	1		
Death in family			.06	1		
Mental health of family members			8.9	4	$p = .06$	Controls better
Relationships						
Marital relationship			9.2	5	$p = .09$	Controls better
Emotional climate of home			3.4	4	$p = .009$	Controls better
Sum of scores of family scale	34.4 (Mean for hyperactives)	37.8 (Mean for controls)			$p = .004$	Controls better

marriage. With respect to sibling order, hyperactives were significantly more frequently the eldest ($p = .01$).

CHILD-REARING PRACTICES. Of the child-rearing parameters assessed, including inconsistency, lack of controls, and punitive–authoritative and overprotective styles, only the punitive–authoritative parameter tended to be more marked in families of hyperactive subjects ($p = .07$).

HEALTH OF FAMILY MEMBERS (Tables 12-1 and 12-2). There was no difference in the prevalence of physical illness or deaths in the two groups of families, but parents of hyperactives tended to have more mental-health problems ($p = .06$). Unfortunately, the types of mental-health problems which prevailed were not specifically categorized. However, the severity was categorized on a 5-point scale. "Severe" referred to any condition which required psychiatric hospitalization, psychotic conditions, character disorders with multiple offenses, or drug addiction including alcoholism. "Mild" referred to any neurotic condition.

We see (Table 12-2) that 7 of 41 (17%) families of controls had psychiatric treatment, compared to 18 of 65 (28%) families of hyperac-

TABLE 12-2. Mental Health of Family Members: 10-Year Follow-Up

	Hyperactives (n = 65)		Controls (n = 41)	
	Number	Grouped percent	Number	Grouped percent
Psychiatric treatment for severe mental disorder of both parents	1		0	
Psychiatric treatment for severe mental disorder of one parent or milder disorder of both parents	8	28	3	17
Psychiatric treatment for mild disorder of one parent	9		4	
No treatment but symptoms present on and off in one or both parents	27	41	10	24
Good dynamic integration of both parents	20	31	24	59
Total	65	100	41	100

[a]Significance: $\chi^2 = 7.99$; $df = 2$; $p = .05$.

tives. However, when one examines a history of psychiatric symptoms in family members who received no treatment, we see that 10 of 41 (24%) control families had such symptoms compared to 27 of 65 (41%) hyperactive families. We thus see that the striking difference in the mental health of family members in the two groups lies not in severe psychiatric pathology which reuqires treatment, but in milder symptoms which usually go untreated. Finally, a significantly higher proportion of parents of controls versus hyperactives showed good dynamic integration ($p = .05$).

RELATIONSHIPS. Marital relationships also tended to be worse in families of hyperactives ($p = .09$). However, the two most significant findings indicated that the emotional climate of the home ($p = .009$) and the overall family score ($p = .004$) were considerably worse in families of hyperactives when compared to those of controls. Emotional climate of the home referred to the degree of positive versus negative interactions among family members (e.g., arguments, quiet talks) giving rise to a general level of tension or tranquility.

SEQUENTIAL EVALUATION OF FAMILIES OF HYPERACTIVE SUBJECTS (Table 12-3)

SOCIOCULTURAL PARAMETERS. There appeared to be little change in factors reflecting socioeconomic status during the three assessment periods. Parents' education and work status appear to have changed little although, as one would expect, more mothers were working at the 10-year follow-up period.

CHILD-REARING PRACTICES. Child-rearing practices remained the same in the three time periods except for a less punitive–authoritative approach at the 10-year follow-up.

HEALTH OF FAMILY MEMBERS. Families had experienced more medical illnesses and deaths at 10-year follow-up than at initial or 5-year follow-up. However, the mental health of family members was better at 10-year follow-up than initially. This trend was seen at 5-year, but was not yet significant at that time.

RELATIONSHIPS. Emotional climate of the home, marital relationship, and total family score were not significantly different at the three assessments. However, when one analyzed those families where the hyperactive subjects were no longer at home, we see that at 5-year follow-up, the emotional climate at home was considerably worse than initially or at 10-year follow-up, even though the marital relationship remained unchanged. It would thus seem that the emotional climate of the home improved when the adolescent left.

FAMILIES' CURRENT ASSESSMENT OF YOUNG ADULTS' FUNCTIONING: KATZ SCALE OF PSYCHOPATHOLOGY (Table 12-4)

Only 2 of the 18 parameters tapped by this scale were scored significantly differently by the families of hyperactives versus control subjects. These two items were negativism ($p = .05$) and ability to derive satisfaction ($p = .001$). In both instances, families of hyperactives scored their offspring as doing worse on these parameters than families of control subjects. Other measures, such as belligerence, verbal expansiveness, nervousness, suspiciousness, confusion, hyperactivity, stability, bizarreness, and compulsive in performing household chores, were not scored differently by the two groups.

QUESTIONNAIRE: CURRENT FUNCTIONING AND CONFLICTS (Table 12-5)

There seemed to be no differences in the families' view about their children's futures—that is, their optimism about offspring's future, whether he was making plans for the future, or if these plans were realistic. There were also no differences with regard to whether they thought the child used money wisely. Families of hyperactive subjects perceived that their child worked for his money more than did families of control subjects ($p = .02$).

Main areas of conflict which distinguished the two groups included conflicts around school or work ($p = .01$), tidiness ($p = .02$), and friends (in general, $p = .06$). In each case, families of hyperactive subjects reported more conflicts than those of controls. However, the two groups did not differ with respect to conflicts around drug use, keeping rules, friends of the opposite sex, and noise levels. The sum of the scores on the questionnaire was worse for families of hyperactives than for those of control subjects ($p = .015$).

FAMILIES' RETROSPECTIVE VIEW OF THEIR CHILDREN AT DIFFERENT DEVELOPMENTAL STAGES (Table 12-6)

Comparison of retrospective family ratings of hyperactives versus controls on all parameters (similar to Table 12-6) at all three time periods (i.e., preschool, elementary school, and high school) indicated that families of hyperactives viewed their children as functioning significantly worse on almost all parameters. This was less marked in the preschool period than in the elementary- and high-school periods.

TABLE 12-3. Sequential Evaluation of Families of Hyperactive Subjects (Scored Means, $n = 35$)

	Initial	5-year follow-up	10-year follow-up	F	Direction
Sociocultural parameters					
Mother's level of education	9.25	10.50	9.25		
Father's level of education	10.25	9.00	10.50		
Father's working status (Hollingshead)	3.68	3.44	3.28		
Mother's working status (Hollingshead)	3.00	3.00	3.00		
Mother working	1.77	1.80	1.40	$p = .001$	10-year more than initial and 5-year
Physical qualities of home	4.09	4.33	4.29		
Family size	5.03	5.06	5.12		
Child adopted	1.89	1.89	1.91		
Sibling order	2.45	2.64	2.58		
Child-rearing practices					
Continued presence of mother or stable substitute	4.52	4.68	4.68		
Inconsistent	1.14	1.21	1.21		

Lack controls	3.94	3.96	3.86		
Punitive–authoritative	3.43	3.50	4.07	$p = .003$	10-year better than initial or 5-year
Overprotective	3.83	9.09	3.88		
Health of family members					
Physical illness in family	1.68	1.80	1.40	$p = .001$	10-year more than initial or 5-year
Death in family	1.93	1.89	1.42	$p = .001$	10-year more than initial or 5-year
Mental health of family members	3.25	3.52	3.89	$p = .003$	10-year better than initial but same as 5-year
Relationships					
Marital relationship	3.42	3.30	3.36		
Emotional climate of home	3.01	3.15	3.07		
Total family score	32.65	33.78	34.45		
Subject no longer at home					
Marital relationship	3.16	2.50	3.00		
Emotional climate of home	3.33	2.00	3.16	$p = .007$	5-year worse than initial and 10-year

Note. n represents the number of subjects on whom all measures were obtained at all three time periods.

TABLE 12-4. Current View of Young Adult by His Family: Katz Scale of Psychopathology

	Mean		Significance
	Families of hyperactives ($n = 63$)	Families of controls ($n = 43$)	
Belligerence	6.0	6.3	
Verbal expansiveness	8.0	7.3	
Negativism	16.1	13.9	$p < .05$ (Controls better)
Helplessness	6.3	6.3	
Suspiciousness	5.2	5.6	
Anxiety	6.6	7.4	
Withdrawal	9.2	10.4	
Nervousness	8.1	7.7	
Confusion	3.2	4.4	
Bizarreness	5.8	6.4	
Hyperactivity	6.0	5.1	
Stability	32.1	32.2	
General psychopathology	36.1	34.4	
Performed household chores	33.2	33.8	
Expected to perform household chores	35.3	35.5	
Discrepancy between performance and expectation	10.4	9.6	
Leisure activities	47.4	46.1	
Satisfaction	32.1	27.6	$p < .001$ (Controls better)

PARENTAL CONCERN. We see that the main areas of parental concern shift from medical problems and activity level *per se* in the preschool period to predominantly social concerns in the elementary- and high-school periods. There was no difference in concern with regard to emotional and intellectual concerns or school difficulties during the three periods. Parents tended to seek more help during the elementary-school period than during preschool or high school.

RESTLESSNESS. Most parents of hyperactives see their children as being less restless as they get older, with the high-school period being scored better than preschool or elementary school.

RELATIONSHIPS. Parents of hyperactives perceive their children's relationships with peers and adults to be similar in the elementary- and high-school periods with the exception of teachers. Parents feel their children related to teachers better in elementary school than in high school.

SOCIALLY POSITIVE BEHAVIOR. Again, there was no difference between parents' rating of hyperactives in parameters such as stealing or lying in the elementary- and the high-school periods.

SCHOOLING. No clear-cut picture emerges as to whether the family perceived their hyperactive child as functioning better in the elementary- or high-school period. Some factors were scored better in elementary school (e.g., whether he liked school), while others were scored better in the high-school period (e.g., school behavior and independent homework).

Discussion

ASSESSMENT OF FAMILIES

Generally, our findings suggest that even though families of hyperactives and control subjects were matched for socioeconomic status, the families of hyperactives tended to have more difficulties, mainly in the areas of mental health of family members, marital relationship, and,

TABLE 12-5. Current View of Young Adult by His Family: Questionnaire (Hyperactives: $n = 62$–64; Controls: $n = 41$–42)

	χ^2	df	Significance	Direction
Parent optimistic about child's future	5.1	4		
Child making plans for future	2.9	4		
Are plans realistic?	4.8	4		
Does he use money wisely?	7.5	4		
Works for money	11.6	4	$p = .02$	Hyperactives more
Parents and offspring agree re				
money	6.9	4		
school or work	13.0	4	$p = .01$	Controls more
drug use	5.5	4		
keeping rules	7.4	4		
friends	8.9	4	$p = .06$	Controls more
friends of opposite sex	3.6	4		
tidiness	10.8	4	$p = .02$	Controls more
noise levels	2.9	4		
Sum of scores on general questionnaire	43.78	49.45	$p = .015$	Controls more

TABLE 12-6. Families' Retrospective View of Their Hyperactive Children at Different Developmental Stages $n = 51$)

	Preschool	Elementary school	High school	Sig.	Direction
Sought professional help	1.78	1.04	1.54	$p = .001$	More in elementary than preschool or high school
Areas of parental concern					
Emotional	1.83	1.63	1.70		
Social	1.79	1.58	1.54	$p = .001$	High and elementary school more than preschool
Intellectual	1.95	1.97	1.97		
Medical	1.89	2.00	2.00	$p = .002$	Preschool more than elementary or high school
Activity level	1.50	1.66	1.91	$p = .001$	Preschool more than elementary; elementary more than high school
School					
Restlessness		1.70	1.74		
Sits through meal	2.72	2.90	3.64	$p = .001$	High school better than preschool or elementary

Sleeps well	3.42	3.52	3.84	p = .026	High school better than preschool or elementary
Occupies spare time		3.24	3.64	p = .006	High school better
Relationships					
Peers (generally)		3.28	3.50		
Teachers		3.82	3.56	p = .06	Elementary better
Close continuous friendships with peers		3.14	3.26		
Considerate of others		2.80	3.04		
Socially positive behavior					
Considerate of others' property		3.10	3.26		
Trusted not to steal		4.32	4.40		
Truthful		3.82	3.80		
Schooling					
Did subject like school?		3.11	2.84	p = .09	Elementary better
Academic performance		2.60	2.50		
Grades failed		1.26	1.28		
School behavior		2.83	3.35	p = .01	High school better
Expelled		2.78	2.46	p = .01	Elementary better
Does homework independently		2.34	3.00	p = .001	High school better

most particularly, the emotional climate of the home. Our findings support those of Cantwell,[21] who found increased incidence of psychiatric difficulties in families of hyperactives. However, the severity of these problems, particularly with regard to mental health of family members, appears much milder. It has also been shown that having a disabled child causes a great deal of stress for families.[37] Several studies have linked hyperactivity with greater psychosocial and disorganizational problems in the family.[38-40] Thus, whether the hyperactive child's difficulties were accentuated because of family problems or whether the family's stress was amplified by his disabilities is difficult to evaluate. It is likely that they eventually worked synergistically in causing the situation to deteriorate. This underlines the importance of focusing on both the child's and family's problems in the comprehensive treatment of the condition and thus preventing this negative synergism.

Families of hyperactives tended to use more punitive, authoritative approaches in child rearing than families of control subjects. It is unclear as to what is the origin or effect of this approach. It is hoped that current research in various behavioral strategies with these children will provide useful guidelines to parents as to which approach is more beneficial with their child.

It should be pointed out that even though the questionnaires were similar at initial, 5-year, and 10-year assessments, the interviewers differed. However, all the interviewers were trained in interview style and scoring methods with another interviewer who had made assessments 5 years earlier. It is unfortunate that we lack these sequential measures for families of control subjects. We can, therefore, only discuss changes over time in families of hyperactives and not whether these changes differ from changes in families of control subjects.

In the sequential view of how families of hyperactives function, it is of importance to point out that the punitive child-rearing approach decreased at the 10-year follow-up and the mental health of the family members improved. However, the emotional climate of the home improved only when the hyperactive left home. Other findings which differed at 10-year follow-up, such as more mothers working and more physical illness and death in the family, can be explained by the aging of parents and children. Factors pertaining to socioeconomic status (e.g., fathers' and mothers' education and physical quality of the home) remained stable throughout.

We thus see that though families of hyperactives do not function as well as families of control subjects at 10-year follow-up, they seem to show some improvement when compared to initial and 5-year follow-up measures. This may be due to the decreasing demands of their hyperactive child as he matures and improves or leaves home.

FAMILIES' CURRENT ASSESSMENT OF YOUNG ADULTS' FUNCTIONING

Generally, families of hyperactive and control subjects did not score their offspring differently on the Katz Scale of Psychopathology. This is supported by our own assessment of the subjects, which indicated that although they still had problems, they did not load the psychiatric or antisocial population.[34] Parents of hyperactives did see problems (e.g., in increased negativism and decreased ability to derive satisfaction), but generally they were not significantly more concerned about their children's future than parents of control subjects. We thus see that positive changes in the hyperactives' functioning did register with the families, too. Nonetheless, some conflicts between the hyperactive and his family remained in the areas of school or work, friends, and tidiness, but these tended to be managed fairly well by both the hyperactive and his family, enabling many hyperactives to remain in fairly close contact with their families.

FAMILIES' VIEW OF THEIR CHILDREN AT DIFFERENT DEVELOPMENTAL STAGES

These findings (reported by parents at 10-year follow-up) are subject to all the limitations of retrospective parental reports, and therefore need to be evaluated in that light.[41] At each stage of development, families of hyperactives viewed their children more negatively than did families of controls on social, academic, and hyperkinetic parameters. These differences are particularly pronounced during the elementary- and high-school periods and somewhat less so in the preschool period.

This finding is expected in light of the difficulties these families experienced with their hyperactive children at all developmental stages. However, this does not necessarily represent a general negative halo effect by parents with regard to their hyperactive children. We see that not only do the areas of concern change (e.g., from medical and activity level in the preschool period to social concerns in the elementary- and high-school periods), but that parents can see improvements in various areas of functioning at various developmental stages—for example, improvement of restlessness with age. It is interesting that despite considerable antisocial behavior in hyperactive subjects during adolescence, their parents do not score them differently on this type of behavior in elementary and high school. It may be that some of the antisocial behavior (e.g., lying, stealing) began at home during the elementary-school period and only became a problem in the community during adolescence, and the parents did not distinguish between the two. An alternative explanation may lie in the fact that adolescents are more skilled in keeping such misdeeds from their parents.

It is important to note that families do not view their hyperactive offspring in a static, globally negative light, but perceive changes, positive and negative, on various parameters with time.

SUMMARY

In summary, families of hyperactive children had more difficulties than those of normal controls. These difficulties were mainly in the areas of mental health of family members, marital relationships, and, most particularly, emotional climate of the home. They also tended to use a more punitive–authoritative child-rearing approach to their children. However, in the sequential evaluation of families, we see that this punitive child-rearing tendency decreases at 10-year follow-up. Mental health of family members also improves at 10-year follow-up, as does the emotional climate in the home, the latter only if the hyperactive has moved out. Generally, families of hyperactive subjects tend to improve in their functioning with time, even though they do not equal the functioning of families of matched controls.

Even though families of hyperactives see their offspring as having more difficulties currently than controls, they are on the whole not more pessimistic about their current or future functioning. Conflicts that remain appear tolerable to both families and the hyperactive young adult. Finally, families of hyperactive subjects can, despite many problems with their children, still appreciate shifts in both their achievements and difficulties at each developmental stage. In view of the above findings, more concentrated work with the families of hyperactives as part of the comprehensive treatment of this condition seems highly indicated.

CHAPTER THIRTEEN

LIFE-STYLES AND ILLUSTRATIVE CASE HISTORIES

The strength of a student of men is . . . to study men, their habits, character, mode of life, their behaviour under varied conditions, their vices, their virtues and peculiarities. . . . Every patient that you see is a lesson in much more than the malady from which he suffers.—From "The Student Life," by Sir William Osler, 1849–1919

In our prospective 15-year follow-up study the clinical outcomes of the hyperactive adults fall roughly into three separate categories.[1] First, there are those whose functioning is fairly normal. Second, there are those who continue to have significantly more symptoms of the original syndrome and social, emotional, and interpersonal problems than the matched controls but whose problems are not sufficiently severe to reflect marked psychiatric or antisocial pathology. Finally, there is a third group who clearly are significantly disturbed and require psychiatric hospitalization and/or have been in adult jails.

Even though one can clearly identify these three types of outcome groups at the margins or in the transition between one group and another, there is a great deal of overlap. Therefore, it is misleading and inaccurate to quote what percentage of the hyperactive young adults fall into one group or another. Very rough estimates suggest that 30–40% fall into the fairly normal outcome group, another 40–50% fall into the group with significant hyperactive, social, emotional, and interpersonal problems, and finally, about 10% are seriously psychiatrically disturbed and/or seriously antisocial.

FAIRLY NORMAL OUTCOME GROUP

These subjects may not have totally outgrown all the symptoms of the syndrome, but where these persist they do not significantly impede functioning. The group includes subjects with excellent functioning (e.g., a medical student who got along well with people!) to fairly good functioning with no major complaints and no psychiatric diagnosis.

These subjects generally are working full-time or are still attending full-time university (usually at a postgraduate level). Their work history is fairly stable and such that subjects see an opportunity for future advancement either in their company or in their general area. Some of the work situations involve mechanical or other technical-type training rather than formal academic training. Occasionally work is combined with part-time evening school.

Subjects in this group are living either at home or with friends. A minority live alone. Their living arrangements are fairly stable, with moves not being particularly numerous nor made impulsively. Hyperactive adults with fairly normal adjustment seem to have some long-standing significant friendships with both sexes. They usually have one or more same-sex friends whom they have known for at least several years. The optimally adjusted among them feel close to these friends and can confide intimate problems. Most of the subjects in this group have also had one or more close heterosexual relationships lasting at least several months. They do not feel lonely or isolated from peers. They get along fairly well with both peers and supervisors at work and generally do not have any marked difficulty in their family relationships.

With regard to mood, they are not particularly depressed or anxious. The subjects have normal variations of mood depending on the circumstances and are able to enjoy positive things in their lives. Most will drink socially and have tried marijuana. However, there is no significant drug or alcohol abuse. Similarly, there is no current history of antisocial behavior. This includes the absence of stealing, aggressive acts, or significant numbers of car accidents. Generally, these subjects have fairly good self-esteem and are quite optimistic about their future, about which they have specific goals.

Case Example: Jeffrey

Jeffrey is an example of a hyperactive in this category. He was not considered problem-free. He was atypical for the normal group in that he was living alone and had not yet established a significant relationship with a member of the opposite sex.

Jeffrey was first seen in the Department of Psychiatry of the Montreal Children's Hospital in 1962 when he was 6 years old. He was referred by his parents following a request for this by his school where he was beginning Grade 1. His presenting complaints were as follows:

- Severe restlessness (since he walked he was always on the go)
- Has difficulty paying attention (particularly in class and when he is bored)

- Is disobedient and has no respect or fear of authority
- Fights with other children (since kindergarten he was kept in the classroom during recess to avoid physical fights in the school yard)
- Is preoccupied with keys and locks

During the summer prior to starting Grade 1, his parents had sent him away to camp (perhaps to get a rest from him). He wanted to go to camp, but on arrival he found he had lost the key to his trunk. He became hysterical when the counselors tried to force his trunk open. After that bad beginning he had an unhappy time at camp. His parents explained that he had become preoccupied by locks since age 4 years.

Jeffrey's birth history was normal. His electroencephalogram (EEG) was mildly abnormal. In the resting state it showed a diffuse mixed (sharp and slow) dysrythmia, which on hyperventilation became more evident as a paroxysmal tendency which was not definitely epileptiform. There was some evidence for bitemporal paroxysmal disturbance brought out by hyperventilation. Jeffery's neurological examination was normal, and on the Wechsler Intelligence Scale for Children (WISC) IQ he scored Full Scale 133, Verbal 128, and Performance 132. Jeffrey's parents were middle-class, of Anglo-Saxon origin, and while reasonably well off neither parent had attended university. The father was a successful salesman and the mother a housewife. There were two older brothers, both doing well. The parents owned a house and considered their marriage happy. They separated 9 years later when Jeffrey was in his teens.

Jeffrey was diagnosed at initial evaluation as having the hyperactive syndrome with additional neurotic symptomatology, for example his preoccupation with keys and locks. He was treated with chlorpromazine for 2 years and had individual play therapy for 1½ years, during which time his parents were seen together for counseling. In play therapy, Jeffrey was so restless that he never stayed in the playroom. He would dash to the elevators and press the button to the top floor. His therapist (G. W.) would take the next elevator up, only to find Jeffrey had come down again. He showed marked interest in locks and, unnoticed, managed to appropriate the therapist's keys, which she discovered only when she got home and could not open her front door. His interest in keys was interpreted along analytic lines, but defied interpretation in the sense of not disappearing. Parental counseling included marital therapy, as well as attempts to enable his father to relate more intimately with his youngest son.

FIVE-YEAR FOLLOW-UP: AGE 13½ YEARS

Jeffrey was no longer on chlorpromazine, which had been discontinued when he was 8 years old because it was not useful anymore. He had been suspended from school numerous times for being disruptive and fighting with other children. He was still very restless and distractible (the latter was slightly better) and was doing below-average work at school in spite of very superior intelligence. His Bender–Gestalt was well below his age level. During psychological testing at 5-year follow-up, he pulled out real handcuffs (which a policeman friend had lent him), handcuffed the psychologist testing him, and refused to release her. She had to shamefacedly leave the testing room handcuffed and ask for help. He stole occasionally but was not caught. His fascination with keys (other than the above episode) had abated.

Following the 5-year follow-up, his parents decided to remove him from his school and send him to a private day school, which accepted normal and problem children. After some months there, Jeffrey began to relate extremely well to the principal, who took a special interest in this difficult-to-teach but very bright teenager. In time, Jeffrey's work improved markedly, and while he remained restless his concentration was good whenever he was interested, which happened more and more frequently. He stayed in this private school till age 17 years, and his strong relationship with the principal continued. Toward the end of his school years, Jeffrey was still restless, but his attention span was poor only when he was bored. He was no longer a serious behavior problem, but related better to adults than to children.

TEN-YEAR FOLLOW-UP: AGE 18 YEARS

At 18 years, Jeffrey was in second year at the University of Toronto studying engineering. He still had many arguments with peers but had become somewhat of a leader in sports and was respected for this. He had not tried nonmedical drugs and other than socially did not use alcohol. He had had no court appearances, and no longer stole. He said he was no longer restless, but he had been extremely hard to contact by telephone because, as he pointed out, "I'm always on the go and almost never home." He had friends, but did not confide in them or spend much time with them. He had never had a steady girlfriend.

Jeffrey planned to take a master's degree in engineering, after he had completed his bachelor's degree, to research designs of burglar-alarm systems. He planned eventually to start his own business in this area. He no longer got into the physical fights which had characterized his childhood and early adolescence. In the psychiatric interview, he tended to be superficial, for example dismissing his parents' separation as "no problem." He appeared to be somewhat of a loner who did not complain that this was any problem. His affect was cheerful, and he had clear plans for his future.

FIFTEEN-YEAR FOLLOW-UP: AGE 25 YEARS

Jeffrey was living in Toronto and still hard to contact by telephone since he spent 10–12 hours daily in his car on business. He owned a burglar-alarm company which was doing well. He had not completed his bachelor's degree in engineering, although he had accumulated almost enough credits, because he preferred to be active and working. He had forgotten about his previous plans to continue toward a master's degree.

A few years previously, he told us, he had "always rushed to the scene" of a suspected burglary armed with a gun, for which he had legal permission. Later, after one actual dangerous encounter with an armed thief, he gave this up. He now no longer rushed to the site when an alarm was sounded. Jeffrey had no problem concentrating on his work, but read only short articles, for example, in *Reader's Digest*. He could not concentrate and became impatient with longer books, such as novels. He was living alone and still had not had a steady female friend, but he had started going out with girls. He felt he would eventually get married when he was ready. He had a number of male friends whom he trusted and whom he had known for several years. He generally did not confide personal matters.

Jeffrey offered no complaints and received no psychiatric diagnosis. He was functioning well in his work. His seeming impairment in relating intimately and his reluctance to have a steady female friend were not acknowledged as problems by him. He had some possible continuing symptoms of the syndrome (impatience with reading material), but this was not disabling him or others. His restlessness was well channeled into constructive work. His good outcome, as he put it, was a mixture of being smart and meeting Mr. _____ (the school principal), "who believed in me."

GROUP WITH CONTINUING SYMPTOMS OF THE HYPERACTIVE SYNDROME AND/OR SOCIAL, EMOTIONAL, AND INTERPERSONAL PROBLEMS

Subjects in this group often have one or more symptoms of the hyperactive syndrome, which they feel are impairing their performance in various areas of their life. While they are usually employed, their work is much more unstable when compared to the control group or the first group of hyperactives. They tend to change jobs more frequently. Often these changes are made suddenly on impulse following some disagreement with a peer or supervisor or just getting "fed up." The jobs they occupy are often manual, with little chance for advancement or future career opportunity. There are general statements that the subject would like to get into something else with more of a future, but few specific plans as to how he would proceed.

Many hyperactive adults in this group give a history of frequent moves, often sudden and impulsive and occasionally the result of disagreements with spouses, family members, or roommates. These subjects were therefore usually more difficult to trace and, once traced, more difficult to contact, because of their irregular and unpredictable schedules. They required up to 5-8 calls to set up an appointment, as opposed to 1-2 for the control group. Subjects needed to be reminded of their appointments frequently; otherwise they often missed them without canceling. At times two or three appointments had to be set up for them before they actually came. This was unnecessary for the control group.

This group of hyperactive young adults generally continue to have interpersonal problems. They often lack long-standing, close, or intimate relationships with either sex. They have more casual friendships, but these come and go and tend to be with recreational friends to go out with from time to time as opposed to people the hyperactive adults can rely on or confide in. Heterosexual relationships tend to be brief and not particularly significant. However, a subgroup does develop a significant, sometimes dependent, heterosexual relationship. Often the wife has the role of structuring, organizing, and motivating the subject. When this happens his functioning improves. We have seen several instances where such relationships have resulted in marriages which appear to be working fairly well. Long-term outcome of these marriages is unknown. Once children result from these marriages there is always the concern as to whether the child will also be hyperactive and how best to address this potential problem. Some of these hyperactive subjects feel lonely, but not totally isolated. They often give a picture of continued disputes with peers, supervisors, and family members.

Hyperactive young adults in this group also have more emotional problems. They are more apt to be depressed. Their use of alcohol and marijuana is greater than that of the control group or the hyperactive group having fairly normal outcome. However, they would not generally be classified as being alcoholic or significantly abusing drugs, and their antisocial behavior, if present, is not severe. For example, some of the hyperactives who have mild or probable Antisocial Personality Disorders would be included in this group. They are more prone to physical aggressive acts and tend to get into more fights. These young adults sometimes describe themselves as being short tempered and as "flying off the handle" easily. They also have more car accidents than the control group, and the accidents tend to result in costly damages. Generally, these subjects have poor self-esteem, are not happy with their current life situation, and are not particularly optimistic about being able to change it.

Case Example: Anthony

Anthony is an example of one of the better-functioning hyperactive adults in this group who had continuing symptoms of the syndrome which disabled him to some degree. He was referred to the psychiatry department of the Montreal Children's Hospital in 1962 at age 7 years. His presenting complaints were as follows:

- Severe restlessness since he began to walk
- Poor concentration
- Disobedient, does not listen (teachers "liked" Anthony, but wanted him out of the class)
- Poor speech articulation
- Repeating Grade 1
- Enuresis and occasional encopresis
- Very untidy

Anthony's birth history was uneventful and his EEG and neurological examination were normal. Anthony's WISC IQ (Full Scale) was 115 with marked scatter. He was found to have body-image and visuomotor difficulties. Psychiatric evaluation revealed a friendly, good-looking, 7-year-old boy with speech (i.e., articulation) difficulties who was restless. His mother had been diagnosed as having hysterical traits, but his father did not show antisocial traits. The parents stated they were happily married and there were two older sisters, both doing well. The father was a traveling salesman, the mother a housewife; their ethnic origin was Anglo-Saxon. A diagnosis of hyperactive syndrome was made with indications of some somatoform features (e.g., soiling).

FIVE-YEAR FOLLOW-UP: AGE 14 YEARS

This evaluation had been delayed (he was seen at the very end of the 5-year follow-up evaluation) because Anthony had been away to boarding school for 3 years and we had to wait until he was on holiday. He had received chlorpromazine for only a short period because it was not useful enough and had the disadvantage of sedating him. At 14 years Anthony seemed very immature and was still restless and distractible. His learning difficulties made school success in a regular classroom almost impossible, but Anthony had a "happy-go-lucky" attitude about his failures. There was no stealing or other indication of antisocial behavior, but Anthony had no close friends. His mother felt he was worse because he did not accept responsibility and had no goals for any future. He was very poor at spelling, behind in reading, and found schoolwork boring. He was no longer encopretic or enuretic, and while he lacked any insight into his difficulties he was found to be friendly and likeable. Repeat WISC IQ (Full Scale) was unchanged.

TEN-YEAR FOLLOW-UP: AGE 20 YEARS

Anthony was seen late also for the 10-year follow-up study because his parents had moved overseas, where his father had started a business. We wrote to Anthony there, sending him numerous self-rating scales and a history for him to complete. The former included the California Personality Inventory (CPI), a self-rating scale which all subjects completed. We did not hear from Anthony for 2 years after the forms were mailed and gave up on him as a lost subject. One day Anthony knocked at G. W.'s office door and announced himself and his girlfriend Sally. He said he had come from New Zealand to see us with Sally to let us know that the CPI was a truly crazy test, and there was no way that he could ever complete "500 dumb questions." When asked what he was really doing here, he said he had told us the truth, then gave a report of his past 5 years and agreed to complete the whole 10-year follow-up evaluation.

While still living with his parents overseas, Anthony had refused to continue schooling, but he had completed Grade 9 in Montreal. He worked intermittently at various menial jobs and lived with his parents. (His last job was collecting stray cats and dogs for the local SPCA.) He felt his father looked down on this job even though he had told Anthony that any honest job is OK. "He obviously didn't mean it," Anthony added. "Anyway I got laid off, and since I have ants in my pants I went to New Zealand." He planned to go perhaps to find work, perhaps for a holiday. But there he met Sally, who suggested that he could try mowing people's lawns for some income. Sally and Anthony soon lived together and she helped Anthony settle down. She encouraged him to work hard, and soon he had saved $1500. They borrowed another $1000 and bought a few second-hand lawn mowers. They then employed younger boys to mow lawns, and a year later had saved $5500 and paid back their debts. "I gave up the lawn-mower business because one day I just found it boring and tense, and I wanted to quit and travel. Also, I wanted to see you to show you how crazy this test that you sent me is."

Anthony appeared happy, as impulsive as ever, and had great charm. He had succeeded in getting Sally a job in Montreal, which was extremely difficult at the time, by telling the immigration department that if they did not give her a work permit he would marry her, and then they would have to give her one anyway. They would feel sorry to have made him marry so young. (Sally got her work permit.) Sally turned out to be a bright, quite delightful, stable young woman, who appreciated Anthony's qualities and had a strong influence on him. She made subsequent appointments for him and made sure he was on time for them. They planned to return to New Zealand after a few months in Montreal, but see the world on the way back.

FIFTEEN-YEAR FOLLOW-UP: AGE 25 YEARS

We could not go to New Zealand to interview Anthony, but we were able to meet with his parents, who were visiting Montreal. They had recently visited Anthony in New Zealand and were in close touch with him and with Sally. Anthony was now taking a university degree in communications. It seemed that where he ended up you could enter university as a mature student without completing high school (he had only completed Grade 9). He was pursuing his courses with some difficulties but was passing in spite of concentration problems. He was interested in what he was doing. Anthony and Sally were still living together and were planning on getting married. During this time Sally had had a malignant lump removed from her breast. Anthony's parents stated that he and Sally "had an excellent relationship," and that they had dealt with their grief and anxiety over her diagnosis well. Sally, they stated, still takes charge of organizational family matters and does most of Anthony's writing assignments. The friends they have are made by Sally, but while Anthony lets her take all the initiative with friends he is well liked. His parents feel that in the past year, partly as a result of Sally's medical problems, Anthony has matured greatly. He was described as still impulsive, still very restless, but he listens to Sally. He still talks too much and "has a big mouth." He has occasionally lost part-time jobs because of this. The couple has no debts, and Anthony plans to start an advertising business when he receives his university degree. His father stated he would help him financially but still would not trust him to handle money responsibly. Anthony himself is not close to the friends the couple has, but he feels close to Sally. While Sally has obviously done a great deal for Anthony, it was felt that the relationship is complementary rather than neurotic.

We asked Anthony's parents what they felt were the reasons for Anthony's good outcome, since they were extremely happy about his progress. His father stated, "Even while Anthony was hyperactive and a discipline problem as a child, he was very lovable. In school, he couldn't learn because he felt so inferior. At 17 years we sent him to Switzerland to learn a trade, but this did not work out. At 18 years, we gave him a one-way ticket to New Zealand and said to him, if you want to come back you have to earn the money for your ticket. Sally was the turning point for Anthony. She gave him what we couldn't, confidence in himself and a sense of direction. She had always loved him and even way back believed in his future when we frankly did not. Sally and Anthony are now saving to buy a house, and we send them money toward this, but we always send it to Sally. She keeps the books."

It seemed clear to us that Anthony without his fiancée would not be functioning as well as he is, and would still be having many life difficulties related to the hyperactive syndrome.

GROUP WITH MORE SERIOUS PSYCHIATRIC OR ANTISOCIAL DISTURBANCE

As the heading suggests, this group divides into two subgroups: the psychiatrically disturbed and the antisocially disturbed, with occasionally some overlap. Hyperactive young adults in this group are usually not working on any regular basis. Some have long histories of unemployment and drifting from one job to another. There may also be a history of one or more jail terms for the more antisocial, or several psychiatric hospital admissions for the more psychiatrically disturbed. The jail terms are for crimes which include assault, robbery, breaking and entering, and drug dealing. The psychiatric hospital admissions are for suicide attempts, drug detoxification, and borderline states.

These subjects often live alone. They also tend to move more frequently and impulsively. This is particularly true when they are living with others and interpersonal difficulties arise. Hyperactive adults in this group have serious interpersonal problems. They tend to be socially isolated and friendless. They generally have no close intimate friendships and sometimes lack even casual acquaintances. These subjects often use their acquaintances for personal gains—for example, drugs—or become overly dependent on them and so lose even these contacts. There is usually little contact with their family. However, a small subgroup is overly controlled and enmeshed by the family, with no contacts outside of family members. Generally, the relationships of this group of hyperactives are either nonexistent, superficial, excessively dependent, or very disruptive.

This group of hyperactive young adults have serious emotional difficulties. Some have had serious depressions with suicide attempts requiring psychiatric hospitalization. Others are clearly borderline psychotic, though none have presented with florid psychosis. Some subjects present a pleasant false facade which hides a great deal of hostility and despair. Subjects in this group tend to abuse alcohol and drugs, particularly marijuana and minor tranquilizers. Some have wide-ranging drug use which includes cocaine, methaqualone, and so on. As described previously, the more antisocial subjects have histories of being jailed for assault, armed robbery, breaking and entering, and drug dealing. This group also has more car accidents which are more costly when compared to the control or other hyperactive group. Generally, these subjects have very poor self-esteem. They tend to live from day to day with little or no view to their future, perhaps because their present is often so bleak.

Case Example: William

William is an example of a hyperactive who is emotionally unstable and has an Antisocial Personality Disorder. He was referred to the Department of Psychiatry of the Montreal Children's Hospital in 1964 at the age of 9 years by his parents and school. His main complaints were as follows:

- Fights with other children in the school and neighborhood
- Constantly on the go
- Does not pay attention in school or at home
- Discipline problem in the school to the degree that "unless something is done, we will have to expel him"

William's birth history was abnormal; his mother had had toxemia of pregnancy and his birth weight was 5 pounds. On a neurological examination, William had many abnormal soft signs (uneven muscle size, uneven palpedral fissures, dysarthria, finger apraxia). On the WISC IQ he scored Full Scale 90, Verbal 91, and Performance 90, and he performed at the 8-year level on the Bender–Gestalt. His EEG was normal.

William was a twin, and besides his twin sister there were three other boys in the family. His father was black and his mother white, and the family lived in their own bungalow in a suburb, of which they were proud. The father was a steady factory worker with no antisocial history, who had himself had a very deprived childhood and remembered constantly being beaten. The parents felt that their color difference presented no problem; they were not particularly psychologically minded but wished the best for their children.

William was treated with chlorpromazine (25 mg q.i.d.), which was ineffective, and with dextroamphetamine for some months. He was engaged in individual psychotherapy with a black resident–psychiatrist for 1½ years, and his parents were seen for counseling. Individual therapy for William was useful because previously he had looked down on "blacks" as inferior. Identifying with his therapist, he began to look up to blacks, including his father. Unfortunately, these good results did not last.

FIVE-YEAR FOLLOW-UP: AGE 13½ YEARS

Mother found William worse. He had been expelled from school and the parents had succeeded in getting him back into school through a legal suit. William had few friends and was not accepted by others in the community or at home. He was rebellious to all authority figures, including teachers and parents. He had had sexual intercourse with his girlfriend and was not allowed to see her anymore. The parents, who had been so proud of their home and their acceptance in a white community, felt ashamed of him. Their marriage deteriorated, and there were more fights between them (many around mutual blame for how William "was"), with threats of separation. However, this couple is still together. William was stealing mainly from them, but also from stores, but he had not been caught.

At school, William was not learning and was still restless and had poor concentration, but his biggest difficulties came from being disruptive and undisciplined. He had very poor control of his temper and was very impulsive. His symptoms had not improved.

TEN-YEAR FOLLOW-UP: AGE 20 YEARS

We had lost contact with William and his family for some years. After we traced him he had to be persuaded to come to see us, pointing out correctly that we had never helped him.

William had completed Grade 9 in a practical class in a training school for delinquent adolescents where he spent 2 years because neither his parents nor the school had been able to keep him. He had subsequently been sent west to live with relatives, but came back because he had gotten into trouble for fighting. William stated he had lived in 27 places in his life, and by now owed a considerable amount of money to his father and to others. He had had four car acccidents in the last year, and had appeared before the social welfare court several times for "B and E" (breaking and entering) and once for theft of a car. He had always received suspended sentences. His parents had given up on him, but he was close to his sister. He was very open at the interview and his affect was depressed. He felt unhappy about himself, his relationships, and his future. He confessed that as a child he had been "battered" by his father on numerous occasions, but had felt afraid to tell us in case he was removed from his parents.

FIFTEEN-YEAR FOLLOW-UP: AGE 24 YEARS

William was working steadily at a semiskilled job and had a fair work record, interrupted by jail sentences for breaking and entering and car theft. He was now married and had a 2½-year-old son, John, whom he said he "adored." He had "never touched" his son when angry and felt proud of this. He said he had a good relationship with his wife except when he lost his temper. Unfortunately, this was quite often, and on one occasion he had "put her and John out" and then felt real remorse. She had gone back to her parents for 2 weeks, but later returned to him. His wife felt that William was a "very worthwhile person" but wanted us to do something to reduce his violent temper and his excessive drinking. William had now served time in jail twice and had made three suicide attempts, after one of which he was admitted to a psychiatric hospital for a short period. He had injured others in fights, but never seriously, and felt they had deserved it. He was proud and would let nobody get away with slighting him. He did not want any psychiatric treatment because he felt he had to do something for himself by himself. But he did ask if the black psychiatrist was still with us. In the interview, he related intimately and was honest. He had fairly good insight, and left his interviewer feeling that he might yet pull himself together. He had a relatively good work record and wanted "to go straight."

Six months after the 15-year evaluation his sister called to say she was worried about him. His wife had permanently left him and refused further contact with him. He had quit his job and was missing. We were extremely concerned that he had suicided (knowing that he really had cared for his wife and child). He subsequently contacted his sister, and we have not seen him since.

William had had several strikes against him. He had learning disabilities, low average IQ, and an abnormal neurological examination. He lived in a family of mixed ethnic background and his parents had marital difficulties. He said he had been severely beaten by his father on many occasions. Even at initial intake, the degree of associated conduct disorder was severe, as were the symptoms of the hyperactive syndrome itself.

CONCLUSIONS

The foregoing clinical descriptions shed some light on the discrepant and divergent reports about the outcome of adults who were hyperactive as children. As we see, the outcome is not homogeneous; some hyperactives do well while others do poorly. However, what determines good versus poor outcome? In a recent study it was shown that no one factor or circumstance, but a number of key factors (e.g., characteristics of the child and family, as well as the number and severity of the child's problems), all act together to determine the outcome. For a detailed account of predictive factors, the reader is referred to Chapters 14, 15, 16, and 17.

The three hyperactives whose histories were described were selected to illustrate three different outcome groups in terms of general life functioning. Their presenting problems were very similar, and their initial scores on the Werry–Weiss–Peters Hyperactivity Scale, as well as on aggression, were almost identical. They differed in terms of learning disabilities (Anthony's were the most serious), health of family functioning (Anthony's family was the most stable), and socioeconomic status (private schools were provided for Anthony and Jeffrey, whereas William went to a "training school" for similar problems). These and other factors (such as meeting key people who were helpful to them) certainly affected their final outcome.

It is important, as these case histories indicate, to identify areas of specific difficulties at the various ages which are potentially amenable to various treatments. Finally, we need to be able to identify as early as possible those subjects whose outcome will be seriously impaired but who may be helped if much effort is put into their therapeutic management.

PREDICTIVE FACTORS

Til old experience do attain
To something like prophetic strain.
—From *Il Penseroso*, by Milton, 1608–1674

CHAPTER FOURTEEN

PREDICTIVE FACTORS PERTAINING TO THE CHILD

INTRODUCTION

The importance of follow-up studies lies not only in providing us with a view of the natural history or prognosis of a condition but also in pinpointing which initial or intervening factors predict or affect this outcome. Only a few follow-up studies on children with hyperactivity or Attention Deficit Disorder (ADD) have focused on which factors are most important in predicting outcome. Most of these, to date, have focused on which initial factors affect adolescent outcome, since few have followed the subjects beyond adolescence. Since factors which affect adolescent outcome or prognosis may also be important in predicting adult outcome, the findings of studies predicting adolescent outcome will be included in the discussions.

Several extensive follow-up studies focusing on predictors[1,2,15] have suggested the importance of several factors (e.g., parameters related to the child, family, treatment) acting together and cumulatively in predicting outcome. In the interest of clarity, these factors will be dealt with separately; however, their interactive and additive effect must be constantly kept in mind.

The prognostic factors to be dealt with in the succeeding chapters have broadly been grouped under the following areas:

1. The child, including such measures as age at referral, degree of central nervous system (CNS) abnormality, IQ, and severity of symptoms at referral (e.g., hyperactivity and aggression)

2. The family, including type and degree of parental health or pathology, parent–child relationship, child-rearing practices, overall family functioning, and socioeconomic status

3. Treatment, including its effects on various aspects of outcome (e.g., personal, social, academic, and work) as well as its physiological effects (e.g., growth)

Following the discussion of treatment (usually stimulant drugs) as a predictor of outcome, we will present the comprehensive comparison of adult outcome of hyperactive subjects who did not receive stimulant treatment, subjects who did receive 3–5 years of stimulant treatment during childhood, and their matched normal controls (Chapter 16). After discussing each of the above predictive factors separately, we will show the complexity of their interrelationships in Chapter 17. This chapter will describe which initial measures predict adult outcome in this relatively untreated group of hyperactives (described in Chapter 5).

CHILD'S AGE AT REFERRAL

The age of children referred for symptoms of ADD varies a good deal depending on the setting and source of referral. Thus, school referrals tend to have a more narrow age range, while private-practice or retrospective medical-record data have a wider age range. Nonetheless, most children are 6–12 years of age at referral, with an average being about 8 years of age. The question of whether or not age of diagnosis contributes to outcome remains unclear. Some would argue that early diagnosis results in early treatment and the greater normalization of the child's development, social, cognitive, and emotional.[3] On the other hand, early referral and diagnosis often reflect more severe disturbance and symptomatology tending toward more negative outcome. Thus, Loney et al.[1] showed that age of onset of symptoms correlated with degree of continued inattention in adolescents and illegal drug use. However, no study to date has clearly delineated the prognostic value (if any) of the age at which diagnosis is made.

DEGREE OF CENTRAL NERVOUS SYSTEM ABNORMALITY

Since children with significant neurological abnormalities (e.g., cerebral palsy, epilepsy) are usually excluded from the diagnosis of ADD, we are, of necessity, asking the question: Is mild neurological dysfunction in hyperactive children predictive of their adolescent or adult outcome? Ackerman et al.'s[4] comprehensive study did careful neurological assessments at initial referral and at follow-up during adolescence, and found that initial global scores were not highly predictive of outcome in all three neurological groups—that is, those with positive, negative, or equivocal neurological signs; all three had statistically identical outcomes in Wide Range Achievement Test (WRAT) and Gray Oral Reading, and similar Wechsler Intelligence Scale for Children (WISC) profiles. These findings suggest that initial mild neurological dysfunction has no predictive value for academic adolescent outcome.

However, Loney et al.,[1] in a careful, well-controlled predictive analysis using multiple regression statistics, showed that a history of perinatal complications correlated with reported hyperactivity in adolescents and WRAT arithmetic scores. Interestingly, both child aggression and adolescent delinquency were associated with *fewer* signs of neurological impairment at referral.

The importance of neurological abnormalities at time of diagnosis for future outcome was particularly stressed by Milman.[5] Hyperactive patients with an initial diagnosis of Organic Brain Syndrome (i.e., those with unequivocal neurological impairment) were compared with hyperactive patients diagnosed as having a developmental lag (i.e., those with language, thinking, and psychological impairment, but with fewer or less-constant neurological soft signs). The organic group had a much worse global outcome at late adolescence and young adulthood. This global evaluation was based on parents' impression, patient's self-evaluation, psychiatric diagnosis, and objective data such as academic level reached, social adjustment (dating, engaged, married), current status (employed, student, sheltered workshop, homebound, residential care).

It was not clear if the degree of neurological abnormality of this "organic" group was so significant that today a diagnosis of ADD would not be given. The neurological abnormalities included gross or fine motor incoordination, hypotonia, problems in postural stasis, adventitious movements, overflow movements, confusion in right–left discrimination, problems in tactile discrimination, confusion in body parts, and problems in intersensory transformations. Complicating the picture further is the fact that 16% of the sample had low-average IQ (< 90) and 19% were borderline retarded (average IQ < 69). Low initial IQ also resulted in poor outcome, although one is uncertain if the "organic" group also had lower IQ's.

The correlation between IQ and organic brain dysfunction was more clearly seen in Menkes et al.'s[6] study—a 25-year retrospective follow-up of 14 out of 18 subjects. In this study all but one of the patients whose original IQ scores were over 100 fall into the probable-brain-dysfunction group, and all but one of those with IQ scores below 100 fall into the definite-brain-dysfunction group. Thus, adult outcome was also correlated to IQ and/or neurological dysfunction, with patients having IQ over 90 being self-supporting and only one of 5 subjects with IQ less than 90 being self-supporting.

The importance of CNS abnormalities in children with hyperactivity has been further stressed by researchers working in the area of electroencephaolography. Satterfield,[7] summarizing several of his studies, suggested that hyperactives had low CNS arousal as shown by power-spectral analysis of resting EEG (excessive slow wave and abnormal auditory evoked cortical potentials). Furthermore, the group with this low CNS arousal responded well to stimulant treatment.

Weiss et al.,[8] Zambelli et al.,[9] and White et al.[10] all indicated that the EEG abnormalities persisted in adolescence, though the clinical significance of this finding was neither clear nor strong. Hechtman et al.,[11] in a 10-year prospective follow-up study (discussed in greater detail in Chapter 11), assessed EEG's of hyperactive and control subjects, mean age 19.2 and 18.6 years respectively. These EEG's showed no significant differences in any of the features assessed. Sequential EEG's, available only for the hyperactive subjects, suggested that a much greater proportion were normal at the 10-year follow-up assessment than at the 5-year follow-up assessment and that the normalization tended to take place mainly in late adolescence. This supports the hypothesis that EEG abnormalities of hyperactive persons involve an immature pattern that tends to normalize with age. Correlation between EEG findings at the 10-year follow-up assessment and global outcome measures was not significant. Initial and 5-year EEG's also failed to predict global outcome at 10-year follow-up.

Despite these diverse findings and views, it seems clear that more significant neurological impairment contributes to poorer outcome, though the prognostic influence of mild neurological abnormality (which is more common in hyperactive children) is less certain or clear. Its impact, if present, is probably mild and depends on many other factors such as IQ, socioeconomic status, and family functioning.

IQ OR INTELLIGENCE

As has been seen in Menkes et al.'s[6] study, IQ is often correlated to CNS dysfunction. This is particularly true of significant CNS abnormality. However, whereas the evidence for the influence of neurological dysfunction on eventual adolescent and adult outcome in hyperactive children seems merely suggestive, tenuous, and at times unclear, the evidence for the effect of IQ on eventual outcome is much stronger. Several studies have pointed to the importance of initial IQ of the child for eventual adolescent or adult outcome.

The importance of IQ as a predictor was stressed by Menkes et al.,[6] who showed that it was the only variable from the diagnostic workup which predicted self-support status in adulthood. Weiss et al.,[8] in a prospective 5-year follow-up of hyperactive adolescents, showed that success at school was predicted only by IQ at initial evaluation and to a lesser extent by lower initial scores of hyperactivity and distractibility. Initial IQ however, did not predict overt antisocial behavior at 5-year follow-up, although such behavior was predicted by initially higher aggression scores and more pathological family functioning. Mendelson et al.,[12] too, found no difference in initial IQ between a group of hyperactive adolescents who showed overall behavioral improvement and a group who did not.

In a detailed 5-year prospective follow-up study of academic achievement in a group of hyperactives and a group of normal controls, Minde et al.[13] showed that hyperactives were inferior academically and behaviorally and had lower scores on group IQ tests. However, they also showed that IQ alone was not the only factor responsible. Thus, in a comparison of hyperactives and controls *matched* for IQ, the hyperactives still performed more poorly.

The importance of IQ is seen not only in academic outcome but in global outcome as well. In another study using the same patient population, Minde et al.[14] divided the group into "good" versus "poor" outcome on the basis of number of complaints from mother, the child's ability to relate to parents and peers, his or her handling of authority, possible delinquency, and sexual adjustments. The "good" versus "poor" outcome groups showed initial significant differences on Peterson–Quay Personality Factor Series and aggressivity, and trend differences for positive history of brain damage, IQ, socioeconomic status, mother–child relationship, and overall family scores. Again, IQ in conjunction with other factors affected overall outcome.

Milman[5] pointed out that associated with unsatisfactory global outcome (as measured by pooling parents' impression, patients' self-evaluation, psychiatric diagnosis, and objective data dealing with academic, social, and work achievements) were initial findings of low-average or borderline retarded. This was the case for 41% of the unsatisfactory outcome group. Other initial factors associated with unsatisfactory outcome included multiplicity of behavioral and neuro-psychological findings, learning disabilities, special-class placement, and initial classification of Organic Brain Syndrome. Again the importance of IQ in conjunction with other factors in predicting adult outcome is stressed.

In a later study Loney et al.[15] evaluated, via multiple regression analysis, initial measures in 65 hyperactive subjects which may predict adult outcome at age 21. They found that the most consistent predictor of Schedule for Affective Disorders and Schizophrenia, Lifetime Version (SADS-L)[16] Alcoholism criteria was childhood IQ. Children with lower IQ's at referral reported more Alcoholism criteria as young adults, and they were more likely to be diagnosed as alcoholic. However, low childhood IQ did not predict greater adult drug abuse. Low childhood IQ was also related to more antisocial acts (e.g., shoplifting) and to SADS-L diagnosis of Antisocial Personality Disorder.

In summary, one can say that IQ seems to be a specific predictor of academic achievement[8] and, in conjunction with other factors (e.g., family, socioeconomic status, learning disabilities), a more general predictor of overall adolescent[13] and adult[5,6,15] outcome.

SYMPTOMS AT REFERRAL

There have been several studies which have attempted to evaluate which initial referral symptoms are predictive of adolsecent or adult outcome. Generally the initial referral symptoms that have received the most attention are:

1. Hyperactivity
2. Aggressivity
3. Antisocial behavior
4. Academic status

Hyperactivity

It has been somewhat surprising that initial levels of hyperactivity have been predictive of only a few specific outcome measures and did not generally predict a large number of measures reflecting overall functioning. Specifically, Loney et al.[1] found that initial measures on the hyperactivity factor, which included hyperactivity (e.g., restlessness, running around), inattention (e.g., distractibility, forgetfulness), and judgment deficits (e.g., impulsiveness, immaturity), predicted adolescent academic achievement. Weiss et al.,[8] too, found that adolescents who were succeeding in school tended ($p = .10$) to have lower initial measures of hyperactivity and distractibility. Riddle and Rapoport[3] found that initial measures of hyperactivity predicted later activity and peer rejection in the subjects they followed for 2 years. Most of these studies[1,8] did not find that initial hyperactivity predicted adolescent antisocial behavior. However, Ackerman and her associates[4] showed that at adolescent follow-up at age 14, subjects who had learning disabilities and hyperactivity had more conduct disorders than those with learning disabilities who were hypoactive or normally active. It may well be that the combination of two handicaps—hyperactivity and learning disability—increases the tendency toward adolescent conduct disorder. In terms of adult outcome, Loney et al.[15] showed that the childhood hyperactivity factor was only predictive of antisocial acts against property (e.g., shoplifting and breaking and entering).

In summary, one can say that initial hyperactivity is predictive of adolescent educational achievement[1,8] and hyperactivity. It generally is not associated with significant antisocial outcome but may be related to some milder antisocial behavior in adolescence[4] and adulthood.[15]

Aggression

The importance of initial aggressivity measures as opposed to hyperactivity in predicting adolescent and adult outcomes has long been stressed by Loney[1,15] and her coworkers Langhorne[17] and Kramer.[18] It should be pointed out that the aggression factor in Loney's studies consisted of negative affect (e.g., excitability, irritability), aggressive interpersonal behavior (e.g., fights, won't mind), and control deficits (e.g., delinquent acts, evasion of rules). We thus see that much more than just aggression is involved. Aggression is really coupled with antisocial behavior, giving rise to what today would be termed conduct disorder. Thus, Langhorne and Loney[17] showed that degree of aggression and not hyperactivity at referral significantly predicted self-esteem deficit in adolescence. Kramer and Loney[18] noted that in addition to other measures, the initial aggressive factor was a predictor for adolescent aggression and antisocial behavior (e.g., offenses against persons and property and illegal drug use). As Loney et al.[1] pointed out, the initial aggressivity factor was also involved in predicting adolescent symptoms of hyperactivity and judgment deficit (e.g., impulsivity).

The importance of initial aggression was also stressed by Weiss et al.,[8] who showed that overt antisocial behavior in hyperactive adolescents was associated with significantly higher aggression scores at initial evaluation. Similarly, Minde et al.'s[14] "good" versus "poor" outcome group at adolescence differed on initial and follow-up measures for distractibility, aggression and excitability, but not hyperactivity. In the adult outcome predictive study, Loney et al.[15] showed that childhood aggression is predictive of adult violence in that it is associated with the adult carrying a weapon and fighting with a weapon.

The importance of initial aggressivity in predicting antisocial outcome in adolescence and adulthood is clear. However, as pointed out earlier, often this aggressivity is very linked to antisocial behavior, and it becomes unclear if it is the initial aggressivity or the initial antisocial behavior which is predicting the antisocial outcome.

Initial Antisocial Behavior

Several studies have shown that initial measures of antisocial behavior predict later similar behavior in adolescence and adulthood. Thus, Weiss et al.[8] and Riddle and Rapoport[3] both found that the degree of antisocial behavior at initial referral predicted later similar behavior. As pointed out earlier, Loney et al.'s[1] aggressivity factor had a good deal of antisocial behavior included in it, so all findings of that group linking initial aggressivity and adolescent and adult[15] antisocial behavior may well be related to the initial antisocial component of the aggressivity factor. One study which did not link initial antisocial behavior to adolescent outcome was that of Mendelson et al.[12] These authors found no difference in initial antisocial behavior in their general improved versus their unimproved groups of hyperactive adolescents.

Generally the hyperactive follow-up studies support Robins's[19] findings that childhood aggression and antisocial behavior predict adult antisocial behavior. It must, however, also be stressed (as Robins has done) that most antisocial children do not become antisocial adults, so additional factors must come into play in determining antisocial adult behavior.

Initial Academic Status

One of the few studies that have looked specifically at the predictive value of initial academic status on adolescent outcome was that of Loney and her associates.[1] The initial academic status was measured by an 81-item school intake form completed by the teacher. From the information on the form, past academic functioning was rated on a 5-point scale ranging from poor to excellent. Current reading achievement and arithmetic achievement were rated as satisfactory (grades of A, B, and C), unsatisfactory but improving, and unsatisfactory (grades of D and F). The authors found that initial academic status was only predictive of adolescent academic achievement as measured by the WRAT. However, adolescent academic achievement was not *only* determined by the initial academic status of the child. The child's initial level of hyperactivity, the nature of the parent–child relationship, and the child's response to stimulant medication also affected his or her adolescent academic achievement.

Loney et al.[15] also looked at initial academic problems and their predictive value in adult outcomes with regard to SADS-L[16] Adult Antisocial and Alcoholism criteria; the Iowa Crime and Punishment Survey[20]; and the National Survey on Drug Abuse.[21] Initial academic problems were significantly correlated only with adult subjects who had tried marijuana and inhalants. There was no significant association with the other adult measures outlined. Other workers who had specificially looked at academic status at follow-up during adolescence did not link it with initial academic status. Minde et al.[13] linked it with IQ, and Weiss et al.[8] with IQ and initial hyperactivity and distractibility level.

Ackerman and her associates[4] have also looked at academic performance. They compared three groups (hyperactive, hypoactive, and normoactive) of learning-disabled boys initially and at age 14. As expected, all three groups were behind expected academic levels for their age, but this was not greater for the hyperactive learning-disabled boys. Since learning disability was common to all groups, initial academic status probably did not differ either; therefore it was not looked at as a predictor of adolescent outcome.

We thus see that the few studies that have specifically looked at initial academic status and adolescent or adult outcome suggest that initial academic performance may, in conjunction with other factors, predict later academic achievement. Surprisingly, it has not proved important in predicting adolescent or adult antisocial behavior,[1,15] though it may be associated with some adult drug use.[15]

In summary, one can say that of the factors pertaining to the child that we have examined, IQ, initial aggressivity, and initial antisocial behavior appear important in predicting later outcome. This appears to be true for specific outcome measures (e.g., IQ for academic achievement and initial aggression for adult aggressivity) as well as for overall adolescent and adult functioning.

CHAPTER FIFTEEN

PREDICTIVE FACTORS PERTAINING TO THE FAMILY

The importance of the family in contributing to the positive or negative outcome of a child's condition has long been recognized. In this chapter we will attempt to delineate various parameters of the family, for example, mental health of family members; child-rearing practices, or parent–child relationship; overall family functioning, including marital relationship and emotional climate of the home; and socioeconomic status. The aim is to see how these factors may predict the hyperactive child's adolescent and/or adult outcome.

It should be stressed that there is a great deal of overlap and interrelationship in these different family factors. Thus an emotionally disturbed parent is likely to have a poor parent–child relationship and a stressed marital relationship, and the family functioning as a whole may be impaired. In addition, these family factors act together and cumulatively with the parameters pertaining to the child and to treatment in predicting outcome. However, for the sake of clarity, each aspect will be dealt with separately while keeping in mind their interrelationship and cumulative effects.

MENTAL HEALTH OF FAMILY MEMBERS

Several studies of families of hyperactive children[1,2] (described in detail in the Chapter 12) have shown an increased prevalence of alcoholism, hysteria, and sociopathy in the parents of the hyperactives when compared to matched controls. The authors attempted to link this parental pathology to possible childhood hyperactivity in the parents, thereby providing a genetic link and a suggestion of possible adult outcome of the condition. However, such pathology in the parents may, in fact, affect the hyperactive child's outcome not necessarily by its genetic link but by the disturbed environment the child has to contend with. Unfortunately the authors did not follow these children to see if having a disturbed parent did in fact affect their outcome.

Stewart et al.[3] attempted to make some link between parental pathology and the hyperactive child's outcome by showing that children who were unsocialized–aggressive tended to have fathers who were antisocial and thus might run a higher risk of becoming antisocial themselves. Many of these unsocialized–aggressive children were also hyperactive. In contrast, children who were just hyperactive tended to have fewer parents who were antisocial and were therefore presumably less likely to become antisocial themselves. Though this connection between parental pathology and the hyperactive child's outcome is somewhat weak and speculative, it is there nonetheless. A similar connection was shown by Mendelson et al.,[4] who followed 83 hyperactive children retrospectively into adolescence. They found that the more antisocial hyperactive adolescents (children with more than six antisocial symptoms) were more likely to have a father who had been arrested several times or who had had learning or behavioral problems as a child.

Weiss et al.,[5] in the prospective 5-year follow-up of hyperactives as adolescents, showed that poor mental health of the parents, coupled with a poor mother–child relationship and punitive child-rearing practices, predicted overt antisocial behavior at adolescence. High initial aggressivity in the child was also a factor. Again we see the importance of parental mental health and its interrelationship with the parent–child relationship and child-rearing practices.

Minde et al.[6] divided the same hyperactive adolescent subjects followed by Weiss et al.[5] into "good" versus "poor" outcome groups on the basis of mothers' complaints, child's relationships, possible delinquency, and sexual adjustment. They found generally that families of "good-outcome" children improve over time, while those of "poor-outcome" children deteriorated. This deterioration was seen particularly in emotional climate of the home, child-rearing practices, and total family score, though not in the marital relationship or parental mental health. It is difficult to determine if the families deteriorated because their difficult child did not improve or if the child's poor functioning at follow-up was due to the family's deterioration. Likely the two are very intertwined in the vicious negative cycle which often exists between the hyperactive child and his or her family.

Loney et al.,[7] in their follow-up of 65 hyperactive young adults age 21–23, examined via multiple regression statistics a large number of potential predictors of adult outcome. Among the familial factors which related to parental mental health were excessive parental short temper and parental psychopathology (psychiatric, social, and legal). The former measure was derived from intake forms completed by parents at the time of initial referral and the latter was rated from material in the child's medical chart completed by clinic psychiatrists, psychologists, and social workers. Outcome measures included Schedule for Affective Disorders and Schizophrenia, Lifetime Version (SADS-L)[8] Adult Antisocial and Alcoholism criteria, Iowa Crime and Punishment Survey (CAPS),[9] and National Survey on Drug Abuse.[10] Parental pathology proved a much stronger prediction of outcome than parental short temper. Thus, parental pathology was related to frequent job changes and unemployment but not to other SADS-L antisocial criteria in the young-adult hyperactive. It was also associated with violence and traffic offenses in the SADS-L criteria for alcoholism. In contrast, parental short temper was not related to most outcome measures listed above. There was, however, a negative correlation with drunkenness and fighting with a weapon. Parental pathology as described by Loney *et al.* in this study is so global that it is difficult to pinpoint what type of parental pathology predicts what sort of adult hyperactive outcome measures. This shortcoming somewhat limits the usefulness of the findings.

We thus see that in general there appears to be some evidence that parental psychopathology may influence a more negative outcome in adolescence and adulthood for the hyperactive child. The studies outlined do not, however, give any clear view of what type of parental pathology will give rise to what type of negative outcome. The most specific connection was seen with parental antisocial behavior and the hyperactive adolescent's antisocial outcome.[3,4] Furthermore, how parental pathology may affect this more negative outcome is also not clear. The genetic hypothesis, reviewed in detail in the Chapter 12, is weak. A more attractive suggestion is that parental psychopathology affects the parent–child relationship and the child-rearing practices and that these more directly affect future outcome.

PARENT–CHILD RELATIONSHIP: CHILD-REARING PRACTICES

Few studies have looked at the parent–child relationship in hyperactives from the predictive point of view. The early studies[11] showed that mothers of hyperactive boys were critical, disapproving, unaffectionate, and used severe punishment. The concern was that this type of parenting might be causing the condition. Later workers [12-14] clearly showed that the mothering style was a response to the child's behavior and not a cause of it, since the behavior of the mother changed when the child's performance and behavior altered, for example, on medication.[14,15] Barkley and Cunningham[15] clearly showed that when hyperactive children were on medication, and their compliance improved, mothers were less intrusive and more responsive. However, the level of their interactions did not equal that of normal controls. We thus have a view of some problems in the parent–child interaction with hyperactives, but its prognostic or predictive importance is not clear.

Several studies have redefined aspects of the parent–child interaction into specific types of child-rearing practices and looked at the predictive influence of these practices on adolescent and adult outcome. Thus, Weiss et al.[5] showed that punitive child-rearing practices at initial referral were a factor which, in relation to others, predicted overt antisocial behavior and in the hyperactive adolescents. Loney et al.,[16] too, looked at initial parent–child interactions and how they predicted various adolescent outcomes in hyperactive children. The authors explored four measures of parenting style. Maternal and paternal parameters of love–hostility and autonomy–control were rated on a 7-point scale (e.g., 1, much love; 7, much hostility). These parenting styles were rated from medical, social, psychological, and educational reports found in the child's chart. More initial paternal control was associated, along with other measures, with more adolescent offenses against persons and less negative affect (irritability). (However, it should be pointed out that in an earlier report, Loney et al.[17] showed that hyperactives who were more aggressive at referral and had lower socioeconomic status and *less* controlling fathers had more unsatisfactory outcomes at adolescence, as rated by their mothers and psychologist.) Interestingly, maternal hostility and maternal control were both associated, among other factors, with Wide Range Achievement Test (WRAT) scores at adolescence, in mathematics and spelling respectively.

It was somewhat surprising that parenting style was not a stronger predictor in this study. Loney et al.,[7] however, showed that parental control was a strong, though at times confusing, predictor in the adult (age 21–23) outcome of the 65 hyperactives they had followed to date. For example, on the SADS-L Adult Antisocial criteria, initial excessive parental control was associated with *less* unemployment, job changes, and vagrancy, but with *more* drunkenness. However, on the SADS-L Alcoholism criteria, initial parental control seemed to have no effect on any of the items. In the CAPS excessive initial parental control was linked with those hyperactives who carried a weapon, fought with a weapon, and had an invalid driving license. However, on the National Survey on Drug Abuse initial excessive parental control was predictive of adult use of cocaine, hallucinogens, opiates, sedatives, and stimulants. On the whole it would seem that initial excessive parental control is associated with more negative than positive outcome measures, but no totally consistent pattern emerges. It may be that whether initial parental control has a positive or negative effect on long-term outcome depends on the nature of other factors which interact with it, for example, parental psychopathology, parent–child emotional relationship, and socioeconomic status, to mention just a few.

Werner and Smith[18] also showed the importance of parenting variables in long-term outcome. The authors followed a group of learning-disabled hyperactive children from age 10 and assessed their outcome on achievement, interpersonal, and self-esteem measures at age 18. Three-fourths of the group were found to have poor outcome, and one-fourth were thought to have improved. Parenting variables such as consistency, firmness, and respect for the child differentiated the improved and unimproved groups.

The suggestion that parenting variables may be influenced by other factors (e.g., socioeconomic status) was made by Paternite et al.[19] They showed that low-socioeconomic-status parents of hyperactive children were more lax, easygoing, and inconsistent when compared to their high-socioeconomic-status counterparts. In addition, parenting style was associated with secondary symptoms such as aggressive behavior and low self-esteem.

SOCIOECONOMIC STATUS

We thus see that the families' socioeconomic status may be an important predictive factor. Socioeconomic status can influence parental psychopathology, the parent–child relationship, and the availability of appropriate treatment resources (e.g., special education, counseling, tutoring). However, when this measure is looked at in terms of whether or not it predicts good or poor outcome, findings are contradictory.

Thus, Weiss et al.,[5] in the 5-year prospective study of 64 adolescent hyperactives, found that socioeconomic status was not a predictor variable for succeeding in school, overt antisocial behavior, or emotional adjustment at adolescence. Minde et al.,[6] studying the same subjects as well as 27 others and dividing the group into global "good" versus "poor" outcomes on the basis of criteria outlined earlier, showed that the poor-outcome group was more likely to have an initial measure consistent with a history of brain damage, low IQ, *low socioeconomic status*, poor mother–child relationship, and low family scores.

As stated earlier, Loney et al.[17] too found low socioeconomic status and other factors contributing to unsatisfactory outcome ratings by mothers and psychologists. However, in the extensive predictive study of adolescent outcome, Loney et al.[16] found that low socioeconomic status *per se* only entered (with other factors) into predicting high adolescent hyperactivity as reported by mothers. However, other variables that may be associated with socioeconomic status (i.e., urban vs. rural residence and number of children in the family) did enter into predicting adolescent offenses against property, involvement with illegal drug use, and WRAT achievement scores in arithmetic and spelling. In each case, urban residence and larger number of children in the family were associated with more negative outcome.

In Loney et al.'s[7] adult-outcome predictor study, socioeconomic status in and of itself was a weak predictor. It did not significantly predict any of the items pertaining to SADS-L Adult Antisocial or Alcoholism criteria. In the CAPS it was significant only for the suspended-license item, and on the national drug survey only for stimulant use. Even for these two outcome items, it appeared that the higher the socioeconomic status, the more frequent these occurrences.

It would thus appear that socioeconomic status may not be as strong a predictor of specific outcome measures[5,7,16] as of global outcome.[6,17] Other workers have also pointed out the importance of socioeconomic status in global outcome of the young-adult hyperactive. Milman[20] followed 73 hyperactive patients prospectively. The mean age at follow-up was 19 years. She found that there was a trend (though this did not reach statistical significance) for those of lower socioeconomic status to have poorer global outcomes as measured by parental impressions, patient's self-evaluation, psychiatric diagnosis, and objective data of academic, work, and social functioning.

However, other studies did not find socioeconomic status to be a strong predictor of adolescent- or adult-hyperactive global outcome. Thus, Huessy et al.[21] followed 83 subjects for 8–10 years. These subjects were seen in childhood for behavior disorders and placed on medication. At follow-up, records of community mental-health agencies were consulted and telephone contact was made with guidance counselors, parents, and state departments of mental health, corrections, social welfare, and education. Various areas of outcome (work, social, legal, psychiatric) were rated on the basis of information obtained. Authors then grouped their 15 "best" and "worst" outcome subjects in different income groups, and found no significant difference in the income distribution between the "best" and "worst" outcomes. However, no clear-cut definition of what criteria constituted these outcome groupings is given.

Mellsop,[22] too, found that socioeconomic status at referral did *not* influence the three- to fourfold increase in need for adult psychiatric treatment in people referred to psychiatry in childhood. Similarly, Robins[23] clearly stated that "social class makes little contribution to the prediction of serious adult antisocial behavior" (p. 617). This statement is supported for hyperactives by findings of Weiss et al.[5] and Loney,[7,16] cited earlier, and Satterfield et al.,[24] to be presented now. The latter consulted official arrest records of 110 adolescent boys, mean age 17, and a group of 88 matched normal controls. They divided the hyperactive and control groups into lower, middle, and upper socioeconomic status. Hyperactives in each status had significantly more offenses than controls. However, offender rates did not vary significantly as a function of socioeconomic status in either group.

In summary, one can say that socioeconomic status is not a strong predictor of any particular outcome measure (e.g., adolescent or adult antisocial behavior). It does, however, appear to be a factor in more global outcome.[6,17,20] This suggests that it may well interact with other factors (already outlined) in influencing the overall functioning of hyperactive adolescents and adults.

OVERALL FAMILY FUNCTIONING

In the preceding sections we have dealt separately with various individual aspects of the family to see how these factors might contribute to the eventual adolescent and adult outcomes of hyperactives. However, these family factors do not exist in a vacuum but interact with each other and other factors to determine overall family functioning. It is this global view of the family's functioning and how it may contribute to the outcome of the hyperactive child which will now be addressed.

Weiss et al.[5] indicated that even though overall family rating did not predict hyperactive adolescents' school success or emotional adjustment, it was important in influencing overt antisocial behavior in adolescents. Minde et al.,[6] who studied a larger sample of the same subjects as Weiss, found that overall family scores were initially worse and deteriorated significantly more in the "poor" versus "good" outcome group. In a subsequent study, Weiss et al.[25] compared adolescent outcome in three groups of hyperactive subjects. Group 1 had received at least 3 years of methylphenidate treatment in childhood; Group 2 had received chlorpromazine for at least 18 months to 5 years; and Group 3 was relatively untreated, having received less than 4 months of drug treatment. The authors found that family diagnosis failed to predict outcome of any measure in Groups 2 and 3. However, in Group 1 a good family situation was significantly correlated with good outcome in adolescence as measured by academic achievement, emotional adjustment, and absence of delinquency. The suggestion that outcome may depend on the interaction between emotional stability of the family and drug treatment was also made by Conrad and Insel[26] and Loney et al.[27]

If one grouped together all the family factors (discussed separately) by Loney and coworkers in predicting adolescent[16] and adult[7] outcome, one can see that they enter significantly into almost every global-outcome variable. For example, in adolescence, family factors enter into the prediction of global adolescent aggressive, hyperactive, and delinquent behavior, as well as achievement. In adulthood, family factors enter into some of the SADS-L Adult Antisocial and Alcoholism criteria, some items on the CAPS, and a number of the substances on the National Survey on Drug Abuse. It should be pointed out that intactness of the biological family was not found to be a strong predictor in adolescent or young-adult outcome by Loney et al.,[7,16] Milman,[20] or Mendelson et al.[4] This is in keeping with other authors,[29] who have shown that living in a household with a great deal of marital conflict may be more detrimental in terms of outcome than living in a family where there has been a separation or divorce.

Unlike the previous studies cited,[6,7,16,25] which have all shown the importance of family factors in predicting outcome, Menkes et al.[28] stated that they found no correlation between patients' social adjustment (e.g., being self-supporting, noninstitutionalized) at follow-up and their early home environment being classified as favorable or unfavorable. The authors felt that the global descriptions in both initial and outcome measures represented the sum total of many variables and that this, coupled with their relatively small sample, may account for this result.

In summary, one can state that family factors are important in both overall outcome and some specific outcome measures. One example of a specific connection is that parental history of antisocial behavior appears to influence antisocial behavior in the adolescent outcome. However, more work needs to be done on clarifying how various types of parental pathology and parent–child interactions might affect long-term outcome in hyperactive children. Such clarification would permit more useful interventions with families of hyperactives and, it is hoped, result in more positive outcomes.

CHAPTER SIXTEEN

PREDICTIVE FACTORS
PERTAINING TO TREATMENT

Most of the attention given to treatment as a predictive factor in outcome of hyperactive children has focused on a particular treatment modality—drug therapy—and specifically on stimulant treatment. In this chapter we will briefly review the impact of drug (stimulant) and other therapies (e.g., psychotherapy, counseling, remedial education) on long-term outcome of hyperactive children. We will also present the results of our 10- to 12-year follow-up study in adult outcome of hyperactives who did not receive any stimulant medication in childhood, those who did receive 3–5 years of stimulant medication, and a matched normal control group.

PSYCHOTHERAPY, COUNSELING, REMEDIAL EDUCATION

Few studies have looked at the influence on outcome of treatment which was not drug—particularly stimulant drug—therapy. In some cases, drug and other forms of therapy are combined, but only the influence of drug therapy is looked at. Mendelson et al.[1] indicated that in addition to stimulant-drug treatment, hyperactives they followed were also given supportive psychotherapy, and the parents were given counseling and instructed in the principles of behavior therapy. The frequency and duration of these interventions are not stipulated. Furthermore, the authors state that they were unable to gauge how these other (nondrug) treatments affected the course of the children's problems.

Some of the problems in evaluating the influence on outcome of various therapies were pointed out by Minde et al.[2] They found that the group which received more psychiatric treatment were more aggressive and distractible at initial assessment. These children also scored worse on the neuroticism dimension of the Peterson–Quay checklist.[3] Psychiatric treatment clearly improved the children's rating on this neuroticism, but not on the psychopathic or immature factor at 5-year follow-up during adolescence. Psychiatric treatment did not distinguish the "good" versus "poor" outcome groups, with some of the psychiatrically treated children falling into the good-outcome group while others fell into the poor-outcome group. It is difficult to interpret these results. Was treatment effective since these children were initially worse (e.g., more aggressive, distractible, and neurotic) than the rest of the group and no significant differences were seen at 5-year follow-up? Or was the treatment of inconsistent effectiveness since in some children it resulted in good outcome while in others in poor? It may well be that the effectiveness of psychiatric treatment may depend on other factors—for example, family functioning, child's handicaps—which affect the therapy's influence on good versus poor long-term outcome. Furthermore, some of the difficulties and limitations of doing psychotherapy with hyperactives at various stages of development are described in Chapter 18.

Minde et al.[2] also assessed the effectiveness of remedial help on outcome. Two-thirds of his hyperactive subjects were considered to have learning problems sufficient to benefit from individual or small-group remediation. People carrying out this treatment were interested but not specifically trained in remediation of perceptual problems. At follow-up, authors did not see improvement on any of the psychological tests in the children who received remedial therapy.

Ackerman et al.,[4] too, looked at educational intervention and its effect on academic progress at age 14 in three groups (hyperactive, hypoactive, and normoactive) of learning-disabled boys. Educational intervention ranged from intermittent private tutoring to resource rooms to full-time programs. Moderate to intense educational interventions produced no dramatic long-term results. In fact, boys who received the more-intense programs were further behind academically at age 14 than those in the less-intense programs. However, it must be stressed that the treatment assignment was not random, and boys in the more-intense programs had more initial deficits. One again sees the difficulty in assessing the long-term efficacy of a particular treatment when the level of initial deficit is not controlled. However, in an extensive review on the efficacy of remedial programs in learning-disabled children on longer-term academic outcome, Helper[5] showed that few studies had found long-term benefits from such programs.

Menkes et al.,[6] in the 25-year retrospective follow-up of 18 hyperactive patients, indicated that none of the subjects had received drug therapy. Treatment consisted of support and encouragement to parent and child and environmental manipulation (e.g., more appropriate school placement), in an effort to better meet the child's needs. The authors concluded that there was no correlation between outcome and the amount of treatment the patient received.

On the surface it would appear that psychotherapy, counseling, and remedial help are not particularly predictive of long-term outcome in hyperactive children. As was pointed out, the problem in assessing the long-term impact on outcome of these treatments is that children requiring such interventions have more problems to begin with and are therefore more likely to have poorer outcomes. Well-controlled studies that have matched subjects on severity of initial problems and then assigned them randomly to receive or not receive well-defined qualitatively and quantitatively controlled interventions have not been done. Ethically and clinically such studies are difficult to do, and so we are left with the imperfect findings and clinical impressions outlined above. In light of the frequent negative cycle of school, peer, and family problems faced by many hyperactives, it still seems clinically sound to recommend individual, family, and/or remedial therapy whenever indicated.

DRUG TREATMENT

Most of the studies involving the long-term outcome of drug treatment in hyperactive children have focused on stimulant drugs. A few[2,7] have referred to long-term phenothiazine treatment outcome. More recently,[8] acute drug studies involving tricyclic antidepressants have reached the literature, but no long-term follow-up of hyperactive children treated with these drugs has been reported. We will not repeat here the long-term effects of stimulant treatment on physiological measures such as growth or cardiovascular status, discussed at some length in Chapter 11. Nor will we deal with the link between stimulant treatment in childhood and later adolescent or adult drug or alcohol use or abuse, discussed in considerable detail in Chapter 8.

Weiss et al.[7] compared the adolescent outcome in three groups of hyperactive children: the first had received 3–5 years of methylphenidate treatment (20–50 mg/day); the second had received 18 months to 5 years of chlorpromazine treatment (50–200 mg/day, mean 75 mg); and the third had received no medication during the follow-up period. The three groups were matched for age, IQ, sex, and socioeconomic status. No significant difference in emotional adjustment, delinquency, or academic performance was seen among the three groups. The authors thus showed that long-term treatment in childhood did not significantly affect hyperactive adolescents' outcome. However, it should be pointed out that in those subjects who were on stimulant medication, having a good family situation was significantly correlated with good outcome as defined by academic achievement, absence of delinquency, and emotional adjustment. Thus the interaction of medication and other factors (e.g., family functioning) appears more important in predicting outcome than medication in and of itself. Similar findings were reported by Conrad and Insel[9] and Loney et al.[10]

Loney et al.,[11] in the careful predictive study of hyperactive adolescent outcome, studied stimulant treatment as a predictor. Subjects had been on medication for an average of 29 months (average dose 34 mg/day) during childhood. The child's response to treatment was rated on a 5-point scale from progress notes in the child's chart. Duration of the stimulant medication was also assessed as a predictor. In summary, response to medication was a factor in only three of the many outcome measures in adolescence. Subjects who responded well to medication in childhood had a less negative affect at follow-up, were less involved in nonmedical drug use, and scored better on the Wide Range Achievement Test in reading and arithmetic. Duration of stimulant treatment did not predict any outcome measure.

However, most authors who have examined stimulant treatment in childhood as a predictor of hyperactive adolescent outcome have found no effect, as if the initial benefits of medication cited by many studies somehow do not carry over into positive long-term outcome. Thus Ackerman et al.[4] found that stimulant drug treatment had no dramatic long-term results on academic achievement in their three groups (hyperactive, hypoactive, and normoactive) of learning-disabled boys at age 14. One could argue that the dual handicap or hyperactivity and learning disability militated against the long-term positive effectiveness of the medication. However, Riddle and Rapoport[12] also found no difference in academic achievement between a subgroup of 20 hyperactive boys who had been randomly assigned to receive methylphenidate for 2 years and their total group of 72 hyperactive boys, some of whom were on imipramine.

Blouin et al.[13] compared two groups of hyperactive adolescents. One group had received methylphenidate treatment in childhood (10–60 mg/day, mean 20 mg/day) for 1 month to 7 years (mean 2 years), and the other did not. The two groups matched for age, IQ, and academic achievement at initial assessment. The authors stated that even when good and poor responses were examined separately, no beneficial effect of the drug on academic achievement, intellectual ability, or behavioral ratings was evident.

Charles[14] divided 62 hyperactive children into four groups depending on the length of time they had been on stimulant treatment (ranging less than 6 months, for Group 1, to 4 years, for Group 5). There were no group differences in behavioral, social, or academic outcome measures, suggesting that duration to stimulant intervention did not have a significant effect on outcome.

The seeming ineffectiveness of childhood stimulant medication in influencing adolescent outcome was further shown by Satterfield et al.[15] In a prospective study, the authors compared 110 adolescent hyperactive boys and 88 matched normal controls on serious offenses, as obtained from official arrest records. The hyperactive group had received stimulant treatment for about 2 years and brief counseling. However, this group had significantly more serious arrests and institutionalization for delinquency than the matched normal control group. The considerably more favorable outcome of Satterfield et al.'s[16] 3-year follow-up of hyperactives who received multimodal (medication plus any number of other required interventions, e.g., psychotherapy, therapy for the child and/or parents, family therapy, and educational therapy) presents some suggestion as to why stimulant treatment has not predicted more positive long-term outcome. It is clear that these children have many academic, social, family, and personal problems. All of these difficulties require intervention, and relying on medication alone to ameliorate all these areas now seems unrealistic.

Feldman et al.,[17] who reported outcomes of 81 hyeractives as adolescents and 48 hyperactives as adults, found that only 8% of the hyperactive adolescents and 10% of the hyperactive adults had serious problems. He attributes these relatively positive results to the fact that most of the children were middle class and received comprehensive treatment in a multidisciplinary setting. In fact, over 80% of the subjects received multiple therapies, including medication; only 2% of the adolescents and none of the adults received only medication. This study further supports the need for a comprehensive, multimodal treatment approach to ensure a more positive long-term outcome for hyperactive children.

YOUNG-ADULT OUTCOME OF HYPERACTIVES WHO RECEIVED LONG-TERM STIMULANT TREATMENT IN CHILDHOOD

Few studies have followed stimulant-treated hyperactives into adulthood. Both Feldman et al.[17] and Loney et al.[18] have looked at the adult hyperactives who received stimulant treatment in childhood and compared them to their brothers. However, such a comparison has the advantage and limitation of similar family pathology or stress in the two groups, and it also is comparing affected and nonaffected individuals. In our 10- to 12-year follow-up study of hyperactive young adults, we compared the outcome in hyperactives who had not received any significant stimulant treatment in childhood (described in Chapter 5), hyperactives who had received 3–5 years of sustained stimulant medication (20–50 mg) in childhood, and a matched normal control group. The two groups of hyperactives grew up at different times. The hyperactives who did not receive stimulant treatment were referred in the early and mid-1960s, a time when stimulants were not generally used for hyperactivity in Canada. However, in the late '60s and early '70s, when the second group of hyperactives were referred, methylphenidate was beginning to be used, so these patients received stimulant treatment. The groups thus did not differ in severity of symptoms or family attitudes to medication treatment, but simply reflect the change in the clinic's practice regarding the general use of stimulant medication. Hyperactives who did *not* receive stimulant treatment and their matched control group went through their years of adolescence and young adulthood some 5 years before the stimulant-treated hyperactives. For this reason it was felt that these stimulant-treated hyperactives required their own control group who had gone through adolescence and young adulthood at the same time. To gather such a control group, letters went out to former classmates of the stimulant-treated hyperactives, inviting them to participate in the study. To be accepted into the control group, interested subjects had to meet the following criteria: IQ's of 85 or above; no significant problems academically or behaviorally in school; and while in school, they had to be living at home with at least one parent.

A control group of 20 such subjects was selected. All subjects had extensive assessments. These included:

1. *Biographic data*—for example, school and work histories, living arrangements, and car accidents.

2. *Physiological data*—height, weight, pulse, blood pressure.

3. *Psychological tests*—of cognitive style: Matching Familiar Figures Test (MFFT),[19] Embedded Figures Test (EFT),[20] and Stroop Color–Word Interference Test.[21]

4. *Psychiatric assessments*, including assessment of past and current nonmedical drug use and antisocial behavior. SADS[22] was administered to the stimulant-treated hyperactive group and their control group. Subjects also completed SCL-90,[23] designed to tap classical psychopathology.

5. *Self-esteem* assessment via Davidson-Lang checklist[24] Ziller Self-Other Social Orientation Test,[25] and Area Test.[26]

6. *Social skills* tests, including the Situational Social Skills Inventory[27] (SSI), in written and oral form.

7. *School and employers' questionnaires*, containing almost identical items, sent to high-school guidance offices and subjects' employers.

Statistical analysis included analysis of variance, t-tests, and chi-squares, with the appropriate analysis being used where applicable. It was felt that real differences might exist in the groups and so, in accordance with Lord,[28] we felt it was not reasonable to adjust for them by using covariance.

Results

DEMOGRAPHIC VARIABLES (Table 16-1)

Hyperactive groups, stimulant treated and untreated, matched on IQ and socioeconomic status. The stimulant-treated hyperactives were slightly older (mean age 21.8 years vs. 19.6 years for the untreated hyperactives at follow-up), since some of the measures (e.g., details of drug/alcohol use and antisocial behavior and social-skills and self-esteem tests) were obtained at 12-year rather than at 10-year follow-up as for the untreated hyperactives. Subjects were thus of comparable age for these measures. The normal control subjects for the stimulant-treated hyperactives matched this latter group on age and scioeconomic status but had significantly higher IQ's (115.2 vs. 107.1, $p < .005$). This higher IQ may have affected some of the results. For example, the control group completed more education (13.2 years vs. 11.0 years, $p < .004$), and more of the controls were in school full time or part time. These differences were not seen between stimulant-treated and untreated hyperactives.

MOVES AND LIVING ARRANGEMENTS. Stimulant-treated hyperactives had more moves in the last 10 years when compared to their matched controls (6.5 vs. 0.9, $p < .05$). With regard to living arrangements, the majority of subjects in all groups were still living with parents or relatives. However, significantly more stimulant-treated hyperactives lived with girlfriends and/or wives when compared either to untreated hyperactives ($p < .01$) or controls ($p < .02$). Other types of living arrangements (e.g., living alone or with same-sex friends) were not significantly different for the three groups.

WORK, VOCATIONAL PLANS, DEBTS. Most of the subjects in all three groups stated that they were satisfied with their present job. However, significantly more stimulant-treated hyperactives either had no future vocational plans or lower-status plans when compared to the matched control group ($p < .05$). In addition, significantly more stimulant-treated hyperactives were in debt when compared to their control group (6 vs. 0, $p < .02$), but not in comparison to the untreated hyperactive group.

TABLE 16-1. Demographic Variables

	Hyperactives			Controls	
	Ritalin	Non-Ritalin	Significance	Ritalin	Significance
	($n = 20$)	($n = 64$–68)		($n = 20$)	
Age (years)	21.8	19.6	$p < .01$	21.1	
IQ	107.1	105		115.2	$p < .005$
Socioeconomic states	3.1	3.3		3.2	
Number of moves (last 10 years)	6.5			0.9	$p < .05$
Education completed	11.0	10.4		13.2	$p < .004$
Subject doing School (full and part time)	3	31		11	$p < .05$
Work (full and part time)	11	27		8	
Nothing	5	8		1	
	($n = 14$)	($n = 30$)		($n = 10$)	
Satisfied with present job	12	22		10	
	($n = 20$)	($n = 67$)		($n = 20$)	
Living arrangements					
Parents or relatives	9	48		17	
Alone	3	7		1	
Friend	1	4		0	
Girlfriend/wife	8	5	$p < .01$	1	$p < .02$
Reformatory	0	1		0	
Married	2	2		0	
Marriage plans eventually	16	47		18	
Debts	6	11		0	$p < .02$
Vocational plans (Hollingshead)					
None	6			1	$p < .05$
1	2			9	$p < .05$
2	2			3	
3	8			2	$p < .05$
4	1			2	
5	0			2	
Realistic	12			14	

Note. The Ritalin hyperactive group was comprised of subjects who had had 3–5 years of stimulant therapy in childhood. Control subjects were normals who were matched and compared only to the Ritalin group.

CAR ACCIDENTS. The untreated hyperactive group had significantly more car accidents when compared to the stimulant-treated group (mean 1.5 vs. 0.62, $p < .004$). However, there were no significant differences in cost or damage of the accidents or extent of bodily injury. Circumstances surrounding the accidents (e.g., drug or alcohol use or various emotional states) did not differ in the three groups.

PHYSIOLOGICAL VARIABLES

No significant differences with regard to weight, height, pulse, or blood pressure were seen in the three groups. Measures of parental heights and weights were similar for the stimulant-treated and control group.

PSYCHOLOGICAL TESTS

Of the three cognitive-style tests—MFFT, EFT, and the Stroop test—stimulant-treated hyperactives performed significantly worse on the EFT when compared to the control group, but no differently from the untreated hyperactive group. The other two tests were not significantly different for the three groups.

SCHOOL

There were several significant differences in school performance between stimulant-treated hyperactives and the control group. Significantly more controls were attending junior colleges and universities ($p < .05$), while more of the stimulant-treated hyperactives were not in school. The stimulant-treated hyperactives tended to fail more grades in high school ($p < .1$) and drop out because of poor marks ($p < .08$). Their average academic standing was significantly lower (in the 51–60 range $p < .05$). They also tended to be expelled more often ($p < .07$ u.c.). Generally, these differences were not seen between the stimulant-treated and the untreated hyperactives. The only significant differences between these two groups were that more untreated hyperactives were attending junior college ($p < .03$) and were not in school because of lack of interest ($p < .05$). However, no differences in average academic standing, failing grades, or being expelled or suspended were found.

SCHOOL GUIDANCE QUESTIONNAIRE

Again one sees significance differences between the stimulant-treated hyperactives and their controls but not between treated and untreated hyperactives. Controls were scored significantly better than stimulant-treated hyperactives on doing assigned work adequately, working independently, completing tasks, and mathematics and language ability. The stimulant-treated hyperactives were scored as having more difficulty getting along with teachers and being less welcomed by the same teachers again, when compared to controls. Interestingly, there were no significant differences in getting along with classmates or punctuality. There were no significant differences on *any* of the items between the stimulant-treated and untreated hyperactives.

EMPLOYERS' QUESTIONNAIRE

The employer and school questionnaires contained almost identical items. However, in contrast to the school questionnaire, very few significant differences were seen in the employer questionnaire. Control subjects tended to be scored as working more independently than the stimulant-treated hyperactives. The only other significant finding was that stimulant-treated hyperactives usually got along with co-workers better compared to untreated hyperactives. All other items—for example, being punctual, doing assigned work adequately, getting along with supervisors, completing tasks, and being rehired—were not significantly different for the three groups.

WORK RECORD

In contrast to the employers' questionnaire, on which few differences were seen between the groups, the work record has some interesting findings. Stimulant-treated hyperactives appear to leave school earlier ($p < .028$), spend more time doing nothing ($p < .01$), start working earlier ($p < .05$), and have more jobs ($p < .01$) when compared to the control group. In addition, despite incomes that were not significantly different, the stimulant-treated hyperactive group had greater debts ($p < .06$) when compared to the control group.

There were no significant differences on any of these items between the treated and untreated hyperactives. In a detailed analysis of the last job, it was found that untreated hyperactives had held this last job for a significantly longer period (70 weeks vs. 21 weeks, $p < .001$), and a larger number ($p < .03$) had no problems with concentration when compared to stimulant-treated hyperactives. This in spite of the fact that the percent of the workday that was active was not significantly different for the three groups. There were no differences between the three groups regarding full-time jobs lasting less than 2 months, summer or part-time jobs, and reasons for leaving jobs.

PSYCHIATRIC VARIABLES (Table 16-2)

In comparing stimulant-treated hyperactives and their control group, the hyperactives tended to be hospitalized for psychiatric treatment more often ($p < .07$), and a larger number were diagnosed as having personality disorders (($p < .02$). On the other hand, the untreated hyperactives had more current psychiatric treatment ($p < .02$) and a less positive view of their childhood than the stimulant-treated group ($p < .02$).

Other variables such as subject's mood, complaints, number of friends, presence of psychosis or borderline psychosis, perversions, verbal ability, and ability to relate to the examiner were not significantly different for all three groups. A detailed comparison of suicidal thoughts and attempts between the stimulant-treated hyperactives and the controls showed no differences in this regard between the two groups. Similarly, these two groups showed no differences with regard to the SADS evaluations. On the SCL-90, no significant differences were seen in the mean total scores between the three groups.

ANTISOCIAL BEHAVIOR

There were no significant differences in reported police involvement or type and degree of police involvement for the three groups in past year.

AGGRESSION

Even though the stimulant-treated hyperactives had significantly more severe problems with aggression than the control group ($p < .05$), the untreated hyperactives tended to have more difficulties than the stimulant-treated group ($p < .06$).

DETAILS OF STEALING HISTORY

Significantly more untreated hyperactives stole in elementary school when compared to the stimulant-treated group ($p < .05$). However, there were no differences in the three groups in subjects who stole in high school or currently. There were also no differences between the three groups in reasons for stealing, in severity of thefts, feelings and circumstances surrounding stealing, or reasons for stopping at any of the three time frames.

CURRENT ALCOHOL AND NONMEDICAL DRUG USE

There were no significant differences in the number of subjects in the three groups who used alcohol currently (almost all had in the last 3

TABLE 16-2. Psychiatric Variables

	Hyperactives			Controls	
	Ritalin	Non-Ritalin	Significance	Ritalin	Significance
	(n = 20)	(n = 67)		(n = 20)	
Psychiatric treatment (present)	1	22	p < .02	2	
Ever hospitalized for psychiatric treatment	3			0	p < .07
Desires psychiatric treatment	5	16		6	
Subject's mood					
Abnormal	4	14		1	
Normal with problems	6	19		7	
Normal	10	34		12	
Type of mood abnormality					
Depression	3	20		1	
Depression anxiety	1	7		0	
Anxiety	0	9		0	
Concept of childhood					
Negative	8	28		3	
Intermediate	4	30		6	
Positive	8	10	p < .02	11	
	(n = 20)	(n = 68)		(n = 20)	
Present complaints	18	47		17	
Type of complaints					
Social	11	20		5	
Emotional	9	26		7	
Self-esteem	2	16		1	
Other	13	6	p < .0001	16	
Personality disorders	6	28		0	p < .02
Psychosis (borderline psychotic)	0	4		0	
Perversions	1	6		0	
Friends					
None	1	9		0	
Few	15	33		15	
Several	6	25		5	
Had sexual intercourse	16			6	p < .09

Note. The Ritalin hyperactive group was comprised of subjects who had had 3–5 years of stimulant therapy in childhood. Control subjects were normals who were matched and compared only to the Ritalin group.

months), nor did the extent of this use differ. There was a trend ($p < .05$ u.c.) for more stimulant-treated hyperactives than controls to use marijuana and hashish, and for more of the stimulant-treated group than of both the control and untreated hyperactive groups to use cocaine. There were no significant differences in the extent of current use of these drugs, or the number of subjects using and extent of use of hallucinogens, stimulants, heroin, and barbiturates. Most subjects in all three groups used only alcohol and marijuana, and very few used any of the other drugs.

PAST ALCOHOL AND NONMEDICAL DRUG USE (Table 16-3)

ALCOHOL. Most subjects in all three groups were still using alcohol. The stimulant-treated hyperactives started using alcohol at an earlier age (14.8 years vs. 16.2 years, $p < .03$), and had a longer period of maximum use (25.0 months vs. 10.8 months, $p < .05$), when compared to the untreated group. There were no such differences between the stimulant-treated hyperactives and the control group on these measures. This points out the value of a control group that grew up at the same time as the stimulant-treated hyperactive group. The mean age of maximum use was around 18 years for all groups, and the extent of maximum use was somewhat greater for the stimulant-treated hyperactives compared to their control group, but not in comparison to the untreated hyperactive group.

HASHISH, MARIJUANA. There appear to be no significant differences in the three groups regarding past use of hashish and marijuana. Generally they started using the drug between 15 and 16 years of age, used it most between 17 and 18 years of age, and if they stopped using this drug, this took place between 18 and 19 years. The duration of maximum use was about 1 year. The extent of maximum use was usually slight or moderate, with only a few subjects in each group falling into the abuse category.

HALLUCINOGENS. The picture is similar for these drugs with no significant difference appearing in the three groups. Mean age they started use was about 16 years, with a maximum use at 16–18 years of age, and a duration of maximum ranging from 8 to 13 months. They usually stopped using the drugs at 18–19 years of age, and most used them to slight or moderate extent, though a few (4) in the two hyperactive groups abused hallucinogens.

STIMULANTS. There appeared to be a trend for more stimulant-treated hyperactives to have tried stimulants in the past than the control group (6 vs. 1, $p < .04$ u.c.). There was no difference when comparison was made to the untreated hyperactive group. Again no difference existed between the three groups on age started using the drug (about 17 years), age of maximum use (about 17.5 years), and duration of maximum use (3–9 months). Most of the use was slight (though 5 untreated hyperactives had severe use), and subjects usually stopped using the drug at 17–18 years of age.

COCAINE. Stimulant-treated hyperactives tended to be older (20 vs. 18.9 years, $p < .02$) when they started using cocaine as compared to untreated hyperactives. This age difference persisted through the age of maximum use and age stopped. There were no significant differences in duration of maximum use, which ranged from 3.2 months for the untreated hyperactives to 12–14 months for the control and stimulant-treated groups. Again no significant differences appeared in extent of maximum use.

HEROIN. None of the controls or stimulant-treated hyperactives had used heroin in the past. However, 5 untreated hyperactives had used the drug, 3 to an abusive extent.

BARBITURATES. Again, no significant differences were seen in the three groups regarding past barbiturate use. Use usually began between 16.5 and 18.0 years of age and peaked shortly thereafter, with the duration of maximum use being 1.5–6.3 months.

REASONS FOR DISCONTINUING USE OF NONMEDICAL DRUGS. Generally there were no significant differences between the three groups regarding reasons for discontinuing nonmedical drug use. Most subjects cited drug consequences for most drugs. Lack of funds was cited by some subjects for cocaine and heroin. Legal and social consequences were listed by the untreated hyperactive group for marijuana, halluncinogens, and heroin.

SOCIAL SKILLS

In the oral or behavioral version of the Situational Social Skills Inventory,[27] the control group tended to score better than the stimulant-treated group for situations requiring assertion. No differences were seen in the job interview or heterosocial situation between the two groups. There were no differences between the stimulant-treated and untreated hyperactive groups on any of the behavioral situations. In the written version of the test, where subjects had to select the most appropriate answer from a number of given possibilities, the stimulant-treated hyperactives tended to do a little better than the controls ($p < .06$) and much better than the untreated hyperactives ($p < .01$) in the job interview. There was also a slightly better performance by the

TABLE 16-3. Past Alcohol and Nonmedical Drug Use

	Ever used (not in last 3 months) (n)	Mean age started (years)	Mean age max. use (years)	Duration max. use (months)	Extent of max. use			Mean age stopped (years)
					Mild (n)	Moderate (n)	Abuse/ addiction (n)	
Alcohol								
Controls	1	14.8	18.4	28	10	5	5[a]	
Hyperactives—Rit.	0	14.8[a]	18.3	25[a]	5	2	13[a]	
Hyperactives—Non-Rit.	0	16.2[a]	18.0	10.8[a]	12	6	26	
Sig.		$p < .03$		$p < .05$			$p < .05$	
Hashish and marijuana								
Controls	5	16.3	18.4	11	8	3	1	
Hyperactives—Rit.	5	16.2	18.1	14	7	7	3	19.2
Hyperactives—Non-Rit.	19	15.5	17.6	13.1	17	11	6	18.1
Sig.								
Hallucinogens								
Controls	4	16.7	18	12.7	2	2	0	19
Hyperactives—Rit.	8	16.3	16.5	8.7	4	1	4	18.3
Hyperactives—Non-Rit.	25	16.8	17.2	13.2	16	4	4	18.6
Sig.								

Stimulants								
Controls	1[a]	17.0	17.5	7.5	2	0	0	17.8
Hyperactives—Rit.	6[a]	17.6	17.6	3.2	5	0	1	18.5
Hyperactives—Non-Rit.	10	16.9	17.8	9.8	6	1	5	
Sig. (u.c.)	p < .04							
Cocaine								
Controls	2	18.2	18.6	12	2	0	0	22.0[a]
Hyperactives—Rit.	3	20.0[a]	20.3[a]	14	6	1	1	18.9[a]
Hyperactives—Non-Rit.	7	18.9[a]	18.9[a]	3.2	5	0	2	
Sig.		p < .02	p < .08					p < .001
Heroin								
Controls	0							
Hyperactives—Rit.	0							
Hyperactives—Non-Rit.	5	17.8	19.4	3.7	2	0	3	20.5
Sig.								
Barbiturates								
Controls	1	18.0	18.5	1.5	1	1	0	
Hyperactives—Rit.	3	16.5	16.5	4.6	4	0	0	16.6
Hyperactives—Non-Rit.	6	18.0	18.7	6.3	3	0	2	
Sig.								

[a]Number used to determine significance of variable.

stimulant-treated hyperactives in the assertion choices ($p < .08$) when compared to the untreated hyperactives. There were no significant differences between the three groups on the heterosexual interactions.

SELF-ESTEEM

In the overall scores, there was no significant difference between the stimulant-treated hyperactives and their control group on any of the three self-esteem tests. However, the stimulant-treated hyperactives tended ($p < .08$) to do better on the Ziller Self–Other test when compared to the untreated hyperactive group. No differences were seen in the overall scores of the other two tests.

A more detailed look indicated that on several items on the Davidson–Lang test the stimulant-treated hyperactives rated themselves significantly better than the untreated hyperactives. These items included: intelligent–unintelligent, $p < .001$; fast–slow, $p < .05$; kind–cruel, $p < .04$; friendly–unfriendly, $p < .004$; curious–indifferent, $p < .04$; and respectful–disrespectful, $p < .06$, where the untreated hyperactives rated themselves somewhat better. Interestingly there were no significant differences between the stimulant-treated hyperactives and their control group on any of the items of the Davidson–Lang. On the Ziller Self–Other test, even though the stimulant-treated hyperactives tended to do better on the overall score, on individual items such as flunking and unhappy the untreated hyperactives scored significantly better when compared to the stimulant-treated group ($p < .004 \rightarrow p < .001$). The stimulant-treated group was significantly better on cruel ($p < .02$), and no difference between the two hyperactive groups was seen in unsuccessful. Again no significant differences were seen on *any* of the items between the stimulant-treated hyperactives and their control group.

Discussion

The most striking finding of the study is the repetition pattern of finding significant differences between the stimulant-treated hyperactives and their control group (with the control group almost invariably doing better), but no such differences on the same items between the two hyperactive groups. This is seen in areas such as schooling, school guidance questionnaire, employer questionnaire, work record, debts, personality disorders, and some psychological tests, to mention just a few. There are almost no items where stimulant-treated hyperactives do significantly better than their controls. (More treated hyperactives have had sexual intercourse and some do better on written social skills.)

However, there are several areas in which the stimulant-treated hyperactives seem to do better than their untreated counterparts. These areas include fewer car accidents, seeing their childhood more positively, stealing less in elementary school, and generally having better social skills and self-esteem. They also have less problems with aggression and less need for current psychiatric treatment. We thus see that stimulant treatment in childhood may not eliminate educational, work, and life difficulties, but it may result in less social ostracism, with subsequent better feelings toward others and themselves.

Certain areas which did not show any differences in the three groups are worth mentioning. These included physiological measures of height, weight, blood pressure, and pulse, suggesting that the amount, duration, and time of administration of the stimulants for this group did not significantly affect their growth or cardiovascular status. The heights and weights of the parents of the stimulant-treated hyperactives and their control group were included to provide familial comparison and help detect any significant deviation. None was found.

Another area which failed to show significant differences was that of serious psychopathology. There were no significant differences in the SCL-90 or the incidence of psychosis, borderline psychosis, or perversions. Unfortunately, we have SADS and suicidal data on the stimulant-treated hyperactives and their control group, but not for the untreated hyperactives. These tests were not used by us when the untreated group was seen. Here again no significant differences were found.

Nonetheless, hyperactives, treated and untreated, have more personality disorders when compared to controls. There was a trend ($p < .07$) for the stimulant-treated group to have more psychiatric hospitalization than their control group. Data for the untreated hyperactive group were not available. Thus some increased psychopathology exists in the hyperactive groups. However, serious psychiatric conditions such as psychosis or borderline psychosis were found in relatively few subjects.

Antisocial behavior (in the past year) was also not significantly different for the three groups, suggesting again that hyperactives as a group do not load the antisocial population in adulthood. Current alcohol use was also not different for the three groups, though more stimulant-treated hyperactives than controls used marijuana and cocaine. Past drug and alcohol use suggested that stimulant-treated hyperactives may have been more involved with alcohol and stimulant use in comparison to their controls. However, more untreated hyperactives were involved with heroin. In contrast to Blouin et al.,[13] who found a higher incidence of alcohol use in hyperactive adolescents, our study suggests that stimulant-treated hyperactives as young adults do not currently use more drugs and/or alcohol. The slightly larger number of stimulant-treated hyperactives who currently and in the past used alcohol and nonmedical drugs does not seem to be particularly significant, and generally we would agree with Henker et al.[29] that there is no substantial support for the hypothesis of an association between stimulant treatment and increased use of nonmedical drugs.

It must be stressed that the number of subjects in the Ritalin-treated group was relatively small, particularly when we are dealing with several subgroups. This makes meaningful statistical analysis difficult. Another limitation of the study is that the groups were not completely matched. The control group had somewhat higher IQ's, and the untreated hyperactive group was slightly younger on some measures. The findings, therefore, must be seen in a tentative light awaiting replication with other comparable groups.

In summary, one can say that as young adults, stimulant-treated and untreated hyperactives are fairly similar and significantly different from a matched normal control group. The hyperactives continue to have educational and work difficulties. Their increased residential moves, job changes, and debt may reflect their more impulsive lifestyle. They have more emotional problems and more problems with aggression. However, they do not load the severe psychiatric or antisocial population. Stimulant treatment in childhood seems to have no significant negative effects but may in fact result in less early social ostracism with subsequent better feelings toward others and themselves.

CHAPTER SEVENTEEN

INTERRELATIONSHIP OF VARIOUS PREDICTIVE FACTORS

In the preceding chapters we have presented various factors related to the child, the family, and treatment which may predict or affect long-term outcome for the hyperactive in adolescence or adulthood. For the sake of clarity, we have presented each factor separately, while stressing that there is a great deal of interrelationship among them and that they most probably work together and cumulatively in predicting outcome. To illustrate this interaction we will present the results of our predictive study,[1] in which we selected certain initial assessment measures of our hyperactive subjects (described in detail in Chapter 5) and statistically assessed how predictive they were of certain adult outcome measures.

The *predictive measures* were:

I. *Personal characteristics*
   1. IQ
   2. Hyperactivity
   3. Aggressivity
   4. Emotional stability
   5. Low frustration tolerance

II. *Social–academic parameters*
   1. School performance
   2. Peer relations
   3. Adult relations
   4. Antisocial behavior

III. *Family parameters*
   1. Socioeconomic status
   2. Mental health of family members
   3. Emotional climate of home
   4. Child-rearing practices
      a. Inconsistent
      b. No control
      c. Authoritarian
      d. Overprotective

5. Family rating
6. Age first worked

The *selected outcome measures* at 10-year follow-up in young adulthood were:

I. *Emotional adjustment*
    1. Brief Psychiatric Rating Scale (BPRS)
    2. Personality trait disorders
    3. Peer relationships, friends

II. *School performance*
    1. Grades completed
    2. Academic standing
    3. Grades failed

III. *Work record*
    1. Number of full-time jobs
    2. Percentage of jobs fired
    3. Percentage of jobs laid off
    4. Longest full-time job

IV. *Police involvement*
    1. Number of offenses
    2. Severity of offenses

V. *Car accidents*
    1. Number of accidents
    2. Accidents with bodily injury
    3. Cost of damage

VI. *Nonmedical drug and alcohol use*
    1. Present use
    2. Past use
    3. Extent of use (current)
    4. Extent of maximum use
    5. Number of drugs used

For each set of outcome measures a selection of the theoretically most relevant predictor measures was made for analysis. These measures were analyzed both singly and multiply, that is, via univariate correlation (or analysis of variance) and multivariate stepwise cumulative regression techniques (or discriminant analysis). This provided us with a view of the power of any initial individual variable predicting adult outcome as well as the group of initial variables which together may predict this outcome. The relative predictive power of each variable in the group (or equation) is indicated by the step at which it is entered into the equation, the most powerful entering first. Only those variables which continued to increase the significance of the equation or continued to improve the predictive power of the group were included.

All subjects with missing data greater than 20% were dropped from the analyses. Variables where missing data were less than 10% were estimated using the group mean. When the missing data exceeded 10% and the variable was deemed of sufficient importance to be retained in the analysis, the missing data were replaced with an estimate (using the group mean) and a binary-coded missing-value indicator was added to the predictor list. It has been suggested[2] that this method minimizes loss of information and loss of power and independent of the assumption of randomness of occurrence of missing data.

RESULTS

Emotional Adjustment (Table 17-1)

It is interesting to note to what extent family parameters predict adult emotional adjustment measures. On a univariate basis we see that initially assessed mental health of family is related to adult BPRS[3]

TABLE 17-1. Emotional Adjustment

	Outcome variables								
	BPRS (n = 64)			Friends (n = 64)			Personality disorders (n = 64)		
Predictor variables at initial assessment	U	SE	MC	U	SE	MC	U	SE	MC
Personal characteristics									
Hyperactivity				p < .07	2	p < .01	p < .06	2	p < .001
Aggressivity									
Emotional instability					4	p < .01		4	p < .001
Low frustration tolerance							p < .07	3	p < .001
IQ		3	p < .05		3	p < .01			
Social–academic parameters									
Peer relations									
School performance									
MVI school performance	p < .05	5	p < .05						
Family parameters									
Mental health of family members	p < .05	1	p < .05				p < .007	1	p < .001
Family rating	p < .05	4	p < .05				p < .06		
Emotional climate of home		5	p < .05	p < .05	1	p < .01			

Note. U = univariate; SE = step entered; MC = multivariate (stepwise regression) cumulative; MVI = missing value indicator.

($p < .05$) and personality disorders ($p < .007$). These adult measures are also related to initial overall family rating ($p < .05$ and $p < .06$, respectively), while emotional climate of the home is univariately related to adult friendships ($p < .05$). There is a tendency for some initial personal characteristics to relate univariately to adult measures of emotional adjustment. Thus hyperactivity correlates with friendship ($p < .07$) and adult personality disorders ($p < .06$), while low frustration tolerance tends to relate to personality disorders ($p < .07$).

In the multivariate analysis we see that family parameters combine with IQ to predict adult BPRS scores ($p < .05$) and emotional climate of the home combine with hyperactivity, emotional instability, and IQ to predict adult friendships ($p < .01$). Again, mental health of family members combines with hyperactivity, emotional instability, and low frustration tolerance to predict adult personality disorder ($p < .001$).

It is interesting to note that aggressivity, peer relations, and school performance did not enter into the analysis; however, one must be careful about concluding that they are not important predictors. Their failure to enter the analysis may be due to being highly correlated with variables which did enter. For example, initial aggressivity was highly correlated ($p < .01$) with emotional instability and low frustration tolerance; school performance correlated with initial IQ ($p < .01$) and hyperactivity ($p < .05$); and finally, peer relationships correlated with aggressivity and low frustration tolerance ($p < .01$).

Thus we see that adult emotional adjustment is affected by various initial variables with some—for example, family parameters and certain personality characteristics—playing a more important role.

School Performance (Table 17-2)

In the univariate analysis we see the importance of initial IQ, which is associated with grades completed ($p < .01$), initial socioeconomic status, which relates to academic standing ($p < .06$), and grades failed ($p < .03$), as well as certain child-rearing practices. These include inconsistency, which relates to grades completed ($p < .05$), and overprotectiveness, which relates to grades failed ($p < .03$). There is a trend for initial hyperactivity to be related to adult academic standing ($p < .08$).

In the multivariate stepwise-regression analysis we see that all variables except aggressivity and overall family rating entered the equation for grades completed ($p < .01$). Similarly, school performance, some child-rearing practices, and emotional climate of the home were left out of the equation for academic standing ($p < .01$). Notably *not* included in the predictive equation for grades failed ($p < .001$) were aggressivity, antisocial behavior, and various family parameters including overall family rating, mental health of family members, and emo-

TABLE 17-2. School Performance

Predictor variables at initial assessment	Outcome variables								
	Grades completed			Academic standing			Grades failed		
	U	SE	MC	U	SE	MC	U	SE	MC
Personal characteristics									
IQ	$p < .01$	1	$p < .01$		2	$p < .01$		7	$p < .001$
Hyperactivity		7	$p < .01$	$p < .08$	4	$p < .01$		8	$p < .001$
Aggressivity					3	$p < .01$			
Social–academic parameters									
School performance		8	$p < .01$					6	$p < .001$
MVI school performance					6	$p < .01$	$p < .01$		
Antisocial behavior		6	$p < .01$		5	$p < .01$			
MVI antisocial behavior		2	$p < .01$				$p < .01$	1	
Family parameters									
Socioeconomic status		4	$p < .01$	$p < .06$	1	$p < .01$	$p < .03$	3	$p < .001$
Child-rearing practices									
Inconsistent	$p < .05$	3	$p < .01$		7	$p < .01$		5	$p < .001$
No control		10	$p < .01$						
Authoritarian		9	$p < .01$		10	$p < .01$		4	$p < .001$
Overprotective		11	$p < .01$		9	$p < .01$	$p < .03$	2	$p < .001$
Family rating					8	$p < .01$			
Mental health of family members		12	$p < .01$		11	$p < .01$			
Emotional climate of home		5	$p < .01$						

Note. U = univariate; SE = step entered; MC = multivariate (stepwise regression) cumulative; MVI = missing value indicator.

tional climate of the home. The important role of IQ, socioeconomic status, and various forms of child-rearing practices in predicting adult academic status is striking.

Work Record (Table 17-3)

Univariate analysis indicated that initial relationships with adults are related to work record ($p < .02$); socioeconomic status relates to number of full-time jobs ($p < .05$); and IQ is related to longest full-time job ($p < .05$).

In the multivariate stepwise-regression analysis we see relationships with adults, antisocial behavior, and hyperactivity predicting

TABLE 17-3. Work Record

Predictor variables at initial assessment	Work record (n = 29)			Number of full-time jobs			% Jobs fired			% Jobs laid off			Longest full-time job (weeks)		
	U	SE	MC	U	SE	MC	U	E	MC	U	SE	MC	U	SE	MC
Personal characteristics															
IQ								4	$p < .05$						
Hyperactivity		4	$p < .05$					2	$p < .05$				$p < .05$	1	$p < .05$
Social parameters															
Relationships with adults	$p < .02$	1	$p < .05$					3	$p < .05$						
Peer relations					4	$p < .05$					2	$p < .05$			
Antisocial behavior		2	$p < .05$					6	$p < .05$		3	$p < .05$			
MVI antisocial behavior		3	$p < .05$	$p < .05$	3	$p < .05$		1	$p < .05$		4	$p < .05$			
Family parameters															
Socioeconomic status				$p < .05$	1	$p < .05$					1	$p < .05$			
Age first worked					2	$p < .05$		5	$p < .05$					2	$p < .05$

Note. n = number of subjects working; U = univariate; SE = step entered; MC = multivariate (stepwise regression) cumulative; MVI = missing value indicator.

There were no significant findings for % jobs quit or number of part-time jobs.

work record ($p < .05$), socioeconomic status, age first worked, and peer relations predict number of full-time jobs ($p < .05$). Hyperactivity, IQ, relationships with adults, antisocial behavior, and age first worked all predict percentage of jobs fired ($p < .05$), while socioeconomic status, relationship with adults, and peer relations predict percentage of jobs laid off ($p < .05$). IQ and socioeconomic status are important factors in predicting longest full time job ($p < .05$). We see that percentage of jobs quit and number of part-time jobs had no significant initial predictor variables. It appears that initial measures of relationships with adults and socioeconomic status are important in predicting adult measures related to work record.

Police Involvement (Table 17-4)

The importance of emotional stability (or lack of it) and its relation to various measures of offenses associated with police involvement—for example, number of offenses ($p < .03$), severity of offenses ($p < .01$), and average severity of offenses ($p < .01$)—is striking. Univariate analysis suggest that socioeconomic status ($p < .01$) and IQ ($p < .08$) also relate to number of offenses in adulthood.

In the multivariate stepwise-regression analysis, personal characteristics such as IQ, hyperactivity, and emotional instability; social parameters of peer relations; and the family parameters socioeconomic status, mental health of family members, emotional climate of the home, and the child-rearing practice of overprotectiveness all predict number of offenses ($p < .001$). It is interesting to note that initial measures of aggressivity, antisocial behavior, relationships with adults, and overall family rating did not enter this predictive equation. Aggressivity was highly correlated to emotional stability or lack of it ($p < .01$). This may account for it not entering the equation. However, no such correlations were found for other variables.

In the multivariate stepwise-regression equation predicting severity of offenses ($p < .05$), we see the inclusion of personal characteristics such as aggressivity, emotional instability, and low frustration tolerance; social parameters such as peer and adult relationships; and family parameters including socioeconomic status, mental health of family members, emotional climate of the home and certain child-rearing practices (no control and overprotective). Again, initial antisocial measures and overall family scores are not included.

When examining predictors of average severity of offenses ($p < .05$), we see included personal characteristics such as IQ, aggressivity, hyperactivity, emotional stability, and low frustration tolerance; social parameters such as relationships with adults; and family parame-

TABLE 17-4. Police Involvement

Predictor variables at initial assessment	Outcome variables								
	Number of offenses			Severity of offenses (total)			Severity of offenses (average)		
	U	SE	MC	U	SE	MC	U	SE	MC
Personal characteristics									
IQ	$p < .08$	3	$p < .001$					2	$p < .05$
Aggressivity					9	$p < .05$		4	$p < .05$
Hyperactivity		4	$p < .001$					8	$p < .05$
Emotional instability	$p < .03$	2	$p < .001$	$p < .01$	1	$p < .05$	$p < .01$	1	$p < .05$
Low frustration tolerance					7	$p < .05$		6	$p < .05$
Social parameters									
Antisocial behavior									
MVI antisocial behavior		8	$p < .001$						
Peer relations		7	$p < .001$		10	$p < .05$			
Adult relations					8	$p < .05$		5	$p < .05$
Family parameters									
Socioeconomic status	$p < .01$	1	$p < .001$		2	$p < .05$		3	$p < .05$
Family rating									
Mental health of family members		9	$p < .001$		4	$p < .05$		7	$p < .05$
Emotional climate of home		6	$p < .001$		3	$p < .05$			
Child-rearing practices									
Inconsistent									
No control					5	$p < .05$		10	$p < .05$
Authoritarian									
Overprotective		5	$p < .001$		6	$p < .05$		9	$p < .05$

Note. U = univariate; SE = step entered; MC = multivariate (stepwise regression) cumulative; MVI = missing value indicator.

ters such as socioeconomic status, mental health of family members, and certain child-rearing practices (e.g., no control and overprotective). Again, antisocial behavior is not included.

The importance of initial emotional instability, socioeconomic status, mental health of family members, and certain child-rearing practices is evident in predicting adult antisocial behavior.

Car Accidents (Table 17-5)

Number of accidents and accidents with bodily harm were not associated with any of the initial predictor variables selected. However, cost of damage is univariately associated with low frustration tolerance ($p < .05$) and emotional climate of the home ($p < .05$). The multivariate stepwise-regression analysis includes family parameters of emotional climate of the home and mental health of family members, while personal characteristics included are low frustration tolerance, emotional stability, and aggressivity ($p < .05$). It is interesting to note that hyperactivity and IQ are excluded.

Nonmedical Drug Use (Table 17-6)

None of the initial variables in our analysis were associated with past drug use. Present drug use was associated univariately with mental health of family members ($p < .07$) and multivariately with overall family rating in addition to mental health of family members ($p < .05$).

ALCOHOL

The importance of family parameters is again seen when examining alcohol use. Overall family rating is associated univariately with extent of alcohol use ($p < .06$). It and other initial variables, including hyperactivity, aggressivity, and antisocial behavior, are part of the multivariate stepwise-regression equation predicting extent of alcohol use ($p < .03$). Mental health of family members is part of the equation for extent of maximum alcohol use ($p < .01$).

TABLE 17-5. Car Accidents

Predictor variables at initial assessment	Outcome variable[a]: Cost of damage ($n = 19$)		
	U	SE	MC
Personal characteristics			
Hyperactivity			
Aggressivity		5	$p < .05$
Emotional instability		2	$p < .05$
Low frustration tolerance	$p < .05$	3	$p < .05$
IQ			
Family parameters			
Mental health of family members		4	$p < .05$
Emotional climate of home	$p < .05$	1	$p < .05$

Note. n = number of those who had accidents; U = univariate; SE = step entered; MC = multivariate (stepwise regression) cumulative.

[a]The outcome variables of number of accidents and accidents with bodily injury were not associated with any of the predictor variables and so do not appear here.

TABLE 17-6. Nonmedical Drug Use

Predictor variables at initial assessment	Outcome variables[a]		
	Present drug use (n = 64)		
	U	SE	MC
Personal characteristics			
Hyperactivity			
IQ			
Aggressivity			
Social parameters			
Antisocial behavior			
MVI antisocial behavior		2	$p < .05$
Peer relations			
Family parameters			
Family rating		3	$p < .05$
Mental health of family members	$p < .07$	1	$p < .05$
Emotional climate of home			

	Alcohol[b]					
	Extent of use (n = 49)			Extent of maximum use (n = 49)		
	U	SE	MC	U	SE	MC
Personal characteristics						
Hyperactivity		3	$p < .03$			
IQ						
Aggressivity		5	$p < .03$			
Social parameters						
Antisocial behavior		4	$p < .03$			
MVI antisocial behavior	$p < .08$	2	$p < .03$	$p < .02$	1	$p < .01$
Peer relations						
Family parameters						
Family rating	$p < .06$	1	$p < .03$			
Mental health of family members					2	$p < .01$
Emotional climate of home						

Note. U = univariate; SE = step entered; MC = multivariate (stepwise regression) cumulative; MVI = missing value indicator.

[a]The outcome variable of past drug use was not associated with any of the predictor variables and so does not appear here.

[b]No significant correlation for age first used alsohol or age of maximum use.

	Marijuana/hashish[c]								
	Ever used (n = 49)			Extent of use (n = 49)			Extent of maximum use (n = 49)		
	U	SE	MC	U	SE	MC	U	SE	MC
Personal characteristics									
Hyperactivity									
IQ				$p < .07$	1	$p < .09$			
Aggressivity	$p < .05$	1	$p < .08$						
Social parameters									
Antisocial behavior				4	$p < .09$		$p < .06$	2	$p < .01$
MVI antisocial behavior				3	$p < .09$			3	$p < .01$
Peer relations									
Family parameters									
Family rating							$p < .05$		
Mental health of family members				2	$p < .09$				
Emotional climate of home		2	$p < .08$				$p < .006$	1	$p < .01$

	Other nonmedical drugs: Extent of maximum use[d]								
	Hallucinogens (LSD) (n = 49)			Stimulants (amphetamine) (n = 49)			Barbiturates (Mandrax) (n = 49)		
	U	SE	MC	U	SE	MC	U	SE	MC
Personal characteristics									
IQ	2	$p < .04$		$p < .02$	2	$p < .001$		2	$p < .05$
Hyperactivity					3	$p < .001$			
Aggressivity									
Social parameters									
Antisocial behavior	$p < .02$	1	$p < .04$	$p < .001$	1	$p < .001$			
MVI antisocial behavior									
Peer relations									
Family parameters									
Mental health of family members					4	$p < .001$	$p < .05$	1	$p < .05$
Emotional climate of home									
Family rating									

[c]No significant correlation for age first used marijuana/hashish or age of maximum use.
[d]No significant findings for cocaine or heroin.

MARIJUANA/HASHISH

In the univariate analysis, whether the subject ever used the drug was associated with initial measures of aggressivity ($p < .05$); the extent of marijuana use related to initial IQ ($p < .07$); and the maximum extent of marijuana use related to initial antisocial behavior ($p < .06$), family rating ($p < .05$), and emotional climate of the home ($p < .006$).

In the multivariate stepwise-regression equations, aggressivity and emotional climate of the home marginally ($p < .08$) predicted if marijuana was ever used. IQ, antisocial behavior, and mental health of family members again marginally ($p < .09$) predicted extent of marijuana use, while antisocial behavior and emotional climate of the home combined to predict extent of maximum marijuana use ($p < .01$).

OTHER DRUGS

Generally, few subjects used cocaine or heroin. This may account for the fact that there were no significant findings for these drugs.

Univariate findings showed that with regard to maximum use of hallucinogens, initial antisocial behavior was related ($p < .02$); IQ ($p < .02$) and antisocial behavior ($p < .001$) were associated with maximum stimulant use; and mental health of family members related to barbiturates ($p < .05$).

The multivariate stepwise-regression equations showed that for hallucinogens, antisocial behavior and IQ were predictive ($p < .04$). For stimulant use, antisocial behavior, IQ, hyperactivity, and mental health of family members predictive ($p < .001$), and for barbiturates, mental health of family members and IQ were important predictive factors ($p < .05$).

Peer relations did not enter any equations, but this item was highly correlated with antisocial behavior ($p < .01$), so its absence may not be so significant. In general, initial IQ, antisocial behavior, and mental health of family members were important predictors of alcohol and nonmedical drug use.

DISCUSSION AND SUMMARY

This type of predictive study has a number of limitations. One of the most important is that we have no measure of intervening variables which may affect outcome. Therefore, it must be stressed that the associations outlined between initial factors and adult outcome are not causal in nature. Another limitation is that some measures did not have corroborative data from other sources but relied on subject's reports— for example, nonmedical drug or alcohol abuse and antisocial behavior. Although we did interview parents and send out questionnaries to schools and employers, these external sources were often not familiar with the above areas of the subject's life. Police and court records are not available for minors. We did obtain data from computerized court records for those individuals over 18 years and thus subject to adult courts. These data are helpful but do not entirely overcome the difficulties, since many subjects with antisocial behavior and/or nonmedical drug use may never have had any police or court involvement.

Generally, our findings suggest that any particular adult outcome is not associated with a particular initial variable, but with the additive interaction of personality characteristics and social and family parameters. (See summary Tables 17-7 and 17-8.) Having said that, it must also be stressed that certain predictor variables stand out as being more important than others because they come into almost every outcome measure in a very significant way. This is particularly true of family parameters such as *socioeconomic status* and *mental health of family members*. Thus, in addition to other variables, socioeconomic status is an important factor in educational and work outcomes, as well as police involvement. The importance of socioeconomic status in predicting adult outcome in children with minimal brain dysfunction was also pointed out by Milman.[4] Similarly, mental health of family members entered (with other variables) significantly into adult emotional adjustment, police involvement, and nonmedical drug use. The importance of family parameters in predicting adolescent outcome measure of aggressivity, delinquency, and school performance was shown by Loney et al.[5] Our study suggests that different aspects of these family measures may predict different areas of outcome; for example, socioeconomic status predicts education and work success, while mental health of family members predicts emotional adjustment and nonmedical drug use.

With regard to personal characteristics, IQ enters almost every outcome measure and is particularly important in educational achievement and nonmedical drug use. The importance of IQ in predicting outcome has been shown by many others.[4,5] Loney et al.[5] have also stressed the greater importance of aggressivity versus hyperactivity in predicting adolescent outcome. We see that both factors entered into outcome measures of educational achievement, police involvement, and nonmedical drug use. Hyperactivity without aggressivity was involved in outcome measures of emotional adjustment and work record, while aggressivity (without hyperactivity) was involved in car accidents. It should be pointed out that aggressivity was often highly correlated with emotional stability (or lack of it) and low frustration tolerance.

TABLE 17-7. Initial Predictors of Adult Outcome

1. *Emotional adjustment*
   Personal characteristics
   Hyperactivity
   Emotional stability
   Low frustration tolerance
   IQ
   Family parameters[a]
   Family rating
   Mental health of family members
   Emotional climate of the home

2. *School performance*
   Personal characteristics
   Hyperactivity
   Aggressivity
   IQ[a]
   Social–academic parameters
   School performance
   Antisocial behavior
   Family parameters
   Socioeconomic status[a]
   Mental health of family members
   Emotional climate of the home
   Child-rearing practices[a]

3. *Work record*
   Personal characteristics
   IQ
   Hyperactivity
   Social parameters
   Relationships with adults[a]
   Peer relations
   Antisocial behavior
   Family parameters
   Socioeconomic status[a]
   Other
   Age first worked

4. *Police involvement*
   Personal characteristics
   IQ
   Emotional stability[a]
   Low frustration tolerance
   Aggressivity
   Hyperactivity
   Social parameters
   Peer relations
   Relationships with adults
   (*not* antisocial behavior)
   Family parameters
   Socioeconomic status[a]
   Mental health of family members[a]
   Emotional climate of the home
   Child-rearing practices[a]

5. *Car accidents (cost of damage)*
   Personal characteristics
   Aggressivity
   Emotional stability
   Low frustration tolerance[a]
   (*not* hyperactivity)
   Family parameters
   Emotional climate of the home[a]
   Mental health of family members

6. *Nonmedical drug use*
   Personal characteristics
   Aggressivity
   IQ[a]
   Hyperactivity
   Social parameters
   Antisocial behavior[a]
   Peer relations
   Family parameters
   Mental health of family members[a]
   Emotional climate of the home
   Family rating

[a]Indicates most powerful predictor variables.

TABLE 17-8. Most Important Initial Predictors

1. *Emotional adjustment*
   Family parameters
     Family rating
     Mental health of family members
     Emotional climate of the home

2. *School performance*
   Personal characteristics
     IQ
   Family parameters
     Socioeconomic status
     Child-rearing practices

3. *Work record*
   Social parameters
     Relationships with adults
   Family parameters
     Socioeconomic status

4. *Police involvement*
   Personal characteristics
     Emotional stability
   Family parameters
     Socioeconomic status
     Mental health of family members
     Child-rearing practices

5. *Car accidents (cost of damage)*
   Personal characteristics
     Low frustration tolerance
   Family parameters
     Emotional climate of the home

6. *Nonmedical drug use*
   Personal characteristics
     IQ
   Social parameters
     Antisocial behavior
   Family parameters
     Mental health of family members

Both these initial measures were very important in a number of out-come measures (e.g., emotional adjustment, police involvement, and car accidents). Therefore, the role of this complex of aggressivity, emo-tional instability, and low frustration tolerance cannot be underesti-mated in influencing outcome.

Another predictive concern has been with regard to the role of initial antisocial behavior in predicting outcome. Even though it appears as an important predictor in nonmedical drug use and as a less crucial one in school performance and work record, it does not appear in predicting adult police involvement. This suggests that the combination of emotional instability, low frustration tolerance, and aggressivity may be more important in adult offenses than antisocial behavior in childhood.

The interesting comparison of initial versus adolescent measures in predicting adult outcome has not yet been done.

In summary, even though some initial measures are more impor-tant in predicting particular outcome variables—for example, IQ in predicting education completed; socioeconomic status in predicting work, education, and police involvement—generally our findings point to the importance of several factors such as personality characteristics and family and social parameters all acting together and cumulatively in predicting outcome. This explains why long-term drug studies have generally not resulted in as positive an outcome as was once hoped for. It also points to the need for a multifaceted approach in treating these children.

TREATMENT ISSUES

CHAPTER EIGHTEEN

CLINICAL VIGNETTES OF PSYCHOTHERAPY AT DIFFERENT AGES

The life so short, the craft so long to learn.—From *Aphorism*, by Hippocrates, 460–377 B.C.

In the existing literature on the clinical management of hyperactives, while considerable attention has been given to home management and parental counseling, much less attention has been paid to individual psychotherapy. Since during the course of the long-term follow-up study we gained some clinical experience with using this modality for hyperactives from the preschool years to adulthood, this chapter presents illustrative case vignettes on the use of individual psychotherapy for hyperactives of different ages.

Psychotherapy for hyperactive children, adolescents, and adults is often an important aspect of the total management, particularly for those adjustment problems which are secondary to the primary symptoms of the syndrome or occur in association with them. For example, concurrent neurotic problems of hyperactives, manifestations of low self-esteem, or suicidal risk without clear evidence of depression are not generally responsive to medication. Psychotherapy with hyperactives had certain built-in difficulties, some of which were specific to different age periods.

In an early study in which they compared the efficacy of medication, placebo, and psychotherapy on hyperkinetic and neurotic children, Eisenberg and coworkers[1] showed that hyperkinetic children respond less well than neurotic children to brief individual psychotherapy. While this study does not seem to have been replicated, the clinical impression gained by one of the present authors in treating young hyperactive children with play therapy (often for the purpose of ameliorating secondary or concurrent neurotic symptoms) matched Eisenberg's findings. (We emphasize that these impressions are clinical and are not supported by empirical studies.)

Young hyperactive children were so restless and distractible that they had difficulty engaging in symbolic play. They did generally make a positive relationship with the therapist, which may have helped them to some extent, but they did not stay still long enough and were not reflective enough to "hear" and therefore benefit from explanation, clarification, or interpretation. These young children were treated before stimulants were in use in our clinic. Concomitant use of stimulants might have made them more amenable to play therapy.

CASE EXAMPLE: DERRICK

Derrick is an exmple of a positive and enduring relationship made in childhood during the 2 years of weekly play therapy, for which he was taken on because he had very low self-esteem, cried easily, and sometimes "wished he were dead." The memory the therapist has about the therapy with Derrick is that he usually ran in and out of the playroom, and while in the playroom spent much of the time pretending he and the therapist were racing cars. Derrick and his therapist sat on little chairs which they pushed as fast as possible round and round the room, making loud noises. The therapist usually tired first and does not remember that Derrick ever heard anything she said. However, when play therapy was terminated because Derrick had improved (probably partly as a result of the parent counseling), he was sad and during his last session gave the therapist his "transitional object,"[2] a mink tail, for her to keep.

Sixteen years later Derrick saw the therapist again for 10-year follow-up. He had been away at boarding school and had not been seen in between. He asked hesitantly whether she still had the mink tail. He was delighted that it had been treasured, and said he only wanted it back when his first child was born.

Difficulties were also encountered in individual therapy with adolescents, but these were somewhat different in nature. Their hyperactivity had often improved but they were far behind in school, had difficulties socially, and sometimes had antisocial behaviors. While they could, and did, benefit from psychotherapy, and were at that age where they were literally hungry to understand their own difficulties, they required much more than individual psychotherapy and family counseling. Educational assessment and remediation, social-skills training, and available community resources where skills could be acquired in a somewhat less than normally competitive setting (such as skills in sports or karate) were all necessary. Adolescents often felt themselves to be a complete failure in all aspects in secondary school, a feeling that was usually only reversed if they discovered that they had a special talent (e.g., Ian's talent in helping other adolescents "on drugs"; see Chapter 21) or someone took a particular interest in them (e.g., Jeffrey's principal, see Chapter 13). A broad range of therapeutic input is required to begin to reverse this profound sense of failure which, in the final analysis, can only be reversed by actual success experiences. Psychotherapy is only one of the many inputs which can be helpful to hyperactive adolescents.

During the 10- and 15-year follow-up evaluations, several adult hyperactives requested individual therapy. Four of them were taken on for this, and a few others were taken on for brief counseling. The 4 who participated in what was intended to be long-term psychotherapy will be described briefly.

CASE EXAMPLE: DAVID

David, age 21 years, had been given a tentative diagnosis of Antisocial Personality Disorder with severe residual symptoms of hyperactivity. He requested therapy after his marriage broke up and he was depressed. He was making money by selling cocaine (which he also took). While in therapy he gave up selling and using the drug (he still smoked hash) and found a "square" job at which he earned considerably less. He stayed off cocaine for 4 months and worked well in therapy. Then, suddenly and without notice, he quit therapy by not showing up; telephone contact indicated that he could not give up the excitement of his previous life-style. He came in once more expressing conflict about the various paths for his future. Much later we learned he had gone relatively "straight." It is hard to say if psychotherapy had had some effect on this decision.

CASE EXAMPLE: RANDY

Randy, age 21 years, initiated psychotherapy while in acute crisis, being seriously suicidal. He was abusing several drugs, mainly hallucinogens and hash, was prostituting himself as a gay, and felt hopeless about himself and his future. He wished to come twice weekly and was reliable and on time for sessions. In therapy he improved, and what had seemed like a thought disorder (but was probably related to the concoctions of drugs he consumed) disappeared. He almost completely stopped taking hallucinogens (being warned these were higly dangerous for him) and used only hash. He got a job making sandwiches at a snack bar. He remained socially isolated but was no longer suicidal. After 6 months he stopped therapy and made peace with his mother, with whom he had stopped contact and who lived out west. Against the therapist's advice, he stopped therapy and moved to join his mother. While he had improved, it was felt he would be likely to relapse. The diagnosis was Borderline Personality Disorder.

CASE EXAMPLE: HENRY

Henry came into individual psychotherapy at the age of 24 because of a call from his mother stating she was worried that he was "suicidal." He was living at home, had never held a job longer than 2 months, and had no friends of either sex. He was close to both his parents, and seemed to have no life of his own. He was found to have a moderately severe characterological type of depression and a severely dependent personality. He continued to have learning disabilities.

Henry was in weekly therapy for 1 year. He learned to drive the family car in order to come to sessions, and learned to talk about his own needs and to distinguish the difference between what he thought and felt and what his mother thought and felt. After some months he went to Club Med alone and while there had a brief affair with a young woman. He felt much better on his return and was encouraged enough to find himself a job. He is still working in this job. He discontinued therapy after 1 year; he could not take any more time off work. It was considered that he had improved considerably, but that he remained dependent. He was no longer depressed or suicidal. He still had no stable friends, and continued to have learning disabilities which affected his abilities at work.

CASE EXAMPLE: JIMMY

Jimmy was the 24-year-old son of two professional parents, both university teachers, whose expectations of their children were very high. He came into therapy because he felt depressed and for some time had contemplated suicide. He felt he did not fit in anywhere and had been unable to find a job. He had failed out of university 2 years previously, mainly because of poor study habits, difficulty concentrating, and possibly some remaining learning disabilities, particularly poor organization skills.

Jimmy was very intelligent and unusually introspective. There were no antisocial problems and he had a healthy personality. His difficulties centered not only around his sense of failure (compared to his parents and sibs) but also around his fluctuating self-esteem. On the one hand there was his poor performance, of which he was acutely aware, and he saw his life as a series of failures. He did not wish to live if this continued, and his thoughts of suicide were serious. On the other hand, he believed himself to be gifted and bright, and could not reconcile these divergent internal images of himself.

After 4 months of therapy Jimmy had enough confidence to find himself a job which he felt was interesting and which utilized his abilities. He remained in therapy 1½ years, stopping because he felt much improved. He is still working and wishes to go back to university to finish his MBA. He feels his present job, although interesting, is not sufficiently challenging and does not come up to his best image of himself.

These four cases show the diversity of the problems of the adult hyperactives who ask for treatment. Three of them clearly came into therapy in crisis and had personality disorders. The fourth (Jimmy) was different; his difficulties related to an unstable self-image. He is likely to need more therapy later should he not succeed in all his aims. While some of his problems of self-esteem continue, he clearly benefited from psychotherapy.

More subjects at all ages, but particularly in adulthood, asked for individual therapy than we could take on or find therapists for. It would have been impossible to do a controlled study of the efficacy of psychotherapy because those who wished to have this therapy formed a highly selected group—being either in severe crisis, or, if not in crisis, being stable enough to come regularly for appointments and continue therapy during periods when the sessions were difficult. Responding to psychotherapy requires some degree of being able to see something through, a quality not all of the hyperactive adults had, even in adulthood.

While these individual case reports are interesting, one cannot confuse clinical impressions from a few selected patients with controlled empirical findings. The whole area of therapies other than stimulants and behavior therapies (which have been studied) requires a great deal of further investigation not only for hyperactive adults, but also for hyperactive children and adolescents.

In conclusion, one can say that psychotherapy was at times, and at different ages, of varying degrees of benefit. For several adolescents and adults it seemed to be the only effective modality of treatment for crises (usually with suicidal risk) or for long-standing problems of self-esteem. Different problems of psychotherapy were encountered at different ages. For the preschoolers particularly, their hyperactivity and impulsivity made play therapy almost impossible. A useful medication used concomitantly might have helped. For adolescents individual psychotherapy is usually only one of the various therapeutic inputs which are required. For adults the problems encountered are diverse, and some seek help in crisis. For the latter a crisis-intervention psychotherapeutic model is helpful, particularly if this is given by someone who understands the childhood problems of these adult patients. Often those who seek help in adult life have personality disorders only some aspects of which are reversed by treatment.

CHAPTER NINETEEN

THE EFFICACY OF MEDICATION ON HYPERACTIVE ADOLESCENTS AND ADULTS

Who shall decide, when doctors disagree. . . . ?—From *Epistle to Lord Bathurst*, by Alexander Pope, 1688–1744

It has been clearly demonstrated that stimulants given to children are effective in reducing symptomatology of the hyperactive syndrome at least in the short term, even though no study has as yet demonstrated long-term efficacy. But, as Gittelman[1] pointed out, "It seems that investigators are placing unusual expectations on a treatment: first, it should reverse symptoms that are the primary diagnostic signs; second, it should ameliorate all secondary complications; and third, it should improve eventual functioning. No psychiatric treatment has been shown to have such a rich therapeutic impact" (p. 446).

With respect to hyperactive adolescents and adults, the most systematic and controlled investigations of any treatment are studies of the acute efficacy of stimulant medication. There are relatively few empirical data on the efficacy of other forms of treatment either alone or in combination with stimulants. The lack of research in this area is unfortunate because, as previous chapters have indicated, many hyperactive children become troubled adolescents and adults. As a consequence, this chapter is devoted to a discussion of the existing controlled studies of the efficacy of stimulant medication for adolescents and adults. Some reference to uncontrolled studies involving stimulants and tricyclic medications will also be made.

STIMULANT THERAPY OF HYPERACTIVE ADOLESCENTS

The question arises whether stimulants should be continued or should be stopped for hyperactive adolescents who continue to be disabled by their symptoms and who may by now have additional problems such as poor social relationships, antisocial behaviors, and increasing difficulty keeping up with schoolwork. The reasons for stopping stimulants during or prior to puberty are various.[2] First, in spite of good evidence to the contrary,[3] it is still widely believed that the so-called paradoxical effect will reverse itself sometime in adolescence. Secondly, there is the concern about the growth-suppressant effect of stimulants and the desire to have adolescents (particularly those who are short) off these drugs until they have completed their growth spurt. Thirdly, there is the fear of drug addiction. This has not been reported in childhood, at which time most children make it clear that they do not like their pills (which taste bitter, make them feel different, and so on). For more detail see Chapter 20, which deals with children's reactions to taking medication as perceived by them when they were adults.

The first investigators to demonstrate the efficacy of methylphenidate in an uncontrolled study of 10 adolescents age 13–17 years were MacKay and coworkers,[4] who wished to evaluate "the fine point at which the child's sedation shifts to the more familiar adult reaction of stimulation" (p. 560). In this study the dose ranged from 20 mg to 60 mg daily. All the adolescents improved in school performance, but none improved their perceptual abilities (as judged from the Raven Matrices). Nine of 10 adolescents showed improvement on their EEG's. None showed any signs of addiction. The oldest adolescent in the group (17½ years) reported a transient elevation of mood when the dose was raised but otherwise no reversal of the paradoxical effect was observed.

Safer and Allen[5] studied response to stimulants in three groups: subjects who had started to take stimulants when they were children ($n = 14$); those who started to take stimulants when they were children but continued to take them in adolescence ($n = 13$); and those who started to take stimulants in adolescence ($n = 14$). The differences of treatment outcome between the three groups were studied carefully. It was found that the therapeutic response of stimulants in improving hyperactivity did not significantly change from age 6 to age 16 years. Pretreatment teacher ratings indicated that as a group, adolescents were as inattentive as younger hyperactive children. The mean dose of methylphenidate required to improve classroom behavior was not significantly different for older adolescents from what it was for children. Parental resistance to medication was not related to the age of the child, but adolescents tended to be more reluctant than younger children to take medication. There were no reports of abuse or addiction. Subjects in all three groups performed less well in their second year of medication than in their first year, but there was no significant difference regarding this between the groups. The finding that hyperactive adolescents respond as well as children to stimulants supported earlier clinical reports of Oettinger[6] and Gross and Wilson,[7] as well as the study already described by MacKay and coworkers.[4]

A recent study by Varley[8] established the efficacy of methylphenidate in 16 of 22 adolescents with Attention Deficit Disorder with Hyperactivity (ADD[H]) who had been responders to the drug before adolescence. Twenty-two adolescents (13–18 years, mean age 14 years) took part in a double-blind active drug/placebo crossover design. The median doses of the active drug were 15.6 mg daily in the low-dose condition and 30.9 mg daily in the high-dose condition. Parents and teachers completed the Conners Abbreviated Rating Scale on a daily basis, and also wrote out daily narrative comments on each child, which were rated by the investigators on a 3-point scale. (The raters were blind as to the patients' drug condition.) Results indicated that both low- and high-dose levels of methylphenidate were significantly more effective than placebo on both Parent and Teacher Conners Rating Scales and on the narratives. Differences between high and low dose were seen favoring the higher dose on the narrative scoring of parents and teachers, and a trend was seen favoring the higher dose on the Parent and Teacher Conners Scales. There was (as described in the other studies) no evidence of reversal of effect of stimulants for adolescents. The authors noted that to date no study has demonstrated that such a switch mechanism occurs at puberty. (Whether this occurs in normal children is not clear.) Finally, Varley concluded that his results imply a persistence of symptoms of the hyperactive syndrome in adolescence as well as a persistence of drug effect. No drug abuse or addiction was reported in this or in any of the other studies.

Varley's studies were recently confirmed by Coons and coworkers.[9] In a placebo-controlled study of Ritalin on 19 hyperactive adolescents, the efficacy of the drug as measured by Conners Parent Rating Scale global readings and the Continuous Performance Test was again established.

The evidence is clear that hyperactive adolescents who continue to show symptoms of the hyperactive syndrome will continue to benefit from stimulants. So far, no addiction has been reported. Most investigators have used relatively low doses, which would be less likely to retard growth. Nevertheless, this side effect would have to be very carefully monitored in adolescents treated with stimulants, particularly in those who are short or in whom tallness is an important aspect of their body-image ideal. It has been pointed out by Safer and Allen[5] that adolescents are much more reluctant to take stimulants than are children because, as Gittelman[1] pointed out, "they view this kind of intervention as defining them as deviant, sick or maladjusted" (p. 441).

Recently Gastfriend and coworkers,[10] in an open trial on 12 outpatient adolescents with Attention Deficit Disorder, demonstrated the efficacy of the tricyclic desipramine. Eleven patients reported improvement within 1 month, with any delay in improvement being the result of dose adjustments. It was of interest that these investigators followed their subjects for 6–12 months, during which time improvement was sustained for 6 months in 10 of 12 patients. Dosages by the fourth week ranged from 0.58 mg/kg to 2.63 mg/kg and were adjusted to obtain maximum benefit with minimal side effects. (Mean dose at 4 weeks was 1.57 mg/kg.) Plasma levels varied up to tenfold between patients, and no significant relationship was found between plasma level and dose. Side effects included drowsiness, postural dizziness, weight loss, decreased appetite, headache, insomnia, and racing thoughts, all of which were alleviated by dose adjustments.

The authors noted that at follow-up several months later, 4 patients had their doses increased to 3.5–5.9 mg/kg, in order to maintain efficacy. They also pointed out the need for further investigation of desipramine as an alternative drug for treatment, particularly when the stimulants are not useful. In this study the majority of patients (11 out of 12) had previously been treated with stimulants, either without benefit or with excesssive side effects.

STIMULANT THERAPY OF HYPERACTIVE ADULTS

The literature in this area is as yet limited, and the controlled studies which exist are not in agreement with one another. One of the difficulties is that in the two major controlled studies which will be described, the diagnosis of the hyperactive child syndrome was made retrospectively from the childhood histories of adults who presented at psychiatric clinic with symptoms of impulsivity, restlessness, and poor attention. As yet no study exists which investigates the efficacy of stimulants on hyperactive adults in whom the diagnosis was made during their childhood and who in adult life continue to have symptomatology related at least in part to their original syndrome.

In the early 1970s case reports began to appear in the literature which suggested that stimulants were effective for hyperactive adults. Arnold et al.[11] reported a case of a 22-year-old man who had had no previous psychiatric attention but who presented with symptoms of restlessness, anxiety, and concentration problems. He was treated in a double-blind, placebo-controlled, crossover design, using 15 mg dextroamphetamine as the active drug, given twice daily.

Huessy,[12] in a letter to the editor of the *American Journal of Psychiatry* in 1974, suggested that a large proportion of hyperactive children are psychiatrically handicapped as adults and called for a careful exploration of the possible usefulness of pharmacotherapy. He had himself used imipramine (a tricyclic antidepressant), methylphenidate, and dextroamphetamine in adults who had a typical childhood history of hyperactivity. In a later publication Huessy *et al.*[13] carried out an uncontrolled study of 64 adults (about half of whom were females) retrospectively diagnosed as having Minimal Brain Dysfunction (MBD). The majority had had psychotic episodes, and 31% had made suicide gestures or attempts. They were treated with imipramine (5–150 mg daily), amitriptyline (50–125 mg daily), methylphenidate (15–100 mg daily), and dextroamphetamine (10–30 mg daily). Half of these patients were found to respond positively. While this study can be considered as a pilot study showing a potential for the use of various psychopharmacological agents, much more information would have been provided if there had been more stringent inclusion and exclusion criteria, if a placebo control had been used, and if what constituted "improvement" had been more carefully defined. As Gauthier[14] commented, "The population studied appears somewhat atypical by its majority of women and its predominant middle-class origin" (p. 437).

Mann and Greenspan[15] hypothesized that adults who had MBD as children constitute a distinct adult diagnostic entity, "Adult Brain Dysfunction" (ABD), which may exist alone or with other psychiatric problems. Two cases of ABD were described, both of whom benefited dramatically from low doses of imipramine (25–50 mg daily) in terms of improved concentration and greater ability to respond to psychotherapy. DeVeaugh-Geiss and Joseph[16] reported the case of a 20-year-old male who presented with symptoms of poor concentration, distractibility, motor restlessness, auditory hallucinations of a persecutory nature, and paranoid ideation. A double-blind, placebo-controlled trial of dextroamphetamine, secobarbital, and placebo favored dextroamphetamine, which improved concentration and reduced anxiety and restlessness. The above are optimistic reports but are limited to very few cases, and in all of them the diagnosis was established retrospectively, and several different medications were employed.

The first series of controlled studies of a group of adults retrospectively diagnosed as having had the hyperactive syndrome was carried out by Wood, Wender, and coworkers[17,18] in Salt Lake City, Utah. Initially 15 adults were selected from various outpatient clinics in a catchment area of 200,000; they had prominent symptoms of impulsivity, irritability, inattentiveness, restlessness, and emotional lability. Patients who had schizophrenia, primary affective disorders, Organic Brain Syndrome or mental retardation as diagnosed by the Research Diagnostic Criteria of Spitzer[19] were excluded. Wender designed a self-rating adult questionnaire designed to tap continued symptoms of the childhood condition.

Eleven of 15 subjects found to be suitable were studied by means of a double-blind, crossover technique comparing methylphenidate and placebo. This was followed by an open trial of pemoline and/or tricyclic antidepressants. The majority (9 out of 15 subjects) were middle-class women whose average age was 28.0 years ± 4.5 years. The maximum dose of methylphenidate employed was 60 mg daily. It was found to be significantly superior to placebo on ratings of nervousness, ability to concentrate, temper, emotional lability, and energy level. All 15 subjects were given an open trial of pemoline, amitriptyline, or imipramine after the conclusion of the double-blind study. Eight of the 11 showed a good response to methylphenidate in the double-blind trial. Of the 15 subjects in the open drug trial, 4 subjects responded well to pemoline (5–75 mg daily, mean 37.5 mg, while 2 subjects who had failed to respond to stimulants responded to tricyclic antidepressants. At the end of the open trial, 7–12 months later, 10 of the 15 subjects were judged by the clinician to have had a good overall response. Five subjects were unresponsive. None of the patients receiving methylphenidate showed any tendency to abuse the drug, and significant changes attributable to this drug were not seen on the happy-to-sad dimension of the self-report scale. Two females stopped abusing their children, 2 achieved orgasm for the first time, and 5 reported some improvement in their marriages. Drug and alcohol abuse were controlled in 4 patients on medication. It seemed that those "hyperactive" adults who were responsive to any of the four drugs sometimes showed quite a wide range of improvement.

In their subsequent replication study, Wender and coworkers[20] made three modifications. Firstly they devised operational criteria for the diagnosis of Adult ADD(H) (the Utah Criteria). Schizotypal and Borderline Personality Disorders were added to their exclusion criteria. Secondly they obtained normative data on parents' ratings of the Conners Abbreviated Rating Scale[20] when it is filled out by parents of adults instead of teachers of children. To do this, they obtained a cohort of normal schoolchildren whose grandmothers were asked to describe the children's parents, when the latter had been between ages 6–10 years. The supposition made was that normal children probably had normal parents, and in this way a "psychologically healthy" comparison group would be obtained. Data were obtained on fathers of 211 children and on mothers of 249 children. Thirdly they decided to use pemoline as the active drug instead of methylphenidate, since they felt it had less euphoriant properties and would be less likely to be abused.

Sixty patients met the inclusion criteria and participated in a random-assignment, double-blind, 6-week, parallel trial comparing pemoline and placebo. Their average age was 28.3 years, and females outnumbered males 7:6. Twenty-six of these patients were thought to have been true hyperactives as children, scoring in the upper 9th percentile of the PRS (Parent Rating Scale). Only this subgroup of 26 patients showed a significant response to pemoline as compared to placebo. Pemoline was more effective than placebo in reducing motor activity, attentional problems, hot temper, impulsivity, and stress intolerance. It did not significantly affect inability to complete tasks, impaired interpersonal relationships, and affective lability. The average dose of pemoline used was 65 mg daily.

The above study is important for its carefully constructed Utah Criteria, which have been used and adopted also in other studies to diagnose Adult ADD. It is also important for its standardization of the Abbreviated Conners Rating Scale for the purpose of identifying adults who as children have been hyperactive, and, finally, for the demonstration that pemoline was effective as compared to placebo for those adults who had continued symptoms of ADD and who had been "true hyperactives" as children. The study is somewhat limited by the retrospective diagnosis of the childhood condition, even with all the care taken by the investigators to standardize the childhood scale and select only those adults who scored in the worst 5% of the population. It is unclear why the majority of subjects were females in both studies by these investigators when it is known that most hyperactive children (80%) are boys.

The final study to be described is that of Mattes and coworkers[21] in Long Island, New York. The purpose of the study was: (1) to determine whether ADD(H) is a specific diagnostic entity in adulthood; (2) to evaluate, using a double-blind, crossover design, the efficacy of methylphenidate in adults with evidence of residual ADD(H) ($n = 26$); (3) to evaluate the specificity of drug response by also administering methylphenidate to a control group of patients with similar adult symptoms but no childhood history of ADD(H) ($n = 35$). Subjects were 18–45 years of age and had applied to the Hillside Hospital Outpatient Department for clinical treatment. (A few patients called in response to newspaper notices describing the study.) All patients completed a questionnaire which listed five symptoms (restlessness, difficulty concentrating, excitability, impulsivity, and irritability), rated on a 4-point scale. Only patients who scored at least 2.0 were eligible for further evaluation. (A score of 2.0 was at the 90th percentile in the Hillside outpatient population.) To qualify for the study the patients thus selected were interviewed by a psychiatrist and had to receive a rating of at least 2 on three of the five symptoms listed above. A decision was also made as to whether the patient had had childhood ADD(H), which determined if he or she would be in the experimental or control group. Patients were excluded if they met DSM-III criteria for Schizophrenia, major affective disorder, other psychoses, mental retardation, or Organic Brain Syndrome, or if there was evidence of current drug or alcohol addiction (abuse without addiction was not an exclusion criterion.)

The experimental group consisted of 26 patients, while the control group included 35 patients. The two groups were found to differ on several baseline measures, in addition to the retrospective ADD(H) diagnosis. The experimental group had more childhood antisocial and other symptomatology, more drug abuse, less depressive and anxiety symptomatology, performed more poorly on the Tactual Perception Test, began drinking at an earlier age, and were more stubborn and more restless.

All patients received a 3-week double-blind, crossover trial of methylphenidate and placebo in random order. The mean optimal dosage of methylphenidate was 48.2 mg daily. Results showed that the two groups did not differ significantly in response to medication, and methylphenidate was not superior to placebo in either group. Subdividing patients according to the presence or absence of significant depression or anxiety did not change the negative results. Of the total group, 15–25% improved clinically with methylphenidate compared to placebo, but this was not a homogeneous subgroup. The findings of Wender about the predictive value of a childhood history of severe ADD(H) were not confirmed. The authors had some questions about their certainty of making a retrospective diagnosis of the childhood condition and felt that this was valid with 90% certainty in 2 patients and with 70% certainty in 16 of 26 experimental subjects. One interesting finding of this study was that 8 experimental subjects with a DSM-III diagnosis of drug abuse were significantly helped by methylphenidate compared to placebo. A history of drug abuse appeared to be the best predictor of positive methylphenidate response.

It is not easy to understand the discrepant results of Wender's and Mattes's studies. It is possible, but not likely, that pemoline is a more effective stimulant for adults than methylphenidate. More likely is the possibility that the experimental groups in the two studies differed in some undefined way which is obscured by the potential inaccuracies of a retrospective diagnosis. Patients' attitude toward the use of medication may have been more favorable in Utah than in New York. In order to gain clearer ideas as to whether stimulants are effective for adult patients who have continued problems and who had ADD(H) when they were children, it will be important to see the results of double-blind studies of adults who have been prospectively followed since the diagnosis of ADD(H) was made in childhood. Such a study has not yet been carried out.

When one takes a look at the adults in our prospective study who wished to have treatment and whose psychotherapy or crisis intervention was described, it is hard to see how they would have benefited from stimulants, with the exception of David (see Chapter 18). However, if Jimmy does return to university to finish his MBA, stimulants might well be a help while he is there. There are others in the group who have clear-cut continued problems of the syndrome, but who refused when asked (soon after the 15-year follow-up study was completed) to take any form of medication. The "antidrug" attitude which prevails is a deterrent to doing good research on the efficacy of stimulants for those hyperactive adults who would probably benefit the most.

It is also not clear which medication is most useful for hyperactive adults. Pemoline was found to be useful in one study; the efficacy of methylphenidate was established in one study and not in another. Mattes is currently evaluating Tegretol.[22] As yet, we do not have a final answer. However, past experience of the various personal, social, academic, and work difficulties faced by adult hyperactives would dictate that stimulant medication should be just one part of a multifaceted approach.

THE HYPERACTIVE ADULT
LOOKS BACK

ADULT HYPERACTIVE SUBJECTS' VIEW OF THEIR TREATMENT IN CHILDHOOD AND ADOLESCENCE

I would say that the principal contribution made by my doctor to the forming and possibly the conquest of my illness, was that he encouraged me to believe that I was a respected partner with him in the total undertaking.—From *Anatomy of an Illness as Perceived by the Patient*, by Norman Cousins, 1912–1977

All 61 hyperactive adults (mean age 25.1 years) in our study, whose background characteristics were described in detail in Chapter 5 (pp. 66, 67), during the course of the 15-year follow-up evaluation were systematically probed as to their view of the various treatments they had received in their childhood and adolescence. These hyperactives constituted a relatively untreated group, since comprehensive treatment and remediation were not available. Only some members of the group had had adequate remedial education, family or individual therapy, or a useful medication for any length of time. None had received treatment with methylphenidate.

A second group of 20 methylphenidate-treated hyperactive adults were also probed by means of similar forced-choice questions as to their view of the treatment they had received. This group was younger (mean age 21.8 years) and had received carefully monitored methylphenidate treatment for at least 3 years during their childhood and (in some cases) early adolescence. The background characteristics of these hyperactives were described in detail in Chapter 16 (p. 240).

The subjects were asked whether in their view any aspect of their management was helpful, ineffective, or harmful. They were also questioned as to what factors, other than treatment, they considered helpful or harmful during the course of their childhood and adolescence. With respect to drug therapy, subjects were asked about their feelings during childhood related to *taking* medication, *efficacy*, or *harmfulness* of the medication, how the medication had helped, and the side effects which they had had. Both groups of hyperactive subjects were probed with respect to the above questions during the course of structured interviews carried out by the two psychiatrists (G. W. and L. H.). Most of the questions were asked in the form of forced choices, which always included the category "other reasons," so that the subjects could give spontaneous answers which were not covered in the forced choices. Some questions were left open-ended from the start, for example: "Knowing what you know now, what kind of help for your difficulties would you like to have had as you were growing up?"

We found that the hyperactive adults remembered the various treatments they had received during their childhood fairly well; in other words, their reports corresponded well with our records as to types of treatment they had received. They were much less accurate, as might be expected, with respect to details of medications received, such as which drug was given, the dose, the duration of treatment, why the drug was discontinued, and so on.

The responses to the questions regarding what aspects of treatment or other factors were most helpful and most harmful are listed in Tables 20-1 and 20-2. In appraising these responses it becomes clear that, even in the methylphenidate-treated group, aside from maturation, *significant people* (mainly parents, but also teachers and friends) were seen to be most helpful; and significant people were also seen as most harmful by some hyperactives. Methylphenidate treatment was seen as being the most helpful aspect of treatment in 4 of 20 (20%) hyperactives treated with this medication during their childhood; in contrast, only 1 of 37 hyperactives treated with chlorpromazine considered this treatment as the most effective received.

TABLE 20-1. Responses to Question "What Did You Consider Most Helpful When You Were Growing Up in Overcoming Your Difficulties?"

	Group not treated with methylphenidate ($n = 61$)	Group treated with methylphenidate ($n = 20$)
Parents	12	7
Teachers (or other significant persons—tutors, grandparents, friends)	14	3
Maturation	14	4
Medication	1	4
Professional help other than medication	4	1

TABLE 20-2. Responses to Question "What Did You Consider to Be a Hindrance to You (i.e., Harmful) as You Were Growing Up in Trying to Overcome Difficulties?"

	Group not treated with methylphenidate ($n = 61$)	Group treated with methylphenidate ($n = 20$)
Parents	31	7
Some teachers and some friends	46	12
Maturation	3	2
Medication	8	5
Professional help other than medication	2	2

TYPES OF COMMENTS MADE REGARDING PARENTS

The most typical types of comments made about how parents had been helpful to hyperactives were:

- "My parents [or my mother or father] understood me and managed to put up with me when others didn't."
- "My father was always behind me, backing me."
- "My parents generally made me feel that they believed in me."

When parents were seen to be harmful, typical comments were:

- "My father was never home."
- "They were always critical, always on my back."

In general parental fights, lack of family closeness, expecting too much, were frequently complained about. A few subjects told us that their fathers had been alcoholic in their childhood; in some cases this had not been previously revealed. Two reported that they had been physically abused; something else which had been hidden from us previously.

TYPES OF COMMENTS MADE REGARDING TEACHERS

Some hyperactives had had very positive experiences with selected teachers or guidance counselors, which several felt to be "turning points" in their lives. In one case this was a school principal. These key people had taken a very caring attitude and had gone out of their way to be helpful in various ways which included extra teaching, involving the hyperactive in extracurricular activities, and so on. Generally a special relationship had existed which was instrumental in producing more successful school performance and was viewed as increasing self-esteem. Specific comments were:

- "Mrs. _____ liked me, she used her free time to work with me and got me interested in _____."
- "Mr. B [a school principal] was the turning point of my life; it is hard to tell you how much he did for me."

Teachers were also seen at times to be harmful. This occurred in general when hyperactives felt they were being scapegoated, personally disliked, or deliberately ignored. Often the hyperactive adult felt he or she couldn't completely blame the teacher:

- "I would hate to have had someone like me in the class."

Negative comments about teachers typically were:

- "My homeroom teacher did not want me in her class and made it very obvious."
- "Many of the teachers I had put me down and made me feel stupid."
- "One teacher had it in for me; I think he really hated me."

Others beside teachers found particularly helpful by the hyperactives included a guidance counselor, a tutor, grandparents (who accepted the hyperactive better than the parents), and friends who stuck by them when many other peers teased them.

TYPES OF COMMENTS MADE ABOUT MATURATION

Maturation was usually seen as an important (and even the single most important) factor in producing positive changes during adolescence and in early adult life. For example, 14 of 61 untreated hyperactive adults considered they had virtually outgrown their symptoms as a result of maturation; this was true of 4 of 20 methylphenidate-treated hyperactive adults. Five hyperactive adults from the two groups combined considered that growing older (i.e., maturation) had worsened their problems. These hyperactives saw themselves as having seriously deteriorated and as more deviant as adults than as children.

TYPES OF RESPONSES REGARDING THE
EFFECT OF MEDICATION

The type of medication, dose, and duration of treatment have been outlined for the relatively untreated group in Chapter 5 (p. 67) and for the methylphenidate-treated group in Chapter 16 (p. 240).

We shall start by describing the response to medication in the 61 hyperactives who had been treated with chlorpromazine or other miscellaneous medications for under 6 months during their childhood. Of the 61 hyperactive adults, 16 considered that their medication had been helpful, 1 considered it to have been "the most effective treatment received," and 8 considered it to have been harmful to them. The reason given for medication (chlorpromazine) being helpful was nearly always "it calmed me down." Reasons given for medication (chlorpromazine) having been harmful varied and included a balance of factors related to lack of efficacy and the following negative aspects of taking pills:

1. Side effects (with chlorpromazine the comment was: "It made me sleepy").
2. Embarrassment (teachers commenting in front of the whole class, "Jimmy, did you forget to take your pill this morning? You are not behaving").
3. Feeling different (the idea that if they had to take pills, something weird was wrong with them, but they did not know what).
4. The bitter taste.

No subjects felt that their medication had done them any physical harm.

With respect to the group of 20 hyperactives who had received methylphenidate for 3–6 years, 4 of them considered medication to have been the single most important factor in their childhood in overcoming problems. (This compares to 1 in 61 hyperactives in the non-methylphenidate-treated group.) Methylphenidate was seen to be helpful in various degrees by 11 of the 20 hyperactives (this excludes the 4 who felt it was *the* most helpful treatment). It was considered to be relatively ineffective and harmful by 5 subjects; reasons for this will be discussed in detail later. The 16 hyperactives who considered that methylphenidate was very helpful or somewhat helpful gave the following reasons for the pill's efficacy (some gave more than one):

- "They calmed me down." (8)
- "They helped me concentrate." (4)
- "They made me less restless." (5)
- "They helped me behave better." (1)
- "They made me learn better at school." (1)

The 5 subjects who found that methylphenidate was relatively ineffective and harmful gave reasons fairly similar to those given for chlorpromazine:

1. Side effects. These were different for methylphenidate than for chlorpromazine. Typical comments were:
   - "They made me not eat." (6)
   - "They made me tired" (or listless, withdrawn, drowsy; or took pleasure out of life). (6)
   - "I could have been tall instead of short, fat, and dumpy." (Both parents were also short.)

2. Embarrassment.
   - "I felt embarrassed in front of other kids and in the family."
   - "Kids at school laughed at me for having to take pills."
   - "The teacher would ask, 'Did you take your pills today?'" (3)

3. Feeling different (3)
   - "I felt rotten about having to take pills; why me? I had no insight into why."
   - "I didn't mind when I was younger, but as I got older and understood more, I hated it."
   - "They were a bad trip for me all those years. I felt different to the other kids."

4. Expressions of resentment about having had to take medication without reasons being able to be given for the resentment (6)
   - "I hated taking them." (Several said this.)
   - "I just felt I didn't want to take them even though they helped."

Some of the above negative comments were made by subjects who had also felt they had benefited from the medication. These had mixed feelings; as a previous generation felt about castor oil, "I hated it, but it was good for me."

All 81 subjects were asked the open-ended question, "Knowing what you know now, what kind of help would you like to have received in your childhood?" Most subjects wanted more of whatever modality of help they had had and found useful. These included:

1. More individual psychotherapy
   - "Dr. _____ helped me to feel more adult, as though I had more power to change things . . . ."
   - "Dr. _____ made me feel better. I was very taken with her; if I could have had more of those sessions, it would have helped me."

2. More individual tutoring and remedial education. For one hyperactive the guidance counselor gave extra tutoring which was seen as a turning point toward more mastery of the learning process. In another case a tutor who was not a teacher himself helped the hyperactive by working a great deal with him to pass his matrics (final exams) even though he had been far behind in his education.

3. More family counseling. Many subjects said that they felt this had helped their parents to understand them and to interact more constructively with them.

4. More clarification of the problem. Subjects complained that they had never really understood what was wrong with them and neither had their parents.

IMPRESSIONS FROM THE SUBJECTS' RESPONSES

It is clear that the hyperactive subjects (even those treated with a useful medication) most valued caring and positive relationships with significant people, mainly parents, which they felt had helped them most with respect to the problems of their childhood. Some selected teachers, others selected tutors, principals, grandparents, or professionals.

Hyperactives who had not been treated with methylphenidate did not view their medication as particularly helpful. Hyperactives who had been treated with methylphenidate viewed medication more positively, and 75% of them knew what aspects of their problems had been ameliorated. Twenty-five of them felt methylphenidate was the most useful help received.

One unexpected finding was the *degree* of negative feeling expressed about having to take medication in childhood. Sometimes this related to side effects, but more commonly it related to embarrassment and feeling different without adequate explanation. Twenty-five percent considered methylphenidate to have been harmful overall. The remainder found the medication beneficial but generally disliked taking it.

One may ask what the reasons are for these negative feelings and whether they are an inevitable part of taking any medication for any condition. In general in the 1960s, while the use of nonmedical drugs was on the increase in adolescents, there was a concomitant "antimedication" reaction, particularly with respect to psychoactive agents for children, on the part of adults in Montreal. This factor and an inherent fear of the possible unknown effects of the medication may have resulted in parents and teachers conveying their negative attitudes about medication to the children.

Similarly, perhaps the physicians in this study did not take enough care to explain to the children why medication was useful, its effects, and its side effects, and did not give the children and adolescents sufficient time to discuss their reaction to taking pills. Perhaps we left the children out of the decision-making process of whether or not to treat with medication. In these ways we might have been able to reduce the negative feelings which the children had about taking methylphenidate. It is, however, impossible to know whether children can be helped not to dislike taking pills. It is well known that in adults, even when medication clearly prolongs life (e.g., antihypertensive agents), compliance is relatively poor, nor is this necessarily a result of any side effects.

SUMMARY

The hyperactives in our study did not have the opportunity for optimal treatment because resources for this were unavailable. Hyperactive adults indicated that:

1. They considered methylphenidate in general more effective than other medications such as chlorpromazine.

2. Taking medication was associated with many negative feelings.

3. Significant people were generally seen as having been most helpful in facilitating improvement in the childhood condition.

4. They required more information and an opportunity for frank discussion as to what was "wrong with them" and what the medication might do for them.

5. They would have liked to have had available when they needed it: adequate remedial education; tutoring; cognitive therapy (some had had this therapy for some months); individual psychotherapy and family counseling. This comprehensive, multimodality type of therapy was accurately perceived by the adult hyperactives to have been potentially of help to them when they were children, for a condition which has so many areas of deficits.

LOOKING BACK: REMINISCENCES FROM CHILDHOOD AND ADOLESCENCE

IAN MURRAY

Ian Murray was a subject in our 15-year follow-up study of hyperactive children, and we have seen him develop over a period of 20 years. He is now 27 years old and works in a residential treatment center for disturbed children, where he is highly regarded in the field for his special ability to understand and reach children. He plans to finish his degree and apply to medical school.

Ian has written an account of his subjective experiences as a child and adolescent growing up with problems of hyperactivity. We chose him for this in part because his course and outcome were relatively typical of other hyperactive youngsters we had followed, and most importantly, because we believed he would be both capable and willing to undertake this difficult task, which required both skill and courage.

During his childhood Ian was learning disabled, hyperactive, and noncompliant; during his adolescence he engaged in moderate antisocial behavior. Certain fortuitous circumstances helped to change his course from an antisocial to a prosocial one. Like other hyperactive children we have followed into adulthood, Ian had certain personality strengths unique to him. We felt that he had unusual psychological insight and self-awareness, perhaps inherent in him but also acquired both from the voluminous novels he read as an adolescent (once he had mastered sufficient reading skills) and from his association with professionals in the field. Ian held strong views which he articulated eloquently. For these reasons we guessed and then discovered that Ian could successfully describe his childhood experiences in writing, in such a way that readers could share them and understand what it feels like for a child and for an adolescent to grow up being different.

Professionals in the field will appreciate Ian's account of his subjective experience of school failure, social ostracism, referral to a psychiatry depart-

In the interest of protecting the privacy of individuals, most names and identifying details have been altered.

ment, being tested and retested without anyone explaining the results, and finally being a subjection a long-term follow-up study. But they will also appreciate what the external world looks like to a child who is not meeting expected standards, since some encounters were experienced by him as helpful and others were not.

Chapter 10 dealing with social skills and self-esteem concluded, based on results from various tests and rating scales, that adults who had been hyperactive in childhood scored significantly worse than normal controls. Problems in these areas continued in many, even when symptoms of the syndrome had disappeared. The human and developmental aspects of these difficulties are pinpointed by Ian's statement, "My dignity and self-esteem rested on my ability to conceal from anyone that there was anything wrong with me." Since in his childhood Ian never did understand what was wrong with him, believing it to be stupidity, and since his behavior "precluded being able to slip by unnoticed," the good sense of self he attempted to maintain was precarious. Perhaps for Ian a permanent sense of failure was nevertheless avoided by the interplay of his personal qualities, the skilled intervention of interested persons, and, finally, being hired in jobs he valued and in which he was valued.

To Dorothy Ross Till, Dr. Weiss, and my mother and father

I heard on the radio the other day that the graduating class from my old high school is holding its tenth reunion this month. Most of my former classmates are no longer living in Montreal, having left to pursue careers in others parts of Canada or the United States as opportunities for success have been displaced west and southward.

At a time in life when those tasks of consolidation and integration, fundamental to the shedding of excess anxieties, self-doubts, and distant yearnings, should have already taken place, I find myself alone, secretly incomplete. I am not sure why the radio message should bother me so much, except for the feeling that once again I have fallen behind; maybe it's that I never caught up in the first place, or ever will.

The sequence of my development has been incongruous at best, chaotic at worst. Growing up in an environment that nurtured and imbued the idea of professional success, I was left in a paradoxical dilemma, since as a child success eluded me, and I was unable to decipher those elements which make a person whole, complete, and which I seemed to lack. Our most precious human resource is our brain, the organ of "intelligence." In a child's eyes this can become an either/or proposition. You are "dumb" or "smart"; the in-betweens only come later with experience, at a time when one is able to see the shortcomings of such a rigid system which defines a child as a success or failure. Only to some degree did I become aware of the fallacy before I was hardened by the unfulfilled expectations others had of me, and the negative labels that followed me as I was molding my self-image through the eyes of others.

I still ask myself, if a child is born to a milieu and his constitution is different from those around him although it is not seen clearly by him or by others as such, at least at the beginning, what happens when he is confronted by the uninhibited unleashing of his own impulses counterpointed by negative external judgments that time after time bear down on him? This causes him either to hold in suspicion his own abilities or to stop believing in those things which define him as good or bad. However, I also ask myself why *should* accommodation be made for children who go beyond the accepted limits, particularly when their breaking of accepted rules appears deliberate and ungrateful.

I did better in my final year in high school than at any other time in my public-school career, though I did not graduate. So I knew they would not be sending me an invitation to the reunion.

During the course of my last year in high school, it was not necessary for me to prove any longer that I could measure up to the expectations that others had. Like a marathon in which I was the only runner, the race was only with myself against the unknown obstacles of the environment. But I was winning the race at the time since I had been accepted into university without having to complete high school, and was working part time as a youth worker in a hospital-based crisis clinic. Being the youngest staff member, I flourished in the status it brought. This experience was a turning point in my life, the single most important affirmation of my abilities. But though chance (or fate) played a decisive role, I had prepared for this kind of opportunity for a couple of years, quietly amassing experiences and gaining self-taught knowledge which began to bring me some esteem, albeit fragile, so that I dared to take more risks, and thus was able to manipulate the odds to ensure a better chance of success.

Looking back, I was fortunate to have spent my formative adolescent years in a cultural time phase (the late 1960s and early '70s) when my defiance in high school could be justified by the generalized social and political disobedience ubiquitous during that era, so that my rebellion was not viewed only as my personal and educational failure. In this way I was saved a "special-education" class, which at that time would have expected too little and put a final seal on my already existing sense of incompleteness. Instead, I held on tenaciously to my jeans, long hair, and suburban rebelliousness along with my peers. The ideals and values which were to become fundamental to my growth as an individual took root in the quiet despair never externalized or even thought out during the comings and goings of my adolescence. An awkward credo which I had written for myself when I was 14 served as my own "bloody truth": "To conceive of what you desire is to experience what you possess." Whatever this meant to me, I hung onto it fiercely.

Ironically, while being far behind in school achievement, I was in some ways more mature than my peers. But I underestimated my difficulties in the academic sphere. I went away to a small out-of-town university, and stuck it out for 1 year, scraping by academically and socially. I came back to Montreal for another year and a half to work in the crisis clinic before returning to a second university for another 2 years. I did better this time, receiving A's in some subjects and failing to complete others. Problems of organization and distractibility were still present, and their existence had been denied by me. Although I did not receive a degree, I recognized during this time that I had the ability to complete university and in all probability would not have to relinquish the career I had chosen, which required academic accreditation. For many years before, I had felt suspended in limbo, while others were observing the natural progression of my "hyperactivity." . . .

The town of Abbotsville, where I was born, was an established community nestled just outside Montreal city limits, purposely designed and circuitously arranged so as to cushion, lessen, the impact of urban living. It used to be called a "model city." An upper-middle-class suburb, its streets, parks, and intersections beckoned quiet, stable relationships. The routines seemed prearranged and curiously adept. I was the youngest of three, and we spent our time and rituals in the same manner as everyone else: work, church, school, polite neighborliness, and family togetherness. My father and mother assumed their roles without obvious hesitation. Mother had been a teacher for 6 years before getting married and my father was a chartered accountant. My mother did not work and my parents were always there, ready in a well-organized responsible manner. In retrospect, I realize it was hard for them to understand what was going on with me, or to have any confidence in my ultimate future.

I was born on Labor Day several days earlier than expected. Mom says that during my first 6 months I was a good, happy baby, waiting quietly in my crib for her to come to me. Our baby-sitter swears I was sitting up watching TV by 4 months. Then from a crawling position I ran, and we were off. My brother, David, was 2½ years older and my sister, Andrea, 6 years older than I. I was all over the house, into their things, into pots and pans, and Mom soon realized I could not be left alone. Darting here, there, and anywhere, I didn't like playing with toys, preferring to explore on my own.

The telephone rings—the neighbor across the street is calling to let my mother know I'm running down the street without clothes. Pursuit begins. It ends with my parents deciding to put me in a harness, which my Mom attaches to a long lead tied to the railing outside the house. The same neighbor calls again to let her know I am at the side of the house pillaging through the garbage cans, eating scraps. Mom decides to take me with her whenever she can. We go shopping together, since David and Andrea are in school. She wants to try on a dress and, taking me into the fitting room, she forgets for a minute I'm there. Looking around, I'm gone but she can hear muffled shouts, then giggles. I am crawling under the other fitting-room curtains surprising the clients. Embarrassed, red-faced, Mom takes me home.

My brother David's kindergarten class is having an open house. Rather than leave me home, Mom decides to bring me along. Charging around the classroom, I am fascinated by all the new things there are. Trying to be in two places at the same time, Mom smiles with tense lips and suppressed anger as she attempts to grab hold of me and pay attention to the performance at the same time. Finally, one of the fathers scoops me up and places me on his lap with a firm grip.

My own kindergarten experience passed relatively unnoticed by either school or my parents. It was only half days and this seemed to give enough of a break for me to pass unnoticed. The complaints didn't start until my first year of grade school.

The Grade 1 teacher, Mr. Roach, was a particularly severe disciplinarian, who had a variety of techniques for punishing misbehavior. I remember standing for what seemed like hours at my desk with arms outstretched and a book in each hand. At other times, a few of us would be lined up in a row beside his desk awaiting the arrival of a whack with his wooden ruler on our knuckles. A story that circulated for several years after he was dismissed was how he had sent one pupil, no longer there, to the hospital with a fractured wrist . . . That year with Mr. Roach I spent most of my time in the corridors pacing back and forth between some invisible boundary listening to the waves of sound from different classrooms rise and fall.

The days are overcast, cold, steel gray. I don't seem to know what's going on at school. I'm failing everything. The principal requests testing, which is carried out by the school-board psychologist, Mr. Ken Murray (no relation!). I liked him from the day he came to get me from the class. Holding my hand, he escorted me to a small office reserved for such things, I imagine. I wasn't told the results, but Mrs. Richards, the principal, is recommending to my mother that I repeat Grade 1 and in the meantime she's going to give her special puzzles and games to play with me at home. David wants to know, snickering, if there are any three or four-piece puzzles he can work on too.

I thought it was going to be a regular checkup. Our pediatrician, Dr. O'Neill, is talking to my mother outside the examination room. Straining to hear what they are saying, I quickly maneuver myself down from the table in my underwear, trying not to crinkle the wax-like tissue paper covering the examination bench. By the doorway I can hear Dr. O'Neill suggesting to my mother that I be referred to the Montreal Children's Hospital for further testing concerning my _____. I can't hear what. "How come I have to go to the hospital?" I asked my mother on our way home in the taxi. "So that we can understand why you are having so much trouble at school," she replied. Nervously, I refrain from more questions.

The hospital is humming with people and activity. They seem to bump into each other as crowds cluster around doorways and benches. Past wards and on elevators, the chorus is broken by voices over loudspeakers announcing that Doctor *this* is immediately required in department *that*. The corridors are flooded by soft urine-like yellow lighting, as we make our way to the Department of Psychiatry on the fifth floor and reach Dr. Werry's office. He greets us and then asks if I mind sitting outside his office while he speaks to Mom. He hands me crayons and paper. Waiting patiently, I draw a picture of a house and lawn with flowers. Soon I am called in too. Dr. Werry is wearing a long white coat and he asks me a lot of questions. I am not sure what he is getting at, but I feel comfortable and like his warm manner. I feel important trying to answer his questions. I went back several more times that year, doing more and more tests, which left me more confused, wondering what was happening. On one occasion I was taken into a room in front of a lot of doctors and Dr. Werry was asking me all the same questions over again. He then asked me to write words I could spell onto a blackboard. I don't know if I can spell any words, but all the doctors look pleased.

I am back at the hospital again; my Mom tells me it is for an "EEG." Dr. Werry isn't around, but they have me sit on a chair as they begin to tape long wires to my head; first they wash these spots with what smells to me like alcohol, just like at Dr. O'Neill's before I get a needle. So I know they are going to stick the wires into my brain, but they say it won't hurt. They ask me to lie down and I see queer-looking pens squiggle outlines and mountain-type shapes on long strips of paper. They tell me to keep still; I can't do it; I want to go home.

During the summer the school psychologist recommends that I attend a camp he has set up which has a special section for children like me, so that he can observe me more carefully. My parents send my unwilling brother along with me because I am only 7. He was more homesick than I was.

I start Grade 1 over, and Rosemary wants to know why I flunked. She thinks "it's weird," and so do the other kids. I don't know what to answer so at lunch I tell my mother that the kids at school are teasing me. She instructs me to tell them that "it's none of their business; they don't know anything about it." For me it's easier to just punch them out.

Dr. Werry has given my mother a large plastic container to pee into every night. The hospital wants a week's supply. Every evening she holds the bottle out steadily for me in the bathroom, looking serious, purposeful, and hopeful. Being the first up in the morning, I set the table while my Dad is shaving. This morning I am momentarily halted by the specimen bottle wrapped in a brown paper bag beside my father's place. I carefully set the dishes around it. He is to take it to work and drop it off at the hospital in his lunch hour. That day, he comes home apologetic; he had left it in the train by accident. We all laughed, wondering who took it and if they would know what it was.

Mrs. Rowe is my new Grade 1 teacher. Kindly and near retirement, she lives close to the school. I like her a lot as she encourages every success and I feel proud helping her when I can. Arithmetic is going much better because now I understand most of the concepts being taught. No longer do I have to hesitate when we have a quiz to do. Mom has bought the "Dick and Jane" reader so that she can drill it into me each night. Drill, drill, drill it in; this is how she was shown to teach. The hospital wants to know how things are going; I hear my mother tell Dr. Werry on the phone, "Homework is a 'battle royal.' He likes to play checkers, but he cheats." Twenty years later, perusing my research chart, I read a note from Mrs. Rowe which says:

Ian is very bossy in class, and needs to be in control with the other kids. He has great difficulty making or keeping friends. Most of the kids in class think he tries to get them into trouble. Would love to take charge, quite the organizer. Inattentiveness and now nonconformity are always disruptive to any class. One is always aware of his presence which, if allowed, could become unpleasant to the other pupils. Ian is an attention seeker whether by fair means or foul. He can be an extremely polite and helpful child and gets along much better with adults than children. He wants affection and is usually responsive. He has a lot of personality.

Dr. Werry has sent pills [chlorpromazine] to my mother for me to take. They are kept in a manilla envelope in the cupboard over the fridge.

Each morning I eat one before going to school. They taste awful. You are not supposed to eat them: "Swallow it whole," I am told. I'd rather eat them. One day I see Mrs. Rowe on the way to school. I ask her if I'm doing better since I am taking pills. "They must be 'good boy pills,'" she says. In my research chart I read Mrs. Rowe's comment: "Since on medication, Ian now has a desire to be good. But he still fights constantly and his work and play patterns are chaotic. Ian has not applied himself, but I feel he is a bright child and should be above average when he finally settles down."

In any case, I got better marks that year, and passed. I felt great.

"You're not special," snaps my Grade 2 teacher when I ask her for extra arithmetic stencils. I am frequently out in the halls again. This time by the staircase, standing in a corner, confined but restless, I find a round flat plate covering a hole. I pretend to unbolt it, spinning it endlessly round and round with my finger. I didn't really expect to loosen it. Beside me there is a wire mesh door leading to a small staircase fenced in by the same braid-like wire. It leads to a small boiler room I think. I imagine myself locked up in whatever is behind the door, free to do what I want.

Throughout grade school some teachers made sincere efforts to help, others opted to pass me over, demanding little, expecting even less, and hoping for my eventual classroom conformity which would not undermine the rights of others. Rote phrases I hear throughout my childhood are "Slow down, Ian," or "Now remember, Ian, you are fooling nobody but yourself." They were wrong. I never wanted to fool myself and I did not know how to slow down.

Often I am sent out of the class for disruptive behavior, and to the principal's office. This happens so often that the countertop outside her office acts as a kind of growth chart for me as I wait on the bench. It soon becomes a matter of survival, as I become hardened to punishment or harsh words. Deep down I know they are right. I don't fit in, but I cannot change it. I must find an alternative. This was not a well-thought-out decision or anything like that. I knew that I had fallen so far behind the others that no amount of catching up would change the perceptions or expectations others had of me.

In a manner of speaking I was the class clown. I could break the monotony of the daily routines with witty comments or antics. The relief was at times welcomed even by the teachers. This occasional approval encouraged me to greater acts of daring. But for some reason I was terrible at gauging just how far I could go before the final "get out" shot across the room, stopping me in mid-action or sentence. On this occasion, I am again sent to the principal's office; this time she decides to give me the strap.

I tried, but I could not hold it in as the leather strap curled up and cracked on my hand. I had never seen Mrs. Richards look that way before as she gave it to me four times on each hand. I wished I had worn my corduroys; how could I return to my class with the noticeable spots dribbled on my pants? I'll punch anyone who says anything, I promise myself. A lull falls over the class as I make my entrance and return to my desk, which I notice is not where it was. Mrs. Dean has moved me to the front, right beside her. I try not to look at anyone as I walk through the classroom. Silently to myself I dare anyone to say anything about my wet pants.

I feel drained. My pants are almost dry. I wonder if the principal will call and tell my mother I got the strap today, so I take the long route home so that I can think up excuses and why I couldn't help it. As I am strolling along I see Warren Tisdale on the other side of the street, who greets me in a friendly way. Warren, the son of a neurosurgeon, is the top student in the class, naturally well behaved and likeable. I look the other way, pretending I haven't seen him.

Rounding the corner to my street, I slow down even further, preparing for what might come if the principal has really called home. Opening the front door, it's very quiet as I step in. Mother is spread out on the couch with sections of the newspaper delicately balanced over her. She is barely asleep, but seems relaxed. She often naps this way in the afternoons when nobody's home. Most likely if she doesn't say anything now I'll be okay. I say "Hi" in a tone which I am sure will betray my guilt. Mom greets me and closes her eyes again. "Phew!" I shoot upstairs to change. I see Andrea and David talking seriously to each other. I feel left out and cheated when they share secrets or activities. Suddenly, Andrea bellows out that someone has been in her room because things are not as she left them. "Look, even my drawers have been gone through. Ian, it's you. Who else could it be? Stay out of my goddam room, do you understand? I can't keep anything without you getting your grubby little fingers on it." I refuse to admit my culpability and adamantly swear up and down I wasn't in her room. Besides, it could have been someone else. Better see what's on TV.

Sharing a small bedroom, David and I maintain an uneasy alliance which frequently erupts into full-scale skirmishes, until Dad would come into the room to rescue us, belt in hand. Mom would make sure the windows were closed so that the whole street wouldn't hear us. She would always "lock" the windows (I was never sure why) before Dad strapped us.

Falling asleep was never easy for me when I was younger. It's not that I wasn't tired or was resistant to the idea, it always seemed there was something more to do. That night, before David came to bed, I lay awake recalling the events of the day. I realized as never before that I did not fit in, not at home, nor at school. For the first time, that night I began to swell up inside with sadness, a kind of remorse. What was the matter with me? I didn't look different. I wasn't missing an arm or a leg. I wasn't deaf or blind. Maybe I was just dumb, because they hadn't found anything wrong at the hospital as far as I could tell. You would think with all those tests and a whole week's supply of urine, they would have discovered something and fixed what was wrong. I hadn't heard from them for a long time so I guessed there was nothing more to be done.

So if that's it, if I am just plain stupid, there was no way that I would let on to anyone that this was the case. I promised myself never to cry in front of others again. If only I could just make a couple of friends, I'd be alright. I know that none of the kids would dare tease me about my stupidness for fear of being punched. On the playground they often followed the games I initiated. Sometimes even the teachers enjoyed my ideas. For now I would have to get by with that.

I was now in Grade 4 and could distinguish right from left because I had a small vertical nick on my left hand from an accident the previous summer. My mother tried extra tutoring for me because I couldn't keep up with the schoolwork, but this did not work out. Both my tutor and I would rather have been elsewhere, neither one of us being motivated. I was given a special exercise book which had "Montreal Children's Hospital Learning Clinic" stamped on it. At the end of the year I stole it and put it in my bedroom closet. Sometimes I secretly pulled it out to try to do the exercises myself, but with no luck. Even years later I didn't understand it.

In the summer, after Grade 4, I heard my mother call Dr. Sam Rabinovitch of the Montreal Children's Hospital Learning Clinic. They had a special program for kids like me. I was really curious as I hadn't run across others like myself before, who failed everything and always got into trouble. The idea teased and repulsed me at the same time. I didn't dare come right out and ask, but I was filled with hope and fear at the thought that somebody might help me do better in school. Would I live there? I was certain I would do very well. No, I couldn't go; that would be giving in. All they had done for me in the past was give me tests that made me feel retarded and send me home again. I was debating this whole thing back and forth, finally bursting out to my mother, "You're not planning to send me to the hospital, are you?" She replied, "Well, I called the MCH Learning Clinic and they have a 2-year waiting list." That took care of that.

Walking smartly to school the first day, in brand new clothes for Grade 5, I said to myself, as I was careful to step on every crack, that this year things were going to be different. I said that every year. The teachers felt sorry for my parents; every subject seemed beyond me. They suggested that we should concentrate just on what I could do and forget about the rest, and told them not to expect too much. Forget about math, for they said I had a severe perceptuomotor problem. I wondered what that was.

My dignity and self-esteem rested on my ability to conceal from anyone that there was something wrong with me. This strange dishonesty had stuck with me since my early years, and was even applied to my teachers, who each year seemed unprepared for what was in store for them. Unfortunately, my hyperactivity precluded being able to slip by unnoticed. The calls home would inevitably start coming by the first week of October. I still could not read phonetically and my teacher offered to help me after school. The boys at school were into the Hardy Boys books and talked about their adventures. I asked my mother to read to me in the evening so I could know what they were talking about. I pretended I read the same books.

They arrived unannounced. I was sitting in class when the office monitor came to get me. I thought I was in trouble for something again. Trying to think what it was that I did and coming up with nothing, I followed the monitor to the office quietly, staying a step behind so I could think over any excuses that might work, even though I couldn't remember what I had done.

I was relieved to find two visitors with friendly smiles waiting for me on the bench in the office. They explained they were from McGill University and wondered if I might be interested in going with them to do a short test. Happy to be out of class, not in trouble, I agreed.

They took me to an empty classroom where they had set up a machine [authors' note: the CPT] that was plugged into a socket. They looked like a young married couple. She was blond and plainly dressed; he was wearing a sports jacket with a red bow tie that overshadowed his face. I asked if they were married. They looked at each other grimacing, and said no. The machine had a small window in the center of the metal box that appeared homemade; the window was out of proportion for such a large container and no glass was covering it. They had fashioned a paper roller on some kind of mechanical belt. I was instructed to take note of the symbols, numbers, and letters that were passing around the window, and to tap each time on what appeared to be telegraph transmitter, a symbol that corresponded to the one they wanted. This went on for a long time. I sighed in frustration after a while, but tried to catch all the correct symbols as it seemed easy enough to do. Sometimes the correct symbol would come by, but I wouldn't have enough time to tap before it would pass on to the next.

The roller went faster and faster, slowing down again for a moment then speeding up until I didn't care anymore. Turning to his partner, he whispered, "It just goes right by him." I tapped quickly, not looking up, thinking I had missed a few. She didn't say anything. We finished after school was over and they offered me a lift home. Secretly, I still held out hope that all would be clear one day, and they might have the answer. These two young people held out hope because their instrument had so clearly demonstrated my stupidity. They were friendly and after we finished, they gave me a lift back home. Dropping me off at my front door, they wished me luck and goodbye.

The next day I was scared to go to school because after this test everyone must know about my stupidity. I thought my teacher, Miss Clayton, looked at me longer than usual, but otherwise nothing was new. She starts to read aloud from *The Last of the Mohicans*, Chapter 6. I like the idea of running through the dense forest with just a loincloth around my waist, relying on my own prowess to survive. Looking out of the window I imagine the world is ending, everything is left intact but the people are gone. I am free to explore as I wish, so I take off in a car . . . All of a sudden, this daydream is interrupted by Miss Clayton asking me for my homework. The whole class is silent, looking at me. The homework is not done. I want to cry, but in Grade 3 I had made a vow not to cry in front of others ever again. I control myself. She instructs the rest of the class to continue working and tells me that this cannot go on, that I am so far behind the others, how can I expect to understand what's going on.

Eventually, teachers stopped expecting me to do homework, and for better or worse the tension eased.

The boundaries beyond the walls and halls of school become my classroom. It was here that I could influence and change the perceptions others had of me. Frequently this left fighting as the only means to establish ground previously lost in school. I didn't have to extend from anything specific said or done in class. I ran and played with a vigor that any time could erupt in a misunderstanding that led to fists. But I never held grudges; when it was over I quickly forgot the matter.

Carla invited me to her house today. We weren't really friends, but I was accustomed to brief friendships that usually involved kids in my class. Carla was skinny with boney knees and buckteeth which she always pressed over her lips after she smiled. She was quiet and never said much in class unless asked, and didn't appear to have any friends. Her house was a large, opulent one with a spacious front lawn and a weeping willow off to one side. Inside, she led me to the rec room. I had become quiet and didn't know what to say. We had never talked much before. Gazing around, I noticed an upright piano. I asked her if she knew how to play. After coaxing her, without further hesitation she sat down and played. Her two hands sprung forth a melody that left me awestruck and soothed. Carla told me it was Beethoven.

I hear David talking to my parents. He wants to go to boarding school and they eventually agree. I wonder for a moment if I have something to do with his wanting to leave. Andrea is planning to go to college for a fine arts program. There's a lot of talk about Vietnam, "hippies," the civil rights movement, drugs in the community. Parents are beginning to worry and kids are questioning the values and morality of their parents. Looking around, they want things they see as wrong to be changed; the protest gathers momentum, and I feel that there is no stopping it.

I sneak into Andrea's room, which is always filled with mature, adult-like things. Her wall is covered with posters, her desk and shelves lined with books. I find *Catcher in the Rye* by Salinger; thumbing through it I realize it is about a boy in trouble. I can't pass it up. I keep going back to it, wondering if I might be able to read it. I take the book back to my room. Sentence by sentence, page by page, a new world opens up to me. This is what I have been waiting for. It's a struggle, but the payoff is enormous. Emotionally, the book compels me to pay attention and not lose track. I go over it again and again. I discover that I can read. I return to Andrea's room and find John Howard Griffin's *Black Like Me*. I read it through.

I'm now in Grade 7 and my body is changing, something both welcome and strange. Mrs. Wilson was the best teacher I ever had. Although strict, she was encouraging and supportive. She understood what I could and couldn't do. I was never thrown out of class; instead she kept me after school and I would help her clean up, set things up for the next day. She got to know me and sensed that I wanted to please, that I craved for sincere, positive feedback. She encouraged me to buy a camera, and I found one for $2.50 at our church bazaar. It looked like an expensive one, but the pictures came out hazy, misted over like steam. She arranged to repair it and asked me to be chief photographer on the school newspaper which she ran. As a result of this new activity I saw my photos of school events prominently displayed on the bulletin board outside my classroom. This gave me satisfaction and also gave me a break from the classroom, since I had to cover various activities going on in the school.

"We've got some difficult days ahead. Like anybody, I'd like to live a long life but that doesn't really matter to me now. Because I've been to the mountain top." Martin Luther King is murdered. Watching the news, hearing his last speech, I cry softly—the first time since I was 9 years old.

I wasn't told until the night before that a new research psychiatrist, Dr. Minde, and a psychologist were coming to the house to see how things were going and to administer more tests. I resented having to feel dimwitted again—"Why do they keep coming back?" Arriving early the next morning, I am ready for them. Thinking they might like to see my room, I fix it up, carefully displaying those things which show me off as a unique person. The books I have been reading are there on the desk in plain view. Dr. Minde is talking to my mother in the living room while Miss Smith takes me into the kitchen to begin testing. I can hear them talking since the kitchen is right beside the living room. Straining to listen, at the same time I distractedly complete the tests. Afterward, we all talk together for a while. Mother tells Dr. Minde that I'm in scouts, have friends now, and had a large birthday party. Everyone is pleased, excited. Dr. Minde mentions that there is a new pill, Ritalin, that might help me, and I agree to try it. They leave without seeing my room, and I never told tham that I had begun to read. That night, I hear Mom tell Dad that I may not go far academically, but I will get a lot out of life socially. I take Ritalin in the morning and at lunch; it really does settle me, but I feel deadened; I don't like its effects. Soon I invent innovative ways not to swallow the pill; instead I let them pile up in my pocket. Six weeks later I stop pretending I'm taking them. "I don't like the idea of taking drugs!" I inform my mother.

I continue my own reading. Often I have to refer to the dictionary, but the books make me wide-eyed with discovery. I have so many questions. Authors like Langston Hughes, Gordon Parks, James Baldwin, Malcolm X, are talking to me. "One flew east, one flew west and one flew over the cuckoo's nest." Ken Kesey's novel is more difficult for me so I use the dictionary often. Characters jump out at me, and I begin to conceptualize on a level I never thought possible. My education has begun.

Adjusting to high school was easier for me than for my parents. Slipping in and out of the mainstream, making new friends, socializing, getting in on—not afraid to find out about drugs and other things. My hair is getting longer, my defiance deeper, stronger, more impulsively confident. The teachers' complaints are once again sounding loud and clear. This time my mother has not one but seven teachers to contend with. Increasingly they don't want me in their class. Mr. Banning is on the phone to my mother. He sympathizes with the difficulties she has to deal with. He doesn't see how I'm going to succeed. He suspects I'm on drugs.

In the center of town Bernard's drugstore is the gathering place for the elite of our suburb's fringe. I manage to gain admission to this unlikely social hierarchy made of people of all ages, where I learn the knowhow of the drug scene, and where I engage with others in endless conversations about things which matter to me.

The student council president wants to know if I would be interested in their attempt to form an association of councils from across the city, to formulate ideas for change to the school board. I'd be a kind of special advisor. I agree to participate, but the year ends and I have failed Grade 9. My future seems dim. I now split for weekends at a time. My guilt is heightened by the absence, whether intentional or not, of severe confrontation by my parents. Sensing their concern, apprehension at my wanderings, I hold myself in, never stepping too far out.

"Ian, it's 8 o'clock, time to get up. You'll be late. *Ian!*" Mom shouts even louder from downstairs, "Get up." "I'm not going to school," I holler back as the radio, which has been on all night, blares out "Everyday People" by Sly and the Family Stone. "I've had it with school; I'm quitting, I'm going out west to work." Mr. James, the new vice-principal, advises my mother that I might as well leave as I'm not getting anywhere and would be better off finding a job.

Dr. Minde asks to see me. I figure Mom has called him, desperate, afraid I'm going to leave home. I don't want to see him. After pleading with me, I finally agree, "but don't expect me to change my mind," I tell her as I walk out the door. I take the wrong bus by mistake, but arrive on the street his office is on anyway. The address I have written down shows it must be a few blocks away, except I don't know which direction to go. Looking at the numbers on the buildings, houses, and high rises, I determine it must be this way. Wait a minute, the numbers are changing. I turn back, looking to the other side to see if those are the right sequence. Ah, I got it. No, they're changing again. It's getting late. I don't have a watch, but I've been going up and down, across these blocks now for a long time. Finally, I ask someone. He doesn't know where I want to go. Over there, I think. I see what looks like a medical building. The numbers don't match, but I go in anyway. The names and office numbers swirl around as I race my eyes up and down the board looking for his number. I'm getting really angry at myself. I decide to pick a direction and just walk, paying no attention to the numbers. Ah, I found it. Almost 1 hour late, I take the elevator up to his office.

Knocking on the door, I can hear him put down the phone as he fully swings open the double doors to his small office. "I've just been on the phone to your mummy," he says, "asking if you had left or maybe had forgotten about our appointment." I tell him I took the wrong bus. "Did the address numbers confuse you?" he wants to know. "No," I reply firmly. Sitting across from me he rather naturally looks perturbed at my long hair, off-handed views, and monosyllabic answers.

Asking me about school and home, he uses expressions like "restless, fidgety, unable to pay attention." Looking at his watch, he says he wanted to spend more time with me, but because I was late, he can't— another patient is already waiting for him. So why, I ask myself, all these years of failing, of being suspended, tested and retested, all for such innocuous-sounding problems?

At the same time, creeping up on me like a virus, spreading insidiously throughout my body—at first just a nagging ache, then full-blown uncontrollable poison—like a heavy weight of total helplessness, dragging me down, moving its ugly force against mine. Two passions— to quit school and leave or end it all are juxaposed in awkward balance.

Perhaps sensing what's going on, Mom is on the phone to the new guidance counselor, Dorothy Ross Till. I can hear her saying that I'm refusing to go back to school, this is really it. She is crying between the wheezing of her asthma.

"You're here to see me?" asks Dorothy. "Yeah," I mutter blasé, cold. To my surprise she indicates that she wants to work with me, to take me on. It's her first year and I sense she likes me. My God, does she have to be so direct as she figures out a schedule for me for next year if I decide to go back? There's no sense in taking maths and you'll need a tutor in most subjects. "There is no way I'm going back if I have to repeat Grade 9," I tell her. "You'll just have to forget the whole thing if that's what I have to do." "No," she says, "I think you can take most of your courses in Grade 10. English, French, history, biology. But you'll need a tutor." I can't believe it. How is she going to pull this off? She also has the school records and IQ tests from Grade 1. She goes over it with me, not telling me the exact scores, but the ranges they're in. A lot of discrepancies, a perceptuomotor deficit—the world isn't coming to an end. You've missed a lot, but you can catch up if you work hard. But there's a problem. Mr. James will only take you back if you get some testing done at the McGill Learning Clinic and a covering letter stating that you have the ability to make it and will get tutoring.

The testing takes three days. I am told that judging from my perceptuomotor skills, I wouldn't have the aptitude for working with my hands. So this rules out vocational school. The learning clinic is starting a summer program which might help me, and Dorothy agrees to take me to the organizational meeting. It ends up that my social and verbal skills are higher than the other kids in the summer program so they have nothing to offer me. Attending this meeting with Dorothy, I appreciate the enormous effort she has made on my behalf, not a small part of which was influencing the school to make an accommodation to allow me to proceed to Grade 10.

I return to school. My new tutor, Paul, and I are becoming good friends. I see him twice a week, and can't believe how fast I am catching up. We started on Grade 4 math and already we're up to Grade 8. He's going to help me with biology and history as well, as I plan to write the provincial matric exams. My French is going well too, and it looks as if I will succeed in my final exams. I still take off from school quite a lot, but Dorothy smooths things over. Together, she and I make plans for university. I succeed in getting a part-time job at the recreation center; it pays $2.50 an hour.

I have this idea to set up a youth clinic in our town. Sandy, who had originally introduced me to the drugstore scene, gave me the idea. The first to explore my sexuality at 14, fumbling along as I did in tame, ignorant pursuit, with her wired on speed, always on the run. Her father used to post ads in the drugstore offering $200 rewards for her return. Her parents were divorced and lived on opposite ends of the same street; she had been shuttled back and forth between them whenever conflicts arose. Later, Sandy suicided, but I remember her as a very good friend and as guiding me in some strange undetermined way toward a path that led somewhere. I had often taken her to the crisis clinic at the hospital, and had come to know several of its staff.

Mustering up my courage, I went back to the hospital crisis clinic and asked them if they had any openings for a volunteer. I figured that I had a chance, as I had gotten to know some youth workers in the field while trying to organize the local youth clinic. I thought my age might deter them from ever considering me, but I must have given the right impressions, said the right things, because I could start in a week, try out for a while, see how things went. This was truly amazing. It wasn't long after that that I was getting paid and assumed a position on staff.

I was on my ten-speed bike not long ago. I rode past my old high school. Slowing down, I noticed my former biology teacher coming out of the side entrance. For an instant I was startled to see how much he had changed. His once stiff black hair was now softer, noticeably gray. No longer bold and upright, he was slouching a little. His briefcase seemed to be leading him as he walked toward the playing field. I realized how much I had changed too, inside I mean. I wanted to say hello, to tell him what I've been doing and still hope to do. But I doubt he would have recognized me—it's been a long time.

POSTSCRIPT: 1993

I have not read my chapter for a number of years now, but I can recall just about every sentiment or theme I was trying to express. Having written about my early problems and thus being forced to define them became very important for me, though its significance really became more apparent as time passed. I became aware in many small ways that the story of my "hyperactivity" was becoming less of a tangled thread in my life and in the way in which it had in my early years entwined so much of my private self. Although I had somewhat reluctantly agreed to write my early reminiscences in the first place, and it had been painful to sit down, organize my thoughts, and see it through to the end, I realized that I had really written the chapter primarily for myself.

It was a challenge, at the time of writing in 1984, to rein in the flood of raw emotion and captive memories that came spilling out in a garble of words and sentences faster than I could organize it or write it down. But, in the end, I felt a kind of liberation of spirit that at least I had revealed a part of myself more or less on my own terms, and not because some person or some event had necessitated the discussion of my problems. I was not sure of the response that might follow the publication of my reminiscences, and I still chose not to inform my close friends of why I had spent so much time writing, though a few years later (through circumstances beyond my control) some of my former coworkers and friends found out about the chapter.

I am still impressed by the ingenious ways I was able to minimize the significance of that side of me that had been "exposed," but after writing about myself I also felt less burdened by what had been years of academic failure, and attempts at consolidation of those divergent views of myself that came in conflict with each other, at so many points along the way. Possibly, it was because I had a degree of self-awareness from when I was really quite young that my past affected me in ways that may be different from the experience of others who are or were hyperactive. Perhaps what was closer to the surface for me may be a little more buried for others who have experienced similar problems. Obviously, other factors such as the family in which I grew up, and the aspirations realized by many of my peers, may have intensified those conflicts. Not having any real idea of what was wrong with me and why I could not succeed in the important domains of family, school, and the emergent social world outside of the family had always preoccupied and nagged at me with quiet urgency.

I never felt that I had cornered the market on negative experiences, but I could not reconcile my own failure with what appeared to me as growing up in an environment that could not respond to my social and academic needs. The joy of discovery and learning was stifled. How I compensated for this took on some interesting dimensions. I became the master of disguise and compartmentalization when weaving my way around situations that might reveal my very discontinuous development. I had really missed so much in the way of a passage along normal developmental stages that to go back and learn them did not seem realistic. I had this recurring fantasy a few years back of disguising myself and returning to high school to start all over again. This fantasy was soothing to me because I could imagine myself taking on tasks in school, now having a foundation beneath me that represented successful passage up the normal developmental ladder, and graduating at the usual age. Instead, denial and defensiveness were postures that I adopted in my ongoing struggle to maintain an adequate sense of self toward the outside world.

I was on a train some time ago, and sitting across from me was a boy of about 9 years old with his mother. He seemed to be having some difficulty entertaining himself on the long trip and was somewhat loud and boisterous, asking his mother innumerable questions. He seemed to be flitting from one topic to another and restlessly moving about. I was watching curiously, wondering if he possibly had some of the same difficulties I had when I was his age. His mother then pulled some school work out of a carrying case and gave it to him to complete. There was mild protest from the boy, but he settled down to complete the work. I watched him become absorbed in the task, and he was enjoying himself, occasionally looking up to ask his mother for some help but otherwise appearing satisfied, confident, and pleased with his success. I observed him with envy and some sadness.

Even today, I have come to grudgingly accept that to sit down and not let myself get distracted or restless when I study or write takes a great deal of energy to stay focused, especially when I have a deadline to meet—which is more often the case than not. I notice that my respiration goes up and I have to contain many small movements and pauses. I generally don't find the process satisfying or self-reinforcing, and I'm usually not that happy with what I have done until sometimes much later, when I look it over. This is not as true when I read, but I can still miss details that I discover upon rereading. I can't say with any certainty what other people who never had ADHD and who have to complete assignments go through, though I suspect it may be much easier for them. Does the combination of repeated failures in my earlier years without any continuous period of success, missed opportunities to learn, and the battering taken by my sense of self-worth as I endeavored to keep up with my peers account for much of my situation today, or is it entirely constitutional? It is most likely a tangled mixture of many forces, both internal and external.

As I tried to convey in my chapter, the recognition of not fitting in and the emergence of a sense of pessimism started to take shape in Grade 1. I have since learned that as early as Grade 1, hyperactive children experience low self-esteem and sometimes subtle signs of depression. I have no idea if even a theoretically "perfect" family could counteract this. My own home environment was not one in which physical or verbal affection was expressed very often. Both my parents came from families in which open show of feelings was scant. It may have something to do with having an English and Scottish Presbyterian background, but, along with my siblings, I looked and craved for open acknowledgment and affection. I learned over time to pick up on the implied expressions of love and being valued, which I know my parents felt for us in their own way.

In my struggle to understand more fully what was different about me, I have searched for and read an enormous amount of literature about hyperactive children. This has given me glimpses of insight into some of the complexities of the disorder. From the clinical and personal accounts of other children and adults, I have seen parts of myself in their descriptions. This has been very important for me, and has helped to unravel some of the mysteries that plagued me for so long, but not without some danger.

I never did want to conform to a script or myth that was evolving in my early years, when I was one of the subjects in the long-term follow-up study on "hyperactive" children. The way I perceived it then, I felt poked and prodded through many tests, interviews, and what I thought were exams about my intelligence and abilities. I was never told what all the various tests were supposed to measure and whether I had done all right or failed. I was never left with a sense of hope, or a feeling of any clinician's real interest in being a partner with me to help me grow and learn. Rather, the mystification of what was wrong with me was reinforced with each new test, indicating to me that the problem was not yet clear. Perhaps that is why I rebelled against taking Ritalin on a trial basis in Grade 7, since by then I had fashioned a coping style for myself, and I feared that the medication would take it away and not replace it with anything that I thought was worthwhile. There had not been sufficient information shared with me about what the pills would do and would not do, nor was I made a partner in the choice. By taking pills, I feared that my unique, newly developed character and the shaky learning style that I had fashioned would be compromised. When I began the pills on trial, I felt as though I had become more disengaged and did not feel like myself. On looking back, I realize that I had become dysphoric, so I stopped the medication.

I now firmly believe that Ritalin can be helpful for some children and adults with ADHD, but only along with other interventions and when an attempt is made to bring the patients, even if they are children, into the decision-making process. I'm hopeful that this happens much more often today than it did when I was growing up. I have a tremendous affinity for children with ADHD, especially today when it seems that conformity, getting ahead, and the pressure to succeed in ever more complex tasks are more prevalent now than they were in my formative years.

During my adolescence in the late 1960s and early 1970s, I had other ideals and values to aspire to that were outside the mainstream of authority or convention, that transcended achievement and personal success. This, in no small way, allowed me to understand that I *could* learn. These experiences molded my emerging sense of adolescent identity and self-acceptance. I was in an environment that challenged my ideas and forced me to consider what I believed in and why. This helped me to become more introspective and assess my impact on those around me. I learned to modulate my more impulsive reactions of thought and action, and to talk myself out of responding in ways that might be misinterpreted. Even when transgressions did occur later, I could re-enter social situations with the intent of repairing the damage in direct or indirect ways. Therefore, what might have been seen as lability may have been my self-regulation to fix what had happened. I also became adept at concealing my wandering thoughts in social exchanges by mirroring the appropriate social or conversational responses and cues while my mind would really be somewhere else. This compensatory skill was especially effective when the exchange was boring. Yes, I have to accept now that some of my earlier difficulties are still with me, although I have learned to compensate in a variety of ways.

One attribute that is commonly seen in hyperactive children and adults is a tendency to get mad or angry easily. This is not something that is a problem for me. Except for bouts of heightened activity and apparent disorganization when I'm feeling overwhelmed or stressed out, I'm fairly even-tempered. This is not to say that I quell my opinions when I feel strongly or passionate about something; rather, I have matured in slowing down a little bit (that expression still reverberates through my body with disdain) to consider others' perspectives more thoughtfully.

I do value those aspects of myself that can be a little crazy and spontaneous to others at times, and my appreciation of the absurd side of things. Recently, while I was working as a research assistant on a project that was evaluating the social styles of hyperactive children, I asked one of the control subjects what he thought hyperactivity was.

He said, "The hyperactive kid is the kid in the class who always has to be right." I smiled when I remembered that this had been true for me in many ways.

I returned to university shortly after I wrote the chapter; I knew I had to try again. Dr. Weiss was instrumental in helping me come to terms with what I needed to do in order to take the necessary steps to reapply. What had been gnawing inside me for so long—the nagging self-doubts, fear of failure, and phobias about formal education—came to the fore. Dr. Weiss helped me to untangle these feelings and externalize them. I had never before been able to tell anyone about these specific parts about myself, but with her help I could, and I knew she accepted and understood me. This self-disclosure dislodged some of the darkest perceptions I had of myself, and began the process of establishing a healing distance between what was construed as real to me and what were the distortions I had harbored inside for so long.

I remained at university between 1985 and 1990, studying for a BA and working as a research assistant. Campus life had changed since the last time I had been at university, and I was apprehensive but very motivated to stick it out this time because of my age, even though I looked younger than 30. I was pleased to discover that there were a few older students in most of my classes. I also became aware that there appeared to be a much more pressured atmosphere among the students to get good grades, to be looking ahead, and to be thinking about what kind of position and status they wanted to achieve. This was different from my first time, when it seemed that many students wanted more from an education than just good grades. While I was anxious to consolidate what I had learned on my own, the others seemed more preoccupied in just wanting to know what might be asked on an exam and nothing more. Being older, I was less intimidated by the demands of the university environment.

However, some of the same patterns re-emerged for me. I found myself waiting for the last few days to study for exams. Because a lot of things came easily for me and I was reinforced by some of the good grades I received, this was not true for the more complex subjects, such as statistics and anatomy, that required careful preparation and practice. Therefore, I thought that I should try Ritalin. This aroused many feelings for me again. I had always been very stubborn about not seeking out help, even though I harbored this fantasy of having someone stand over me to help me organize what I needed to learn and study for. I thought back to the only ongoing tutoring I had received, in Grade 10, and what a difference it had made. I therefore held my breath and walked into the university health clinic and requested to see the psychiatrist. Fortunately, the psychiatrist was supportive, but perhaps a little suspicious of an adult requesting Ritalin. She spoke to Dr. Weiss, and I got my first prescription for Ritalin since Grade 7.

Taking Ritalin at age 30, I experienced much the same reaction as at age 13. The effects were quite noticeable. I discovered that I had a heightened awareness and ability to focus on what was going on around me, and could more easily filter out extraneous stimuli; however, it was not a panacea. It could not repair years of missed learning, poor study habits, and low self-esteem. I also experienced some side effects that bothered me, such as mild insomnia and a noticeable increase in my heart rate. This became especially true when I took Ritalin to cram for an exam, which compounded the necessary mobilization on my part to neurologically "reef myself up," so to speak, to attack the task at hand. After the first couple of months, I did not take Ritalin on a regular basis, partly because of the side effects, and partly because of those still-lingering fixed beliefs that I did not need help to learn and I could do it on my own. However, I continued to take it before exams or during intensive periods of study. I had always fought against seeing myself as handicapped in any way. I had taken on so many different challenges outside of school and been successful, so why couldn't I succeed on my own? Unfortunately, this got me into trouble with the subjects that required complex organization and rehearsal. My grade point average was affected by this, but I managed to complete my BA. However, not getting into medical school after a couple of attempts produced strong and mixed feelings as I recognized, on the one hand, how much more I needed to do and that I had to give up the idea of medicine, which had for many years been my first choice. But, on the other hand, a career in medicine was no longer as important to me as it had once been. Again, though, those divergent views of myself came into conflict with each other.

In one of my undergraduate courses, the professor was impressed by the range and depth of my knowledge in that subject, and invited me to have lunch with him to talk about furthering my studies in graduate school. Whereas at one time I could become paralyzed with fear that others might "find out" about me, and I was definitely anxious when I knew I had to tell him about myself, it was not as difficult as it used to be. His reaction was telling: He said he would never have guessed, although his research interests were in the area of impulsivity and learning problems!

The professor invited me to join his research team and to work on my honors thesis with him. I was also hired to work as a technician in his neuropsychology assessment lab, which tested children from the surrounding areas. The very first child I had to administer the battery of tests to was a young, quite severely hyperactive girl. Just before the testing was to begin, I was informed that another professor and some of his students would be observing behind the one-way mirror. Unfortunately, the girl was not especially cooperative and was, in fact, almost impossible to contain in the room; she also tried to cheat on many of the tests. I was told afterwards that she often stuck her tongue out at me when I wasn't looking, but would smile at me when I turned to look at her. It was a very long day and I went home exhausted. I thought afterwards that there was obviously some poetic justice to this, and I did not miss the irony of having to administer the CPT. Later, when I became familiar and confident with testing, I always tried to ensure that the children I tested felt good about themselves, that they had tried their best, and that the experience had a positive meaning for them and was fun.

I had taken several courses almost every semester throughout the 5 years I was back at university, and, in addition, at one point was holding down four part-time jobs to support myself. I realized I needed to take a break, and although I had not accomplished everything I wanted to do, it was time to move on for awhile.

I left university and moved to Toronto, where I presently live. I work in a large children's mental health center, where I am a supervisor in the residential treatment services division. I supervise a staff of about 20 who provide multimodal treatment to emotionally disturbed latency-age children. In the interview for the job, one of the psychologists asked me if I thought I might become impulsive at times and how I would handle this. I think he noticed that I was somewhat anxious and had moved from topic to topic. I hesitated, but then told him of some of my early experiences. It really has become easier to talk about myself.

During the years at university, I had experienced intermittent depressions. In contrast, in the past 2 years at work, I have had none. I wondered why this was so, because I had really enjoyed university, had found it challenging, and had made lifelong friends there. I suppose that completing term papers or theses or working for and passing exams will always make me more vulnerable to depression, because these things highlight handicaps I still have. In contrast, I usually feel competent at work.

I am not ready to settle down yet in marriage or in my final career goals, but I have come to terms with who I am, my strengths, and my weaknesses, and I will return to university again one day to complete my graduate studies. I have found that each time I enter the world of formal education, it has become a little more familiar and less like I don't belong. I know that learning is a lifelong journey, whether it is the accumulation of knowledge about things, people, or myself. Sometimes when I am alone in the country, I think of a passage from Ted Hughes that reads:

> The incomprehensible cry from the boughs in the wind
> sets us listening for below words,
> meanings that will not part from the rock.

It beckons me to pay attention, and I don't want to miss anything.

* * * * *

Comments by Dr. Weiss

I have come to know Ian well since his writing of the chapter for our book. I have seen him develop into a competent professional, a supervisor, and a therapist. Most importantly, he is a person with a high level of integrity and creativity. In 1984, when Ian began to write his reminiscences, the project took him months, and he wrote at least five times the amount that he could finally submit. Nine years later, he wrote the "Postscript" independently, and little editing was needed. Ian's story is unfinished—an ongoing journey, but now with a clearer destination.

NEW DEVELOPMENTS IN ATTENTION-DEFICIT HYPERACTIVITY DISORDER

CHAPTER TWENTY-TWO

RECENT BIOLOGICAL AND DIAGNOSTIC ISSUES

There have been many exciting new developments in the area of Attention-Deficit Hyperactivity Disorder (ADHD). Several of these developments have centered in three interrelated areas: evidence for the possible genetic etiology or influence in this condition; neurobiological data suggesting the possible nature of the abnormalities involved; and data indicating that various comorbid conditions, such as Oppositional Defiant Disorder, Conduct Disorder, Anxiety Disorder, and Major Affective Disorder, are important to evaluate and treat in the child with ADHD and his or her family. These three areas are expanded on in this chapter.

GENETIC STUDIES OF CHILDREN WITH ADHD

Four types of studies suggest that genetic factors play a role in this condition: twin, sibling, adoption, and family studies.

Twin Studies

Generally, genetically based disorders should be concordant in twins, and more so in monozygotic (MZ) than in dizygotic (DZ) twins. Recently, a number of twin studies have looked at the concordance of ADHD in twins.

An early study by Lopez[48] compared four pairs of MZ males with six pairs of DZ twins. However, four of the DZ twin pairs were opposite-sex pairs in which the male was hyperactive; this limits the validity of the study. Another small study by Heffron et al.[38] reported on three pairs of MZ twins, all concordant for Attention Deficit Disorder (ADD).

More recently, Goodman and Stevenson[34] studied 570 twins aged 13 years. These authors focused particular attention on 29 MZ and 45 same-sex DZ twin pairs in which at least one twin met criteria for pervasive hyperactivity. MZ twins were more alike than same-sex DZ pairs on objective measures of attentiveness and on parent and teacher ratings of hyperactivity (59% vs. 33%). In their careful study, these authors also explored the possible effects of stereotyping (i.e., the tendency to rate identical twins similarly), adverse family factors (e.g., marital discord, parental criticism, and malaise) and perinatal adversity (e.g., low birth weight). They concluded that genetic effects accounted for approximately half of the explainable variance of hyperactivity and inattentiveness.

In their extensive study of reading-disabled twins in the Colorado Reading Project, Gillis et al.[32] and Gilger et al.[31] attempted to diagnose ADHD in the twins by parental responses on the Diagnostic Interview of Children and Adolescents (DICA[40]). They thus examined 81 MZ and 52 same-sex DZ pairs of a reading-disabled sample of twins. They found that for reading disability, the concordance rate was 84% for MZ twins and 66% for DZ twins. For ADHD, the concordance rate was 81% for MZ twins and 29% for DZ twins. The concordance rate for both reading disability *and* ADHD was 44% for MZ twins and 30% for DZ twins. The data suggest that reading disability and ADHD may have strong though independent genetic components.[31]

Gillis et al.[32] examined the same group of subjects but focused particularly on 37 MZ and 37 same-sex DZ twin pairs where one twin had been diagnosed with ADHD via the DICA. The authors used a basic regression model for analysis and found that 79% of MZ twins and 32% of DZ twins were concordant for ADHD ($p < .001$). Furthermore, adjustment for IQ or reading performance differences did not substantially change the results. The authors thus conclude that the results of this analysis suggest that ADHD is highly heritable.

One of the largest twin studies is currently being carried out by Levy and Hay[47] in Australia. They plan to screen 3400 pairs of twins aged 4–12 years and their siblings, and to determine the perinatal and developmental history as well as the incidence and concordance of ADHD, Conduct Disorder, and Separation Anxiety Disorder. The study is ongoing and current data are still very preliminary.

Various studies have suggested that different symptoms of the ADHD syndrome are heritable. In an early study, Rutter et al.[66] reported that MZ twins were more similar to each other than DZ twins in psychomotor activity. Similarly, Willerman[79] reported heritability of activity scores to be .77 for 54 MZ and DZ twin pairs. Torgensen and Kringlen[75] also found evidence for a genetic component in both activity levels and distractibility.

Stevenson,[72] using multiple regression analysis on data obtained from 91 pairs of MZ twins and 105 pairs of same-sex DZ twins, concluded that results were consistent with a significant genetic contribution to individual differences in activity level and attention abilities.

Recently, Edelbrock and colleagues[25] evaluated 99 MZ and 82 same-sex DZ twin pairs aged 4–15 years via the Child Behavior Checklist (CBCL) completed by parents. They found correlations of .68 (MZ) and .29 (DZ) for attentional problems. Generally, using multiple regression analysis, they found significant genetic influences on competence in school and on all areas of problem behavior. Significant shared environmental influences were detected for participation in activities, quality of social relationship, performance in school, anxiety/depression, and delinquent behavior.

Thus, these twin studies also indicate a greater concordance in MZ than in DZ twins for different components of the ADHD syndrome. This supports the hypothesis that there is a genetic component in this condition.

Siblings and Half Siblings

Welner et al.[78] evaluated 53 hyperactive children and their siblings and compared them to 38 nonhyperactive controls and their siblings. The authors found that the hyperactive child syndrome was more common among the brothers of the hyperactive children than among brothers of controls (26% vs. 9%). Furthermore, the hyperactives and their brothers presented with more symptoms of anxiety and depression than did the controls (16% vs. 6%). The probands, but not their siblings, also presented with more antisocial symptoms than controls. This lends support to a family–genetic risk in this condition, and suggests that hyperactives may also show comorbid conditions of depression and anxiety.

In another early study, Safer[67] compared the incidence of ADHD in 19 full-sibling and 22 half-sibling pairs. Each pair had been raised together by a common mother. One member of each pair was known to have Minimal Brain Dysfunction (MBD), now known as ADHD. Over half (10) of the full-sibling pairs were concordant for ADHD, compared to only 2 of the 22 half-sibling pairs. This significant difference between full and half siblings further supports a genetic component of hyperactivity.

Adoption Studies

Early studies by Morrison and Stewart[56] showed that adoptive relatives of ADHD children are less likely to have ADHD or associated disorders than are biological relatives of such children. In addition, biological relatives of ADHD children perform worse on standardized measures of attention than do adoptive relatives of ADHD children.[1]

In a recent adoption study, Cadoret and Stewart[17] studied 283 adoptees aged 18 to 40. The adoptees were divided into two groups based on whether or not biological parents showed evidence (from adoption agency records) of psychiatric problems or behavioral disturbances. In addition to these evaluations, direct evaluation of adoptees and adoptive parents were performed. The authors concluded that adult adoptees had to have both a biological parent with a history of criminality/delinquency *and* a placement in a lower-socioeconomic-status adoptive home to have an increased likelihood of developing Antisocial Personality Disorder. This suggests that while in general adoptive studies support a genetic component in hyperactivity, there is always an important interplay between genetic and environmental factors.

Thus, in general, adoption studies also support a genetic component in this condition.

Family Studies

Family studies of hyperactive children have been based on the assumption that a genetic component of hyperactivity will be reflected in a higher familial rate of the disorder for probands. Thus, in an early study, Morrison and Stewart[55] found that 20% of hyperactive children had a parent who could be (retrospectively) diagnosed as hyperactive, compared to 5% of their medical controls. Similarly, Cantwell[18] reported that 20% of hyperactive boys in his sample had a parent who could be classified as being hyperactive/antisocial in childhood, as opposed to 2% of the pediatric clinic controls.

However, in addition to an increased rate of hyperactivity in families of hyperactive children, these authors (Morrison and Stewart, as well as Cantwell) found that biological parents of hyperactive children had higher rates of "alcoholism, sociopathy, and hysteria"[18] compared to parents of normal controls. Morrison[54] also found a higher incidence of unipolar but not bipolar affective disorder in the combined second-degree blood relatives of hyperactive children.

These may have been the first signs of the importance of other comorbid conditions in this disorder. The importance of particular comorbid conditions, and their association with specific parental pathology, have been illustrated in studies by Lahey et al.[44] and more recently by Barkley et al.[6]

Lahey et al.[44] compared parental pathology in 6- to 13-year-old children with Conduct Disorder ($n = 37$), with ADHD ($n = 18$), and with both disorders. Parents of children with Conduct Disorder were more likely to abuse substances. In addition, mothers of conduct-disordered children were more often depressed and more frequently had the triad of Antisocial Personality Disorder, substance abuse, and Somatization Disorder. In contrast, parents of children with ADHD only did not have any significant disorders. However, fathers of children with both Conduct Disorder and ADHD were more likely to have a history of aggression, arrest, and imprisonment.

Barkley and colleagues,[6] in their 8-year follow-up of hyperactive children, also collected information on the biological fathers of these children. They found that fathers of hyperactive children, compared to fathers of normal controls, had a history of significantly more antisocial acts, alcohol abuse, police contacts, and arrests. Their job histories were also less stable, and they were generally less financially responsible. The authors concluded that 11% of fathers of hyperactive children met DSM-III-R criteria for Antisocial Personality Disorder, as opposed to 1.6% of fathers of normal control children ($p < .05$). When the authors examined the antisocial acts of fathers of children with hyperactivity, with and without associated Conduct Disorder, they found that the fathers of children with hyperactivity *and* Conduct Disorder had more antisocial acts than those with hyperactivity alone. However, fathers of children who were only hyperactive still had more antisocial acts than fathers of normal controls.

These studies clearly suggest that the combination of ADHD and Conduct Disorder is associated with significant parental pathology. As shown by Cadoret and Stewart[17] in their adoption study described above, genetic and environmental factors may in fact act synergistically to influence antisocial outcome of this condition.

The most extensive family studies to date have been carried out by Biederman and his colleagues.[10,11] In the first of these studies, Biederman et al.[10] compared 73 male ADD probands and 264 of their first-degree relatives to 26 psychiatrically referred but not ADD children and 101 of their first-degree relatives, as well as 26 normal pediatric clinic controls and 92 of their first-degree relatives. The authors used interviewers who were unaware of the children's diagnostic status, and employed structured psychiatric interviews; they also controlled for gender, generation of relative, age of proband, social class, and the intactness of the family. Relatives of ADD probands had higher morbidity risks for ADD (25.1% vs. 5.3% vs. 4.6%, $p < .00001$), antisocial disorders (24.3% vs. 6.9% vs. 4.2%, $p < .00001$), and mood disorders (27.1% vs. 13.9% vs. 3.6%) than did relatives of psychiatric and normal controls. These findings indicated the importance of family–genetic risk factors in ADD.

In a more recent, similar, expanded study of 140 probands, 120 normal controls, and 822 first-degree relatives, Biederman *et al.*[11] found nearly half (49%) of the ADHD subjects had no comorbidity with Conduct Disorder, Major Depression, or multiple Anxiety Disorders. However, compared to controls, ADHD probands were more likely to have these conditions. Similarly, relatives of ADHD probands had a higher risk for ADHD (25% vs. 8%), antisocial disorders, Major Depression (26% vs. 9%), substance dependence, and anxiety disorders. Biederman and colleagues suggest that ADHD and Major Depression may show common familial vulnerabilities, that ADHD and Conduct Disorder may be distinct subtypes, and that ADHD and Anxiety Disorders are transmitted independently in families. The authors conclude that these results extend previous findings indicating family–genetic influences.

Mode of Inheritance

Given the strong evidence of genetic influence in ADHD, several hypotheses have been presented as to the possible mode of genetic transmission. Omenn[61] examined the possibility of sex-linked transmission, given the preponderance of males with the condition. However, the author concluded that this was unlikely because of the high frequency of father-to-son transmissions. Morrison and Stewart[57] suggested a polygenic mode of transmission, but could not substantiate it because of limitations of their sample size. Deutsch *et al.*,[22] studying dysmorphic children with ADHD, stated that the dysmorphic changes were consistent with a single genetic autosomal dominant inheritance. Tests of this model would require larger samples and more definitive diagnoses of both ADHD and dysmorphic phenotypes.

Faraone *et al.*,[28] using the data obtained from subjects and relatives studied by Biederman *et al.*,[11] applied segregation analysis to this data. Specifically, they analyzed the family data with a mixed model as implemented in the computer program POINTER, and a Class A regressive logistic model as implemented in the computer program REGTL. On the basis of their results, they suggest that the familial distribution of DSM-III-R ADHD can be attributed to the effects of a single major gene; they feel that they can reject multifaceted polygenic transmission, nonfamilial environmental transmission, and cultural transmission.

To date, a specific definitive mode of inheritance has as yet not been established, but work in this area is proceeding. However, Pauls[62] points out that diagnostic uncertainty impedes progress in developing genetic models that address the type of genetic transmission involved.

He argues for the importance of longitudinal studies of prospectively identified subjects and careful observation of their offspring as the best way to resolve some of the thorny methodological difficulties of family and genetic studies. Our currently planned study of childhood-diagnosed, prospectively followed hyperactives and their biological offspring is just such a study.

Specific Genetic Abnormality

Recently, Hauser and colleagues[36] at the National Institute of Health have been studying generalized resistance to thyroid hormone (GRTH), which is a rare dominant disorder. Eighteen kindreds, comprising 49 affected and 55 unaffected family members, have been studied. Interviewers unaware of subjects' GRTH status, using structured questionnaires, found that 61% of GRTH patients had ADHD as compared to 13% of unaffected family members. The mutations have been pinpointed in 13 kindreds. The authors suggest that this is the first molecular model of ADHD and may open the door to identifying the specific genetic abnormality in this condition.

An exciting and potentially important genetic finding has been reported by Comings and his colleagues.[21] They discovered that a genetic variant of the dopamine D_2 receptor gene (D_2Al allele) was significantly increased in patients with Tourette's syndrome (44%, $n = 147$), ADHD (46.2%, $n = 104$), autism (54.5%, $n = 33$), alcoholism (42.3%, $n = 104$), and Post-Traumatic Stress Disorder (45.7%, $n = 33$), compared to normal controls (24.5%, $n = 77$). However, the prevalence of this allele was not significantly increased in patients with depression, panic attacks, Parkinson's disease, or obesity. However, since the D_2Al variant is present in fewer than half of the individual's affected, the gene is not thought to be the primary cause of these disorders. The authors suggest that the D_2 receptor gene acts as a gene that can modify the expression (making the symptoms better or worse) of the major gene (yet to be discovered) that causes the condition.

We can thus see that the genetic contribution to ADHD may be complex to unravel, but that important clues are being discovered and followed. It is important to place the role of genetics in proper perspective. Even if the complete genetic makeup of an individual could be determined and our diagnostic assessments were certain, only 50% of an individual's future offspring's ADHD could be predicted. The other 50% might be acccounted for by "environmental" factors, such as events during pregnancy, delivery, diet, toxins (e.g., lead), temperament, and parenting styles. Thus, even though new genetic developments are relevant and interesting, they will not provide all the answers in this important condition.

NEUROBIOLOGICAL DEVELOPMENTS

The neurobiology of ADHD has not been comprehensively worked out. Several excellent recent reviews of the subject[42,53,76,81,82] clearly illustrate the complexity of the area, the divergent findings, and the many questions yet to be resolved. The condition is not unidimensional, and its symptoms involve various interrelated neuroanatomical and neurochemical systems. Thus, it is unlikely that any *one* area or neurochemical system will be found to be solely or primarily involved in the condition. The summary that follows is a brief overview of which neuroanatomical and neurochemical systems may be involved.

Neuroanatomical Systems

Mirsky,[53] in his excellent review entitled "Behavioral and Psychophysiological Markers of Disordered Attention," makes the case that attention has various distinct and separate aspects, such as focusing, executing, sustaining, and shifting attention. Each of these different attentional functions involves different brain regions that are interconnected and organized into a system. The overall attentional system is very widespread and thus vulnerable to damage and dysfunction. Depending on where the damage or dysfunction occurs, different aspects of attention may be affected (see Figure 22-1). Specifically, Mirsky has stated:

... the functions of focusing on environmental events are shared by superior temporal and inferior parietal cortices, as well as by structures that comprise the corpus striatum, including caudate, putamen and globus pallidus. The inferior parietal and corpus striatal regions have strong motor executive function. Considerable amounts of encoding of stimuli are accomplished by the hippocampus, [as well as] essential mnemonic function that seems to be required for some aspects of attention. The capacity to shift from one salient aspect of the environment to another is supported by the prefrontal cortex. Sustaining a focus on some environmental event is the major responsibility of rostral structures, including the tectum, mesopontine reticular formation and midline, and reticular thalamic nuclei.[53] (p. 197)

Thus, it is understandable that over the years a wide variety of brain areas have been implicated in ADHD, as shown by Zametkin and Rapoport[82] in their review of the literature (Table 22-1).

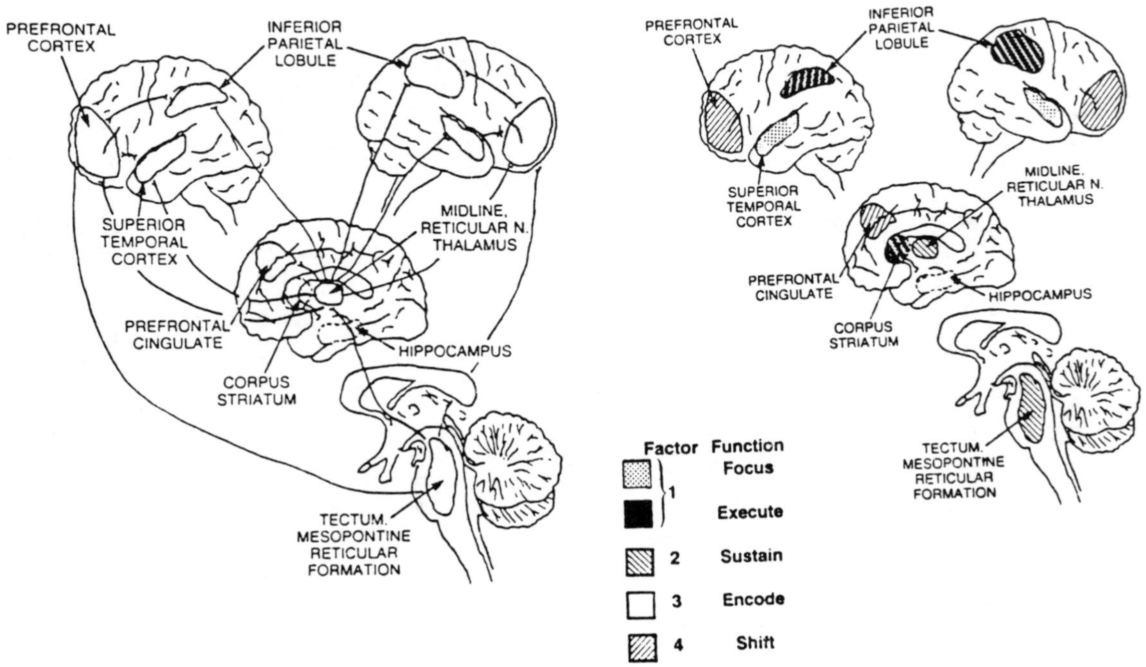
PREFRONTAL CORTEX
INFERIOR PARIETAL LOBULE
SUPERIOR TEMPORAL CORTEX
MIDLINE, RETICULAR N. THALAMUS
PREFRONTAL CINGULATE
HIPPOCAMPUS
CORPUS STRIATUM
TECTUM. MESOPONTINE RETICULAR FORMATION
Factor Function
1 Focus
Execute
2 Sustain
3 Encode
4 Shift
PREFRONTAL CORTEX
INFERIOR PARIETAL LOBULE
SUPERIOR TEMPORAL CORTEX
MIDLINE, RETICULAR N. THALAMUS
PREFRONTAL CINGULATE
HIPPOCAMPUS
CORPUS STRIATUM
TECTUM. MESOPONTINE RETICULAR FORMATION

FIGURE 22-1. Left: Semischematic representation of brain regions involved in attention. Some interconnections among the regions are shown; the connections are conceivably sufficient to support the concept of an attention system. Right: Semischematic representation of brain regions involved in attention, with tentative assignment of functional specializations to the regions. Source: 53.

TABLE 22-1. Neuroanatomical Hypotheses of Dysfunction in ADHD

Investigator	Hypothesis	Test
Laufer, 1957	Diencephalic dysfunction (thalamus, hypothalamus)	HA have lower photometrazol seizure
Knobel et al., 1959	Cortical "overfunctioning"	See text
Satterfield and Dawson, 1971	Decreased levels of reticular activating system excitation	
Wender, 1971, 1972	Decreased sensitivity in limbic areas of positive reinforcement (medial forebrain bundle) (hypothalamus) (NE)	Multiple medication trials
Conners and Eisenberg, 1964	Lack of "cortical inhibitory capacity"	
Dykman et al., 1971	Defect in forbrain inhibitory system over ventral formation + diencephalon	
Hunt et al., 1985	Locus coeruleus dysfunction (hypersensitive alphapostsynaptic receptor)	Clonidine growth hormone response
Lou et al., 1984	Central frontal lobes, anterolateral, posterolateral caudate region	Cerebral blood flow
Gorenstein and Newman, 1980	Dysfunction of medial septum, hippocampus, orbito-frontal cortex	Animal lesion studies
Porrino et al., 1984	Nucleus accumbens	Animal studies, 2-DG studies with low-dose stimulants
Mattes, 1980	Frontal lobe	Speculation
Gualtieri and Hicks, 1985	Frontal lobe	Speculation
Arnold et al., 1977	Nigrostriatal tract	Amphetamine Rx
Chelune et al., 1986	Frontal lobe	Neuropsychiatric testing

Note. HA, hyperactives; NE, norepinephrine; 2-DG, 2-deoxyglucose. Source: 82 (see source for references).

In recent years, the development of sophisticated neuroimaging technology has opened up new ways of investigating neural substrates of behavior and psychopathological conditions. However, few neuroimaging studies involving individuals with ADD or ADHD exist. Shaywitz et al.[70] performed computerized tomography (CT) scans on 35 children with ADD aged 4 to 19. Twenty-seven children matched for age, sex, and IQ, who had scans for other reasons, were used as a contrast group. Using quantitative techniques and "blind" analyses of the CT scans, the authors found no differences in the two groups.

Lou et al.[49] measured cerebral blood flow in 13 subjects aged 6 1/2 to 15 years with developmental dysphasia and/or ADD. The normal comparison group consisted of 9 children aged 7 to 15 years, who were siblings of the dysphasic/ADD children. Lou et al. found no CT differences in the two groups; however, the dysphasic/ADD children showed hypoperfusion in both hemispheres compared to normal controls. Areas of hypoperfusion included periventricular white matter, border zones between major arterial territories, and (in dysphasic subjects) perisylvian regions. All ADD subjects showed hypoperfusion in white matter of frontal lobes and some caudate nuclear regions. Object-naming tasks did not result in any increased blood flow. However, methylphenidate increased perfusion in central regions (e.g., mesencephalon basal ganglia) and decreased perfusion of motor and primary sensory cortical areas. These results need to be evaluated in light of the fact that subject numbers were relatively small, the age ranges were relatively wide (reflecting varied stages of development), and the sample included subjects with developmental dysphasia and mental retardation. Thus, the subjects were not truly representative of most ADD children. Furthermore, the method used did not allow precise localization of the group differences in cerebral blood flow. In addition, the authors were limited in their analysis to one (middle) slice only.

More recently, Lou and colleagues,[50] using similar xenon inhalation techniques, showed hypoperfusion in the striatal regions of children with symptoms of hyperactivity, impulsivity, and inattention. The primary sensory and sensorimotor cortical regions were highly perfused. Methylphenidate increased flow to striatal and posterior periventricular regions and tended to decrease flow to primary sensory regions. Thus, low striatal activity may be involved in these symptoms.

Nasrallah et al.,[59] studying 24 young adults (mean age 23) with a history of hyperactivity in childhood, reported that the hyperactives had increased cortical atrophy compared to 27 male matched normal controls. All subjects with hyperactive symptoms had received stimulant medication in childhood. However, a large proportion of the hyperactive subjects also had a history of significant substance abuse. Therefore, it is unclear if the cortical atrophy found was associated with the hyperactivity, stimulant medication, or secondary to chronic substance use.

Most recently, Zametkin et al.[80] evaluated glucose metabolism in 25 biological parents of hyperactive children. These parents had retrospective histories of childhood hyperactivity but had not received any stimulant medication. The control group consisted of 50 subjects of similar age, sex, and IQ. Glucose metabolism tests were carried out while subjects were performing an auditory attention task (selection of lowest of three tones). The task lasted for 35 minutes. Analyses included computer-assisted measurements and were performed by two "blinded" research assistants. Zametkin *et al.* reported that global glucose metabolism was decreased by 8.1% in the hyperactive adults compared to the controls. Specifically, absolute rates of glucose metabolism in the hyperactives were significantly low in 30 out of 60 brain regions examined, including lateral, frontal, and parietal cortex (bilaterally), medial frontal cortex (including the cingulate), and some subcortical structures (the striatum and the thalamus). When the rates of glucose metabolism were normalized, the only regions with significantly reduced metabolism were the premotor and prefrontal cortex in the left hemisphere. However, since the diagnosis of the subjects in this study was based on retrospective reports, its validity is obviously somewhat compromised.

Additional evidence for possible frontal lobe involvement in ADHD has also come from Chelune *et al.*,[20] who pointed out that the prefrontal regions of the frontal lobes have reciprocal pathways with the reticular formation and the diencephalic structures, which regulate arousal and the ability to suppress responses to task-irrelevant stimuli. Lesions in this area decrease goal-directed activity and the modulation of impulsive behavior. Thus, frontal lobe lesions result in hyperactivity and disturbed higher-level cortical inhibition, with a resulting failure to inhibit inappropriate responses. The authors found partial support for this frontal lobe dysfunction hypothesis by comparing normal controls and children with symptoms of hyperactivity, impulsivity, and inattention on a comprehensive neuropsychological test battery designed to assess the above-described functions.

Since then, Gorenstein *et al.*,[35] Tannock *et al.*,[74] and Everett *et al.*[27] have also shown deficits in children with ADHD that are compatible with frontal lobe dysfunction. Recent reviews by Heilman *et al.*[39] and Benson,[7] which explore a number of syndromes of abnormal mental awareness associated with prefrontal, frontal, and striatal dysfunction, suggest that abnormalities seen in these patients resemble deficits documented in children with ADHD. They thus suggest that the prefrontal and right frontal–striatal systems may be affected in children with ADHD.

We thus see that a number of different areas of the brain have been implicated in this condition. Recently, there has been particular emphasis on the frontal lobes. It is likely that different areas may be associated with different aspects of the syndrome and that the various areas mentioned may be interconnected into a reciprocal modulating system. The questions of which areas may be affected and how these interconnections function are being explored with new neuroimaging tools such as CT scans, magnetic resonance imaging, and positron emission tomography.

Neurochemical Aspects

The hypotheses of the neurochemical systems that may be involved in ADHD come from three general types of studies: neuroanatomical studies of transmitters, nonpharmacological biochemical studies of neurotransmitters and their metabolites, and psychopharmacological studies of neurotransmitters. These studies are well summarized and reviewed by Zametkin and Rapoport[81,82] and Hechtman.[37]

NEUROANATOMICAL STUDIES OF NEUROTRANSMITTERS

Even though some areas of the brain have been clearly associated with certain neurotransmitters, neuroanatomical studies of neurotransmitters have proven to be very complex. The complexity comes from the fact that any particular area can be involved with several different neurotransmitters or can receive projections from various neurotransmitter pathways or nuclei. Thus, there is rarely a one-to-one correspondence between a particular area and a single neurotransmitter exerting exclusive influence on this area.

NONPHARMACOLOGICAL STUDIES OF NEUROTRANSMITTERS AND THEIR METABOLITES

Other studies have compared subjects with ADHD and normal controls with regard to monoamines and their metabolites in urine, plasma, platelets, and (rarely) cerebrospinal fluid. The limitations of such peripheral measures in reflecting an accurate central nervous system neurotransmitter picture are clear. Generally, no consistent differences in any of the peripheral measures of monoamines and their metabolites have been found between ADHD children and normal controls.

PSYCHOPHARMACOLOGICAL STUDIES OF NEUROTRANSMITTERS

Still other studies have looked at a particular psychopharmacological agent, its possible relationship to one or more neurotransmitters, and its clinical effect. From such an analysis, it is then postulated how the drug may work and what the possible underlying problem in the neurotransmitter systems may be. The three types of studies outlined above have given rise to various neurotransmitter hypotheses.

DOPAMINE HYPOTHESIS

The dopamine hypothesis was first proposed by Shaywitz et al.[69,71] following the examination of cerebro spinal fluid dopamine levels in ADHD children, and their work with an animal model of hyperactivity in rats whose brains were depleted of dopamine by injection of hydroxydopamine.

More recently, Schneider and Kovelowski[68] and Roeltgen and Schneider[64] showed that chronic low-dose N-methyl-4-phenyl-1,2,3,6-tetrahydropyridine (MPTP) administered to monkeys caused caudate-frontal dysfunction and cognitive difficulties that were consistent with those seen in children with ADHD. Pilot neurochemical studies on these monkeys have suggested abnormalities in dopamine and norepinephrine metabolism. Moreover, stimulants affect both the dopamine and norepinephrine systems and are very effective in ameliorating this condition. Lou et al.[50] have suggested that methylphenidate activates the dopamine neurons by decreasing the reuptake of dopamine. However, stimulants are also known to have dopamine-releasing effects. These studies clearly suggest dopamine involvement in ADHD.

NORADRENERGIC HYPOTHESIS

The noradrenergic system has been implicated in ADHD in a number of ways. Stimulants, particularly dextroamphetamine, have been shown to release epinephrine in the hypothalamus, and clinical studies have noted that dextroamphetamine and methylphenidate elevate urinary epinephrine excretion by as much as 200%.[26] A norepinephrine agonist, clonidine (an alpha-adrenergic agonist), has been somewhat effective in treating ADHD.[41] Hunt and his colleagues[41] have suggested that the effectiveness of clonidine is mediated by direct stimulation of presynaptic sites to decrease production or release of norepinephrine, and a corresponding increase in postsynaptic noradrenergic sensitivity. Furthermore, the moderate effectiveness of some antidepressants (e.g., desipramine[23]) and of some monoamine oxidase inhibitors also suggests drug-induced changes in the noradrenergic system.

McCraken[52] has thus proposed a two-part model of stimulant action in ADHD in children. He suggests that stimulant medication increases dopamine release and increases adrenergic-mediated inhibition of the noradrenergic locus coeruleus. Thus, he posits involvement of both the dopamine and norepinephrine systems.

SEROTONIN HYPOTHESIS

There is weak evidence for involvement of the serotonergic system in ADHD. Serotonin-depleted animals show increased aggression and hyperactivity. Tricyclic antidepressants and monoamine oxidase inhibitors are moderately effective in ADHD and are known to affect serotonin metabolism. However, hyperactive subjects have shown inconsistent changes in platelet and blood 5-hydroxytryptophan. Furthermore, pharmacological studies involving L-tryptophan, a serotonin precursor,[60] and fenfluramine, which acutely increases and then depletes brain serotonin, have shown no consistent results.

NONSPECIFIC CATECHOLAMINE HYPOTHESIS

It thus becomes clear that not one but several neurotransmitter systems are involved in ADHD—dopamine, norepinephrine, and serotonin. Stimulants, the most effective treatment for most ADHD children, promote catecholamine utilization in the synapse by facilitating synthesis and release of catecholamines and by blocking their reuptake. Furthermore, stimulants appear to inhibit the catabolic enzyme monoamine oxidase. A summary of various neurotransmitter systems and how they may be affected by various drugs has been presented by Zametkin and Rapoport,[81] as shown in Figure 22-2. The interrelationship of the various neurotransmitter systems further undermines the likelihood of the single-neurotransmitter hypotheses' being correct.

Enzymatic regulation of neurotransmitter production and metabolism has also been investigated. Children with ADHD and normal children have shown no significant differences in levels of dopamine-beta-hydroxylase, monoamine oxidase, and catechol-O-methyl-transferase.[16]

OTHER NEUROTRANSMITTERS

One should consider other neurotransmitters that have not been studied in relation to ADHD but may be implicated in the future, such as gamma-aminobutyric acid, which is thought to be predominantly an inhibiting neurotransmitter in the central nervous system, and histamine, which acts both centrally and peripherally.

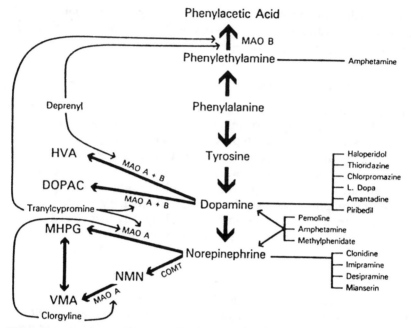

FIGURE 22-2. Presumed effect of drugs that have been studied with hyperactive children. HVA, homovanillic acid; MAO, monoamine oxidase; MHPG, 3-methoxy-5-hydroxyphenylacetic acid; VMA, vanillyl mandelic acid; DOPAC, 3-4-dihydroxyphenylacetic acid. Source: 81.

Neurobiological Aspects: Summary

In general, there has been some progress in the understanding of the neurobiological basis of ADHD. Neuroanatomically, it is clear that the frontal lobes, particularly the prefrontal and striatal areas, play an important role in this condition. Neurotransmitters such as norepinephrine, dopamine, and (to a lesser degree) serotonin are clearly important. However, it is also clear that no one area or neurotransmitter will adequately explain the neuropathology or neurophysiology of this condition. It is much more likely that the condition results from an interaction of various areas of the brain and possibly a number of different neurotransmitters. The variation in the condition with regard to particular symptoms (e.g., ADD[H] vs. ADD only) and their severity, and the association of particular comorbid conditions, may reflect the various areas and neurotransmitter systems involved. Let us hope that recent technological advances, including measures of cerebral blood flow, glucose utilization, and positron-emitting liquids that can quantitate and label specific neurotransmitter receptors, will enable researchers to unravel the complex puzzle of what underlies ADHD.

COMORBIDITY AND SUBGROUPS OF CHILDREN

Children with and without Hyperactivity

The DSM-III classification described two subtypes of ADD: ADD with hyperactivity (ADD[H]), and without (ADD only). Children with ADD(H) exhibited problems of attention, impulsivity, and hyperactivity, while ADD-only children had problems only with attention and impulsivity. DSM-III-R no longer required symptoms in the three domains of attention, hyperactivity, and impulsivity, and ADD only was no longer a separate diagnostic entity, although a nonspecific, undifferentiated ADD category was added. However, the interest in these two subgroups of ADD children has continued. Although some have found few differences between the two groups,[51,65] a number of other studies[4,24,43,45,46] showed that ADD(H) children displayed more conduct-related, aggressive, and oppositional problems. They were more impulsive and distractible and experienced more social rejection when compared to the ADD-only children. In contrast, children with ADD only were more sluggish, lethargic, and daydreamy. They also tended to be more anxious and shy[45,46] and had more symptoms of depression[4] than the ADD(H) children.

The empirical findings are not clear-cut. Some report poor academic achievement in the ADD-only group[24,46] while others do not.[19] Similarly, Frank and Ben Yun[29] suggested that ADD(H) children had more prenatal and perinatal problems than ADD-only youngsters, whereas Barkley et al.[4] found no significant differences between the two groups in this domain. Frank and Ben Yun[29] also found no difference in family history of psychiatric disorders in the two groups. On the other hand, Barkley et al.[4] reported that families of ADD(H) subjects had more aggression, ADD(H), and substance abuse, while families of ADD-only children had more anxiety.

Barkley et al.[5] also compared three dosages (5, 10, and 15 mg b.i.d.) of methylphenidate in ADD(H) and ADD-only youngsters. Generally, both groups were drug responders. However, more ADD-only than ADD(H) subjects were nonresponders (24% vs. 5%), and more of them (35%) responded best to the low dose, whereas more ADD(H) subjects responded best to the high dose (71%).

Given the different behavioral, emotional, familial, and cognitive profiles reported for ADD(H) and ADD-only children, it is conceivable that they may require different treatments. These issues therefore need to be kept in mind in diagnosing and treating these two subtypes of children.

Comorbidity

There is increasing evidence that children with ADHD are often comorbid for a number of other conditions, particularly Oppositional Defiant Disorder and Conduct Disorder, but also Mood and Anxiety Disorders.[14] Epidemiological studies in New Zealand,[2] Puerto Rico,[15] Canada,[73] as well as clinical studies[3,14,58,63] have suggested that the rate of comorbidity in ADHD is on the order of 30–50% for Conduct Disorder, 35–60% for Oppositional Defiant Disorder, 20–30% for Anxiety Disorders, 30% for Mood Disorders, and 20–25% for learning disabilities. Rates are typically higher in clinic-referred than nonreferred children. Despite these high levels of comorbidity, Biederman *et al.*[12] have also reported that close to 50% of ADHD children are not comorbid for other disorders.

Multiple Comorbidity

The fact that children can be comorbid for multiple conditions further complicates the issue. The rate of various multiple comorbidities has been addressed in very few studies. Generally, Oppositional Defiant Disorder and Conduct Disorder are grouped together because of their frequent co-occurrence and because a good proportion of children with the former go on to develop the latter. Biederman *et al.*[12] found that 20% of ADHD and ADD subjects were comorbid for two or more conditions. The number, type, and particular combination of comorbid conditions have significant implications for etiology,[13,73] course,[33,77] and for treatment.[5,63] For example, ADHD youngsters who are comorbid for Conduct Disorder often have family members with Antisocial Personality Disorder, greater family dysfunction, and poorer long-term outcome; as such, they probably require a more comprehensive treatment approach. On the other hand, children with ADHD and Anxiety Disorders have a significantly poorer response to stimulant treatment than do ADHD children without Anxiety Disorders.[63] Similarly, children with ADHD and depression may respond better to tricyclic antidepressants than stimulants.[8,30]

However, the effect of comorbidity on treatment is as yet unclear: For example, Biederman and colleagues[9] conducted a 6-week double-blind placebo controlled study of desipramine for children with

ADHD, who were also comorbid for Conduct Disorder, Major Depression, and Anxiety Disorders. Contrary to their expectations, there was no impact of comorbidity on clinical response to desipramine. Nonetheless, in view of the fact that patients responded well to desipramine, the authors suggest that a tricyclic antidepressant may be superior to a stimulant in cases of ADHD when depression or anxiety is a prominent comorbidity. Therefore, it becomes important to delineate how children with ADHD and various comorbid conditions respond to different treatment approaches, and how treatments may need to be modified to make them more effective for the various comorbid groupings. Course of the condition and eventual outcome may also be affected by particular types of comorbidities.

CHAPTER TWENTY-THREE

MEDICATION TREATMENT
OF ADHD

PREVALENCE OF STIMULANT USE

Stimulant medication (particularly methylphenidate, or Ritalin®) is the most frequently used drug treatment for children with ADHD.[79] As pointed out by Wilens and Biederman,[99] there has been more research on the use of stimulants for ADHD than on any other medication in pediatric psychopharmacology, with more than 900 scientific articles appearing on this topic from 1983 to 1992. The widespread use of stimulant medication in ADHD is in part attributable to the prevalence of this condition, which is estimated to be present in 3–5% of the school-age population,[84] and in part to the efficacy, rapid action, and relative safety of this medication.

The use of stimulants has been steadily increasing over the last 20 years. Gadow[31] estimated that in 1970, 150,000 children were taking stimulant medication; by 1980, that 270,000 to 541,000 elementary school children were receiving stimulants. In 1988, Safer and Krager[79] showed that in the Baltimore area, 6% of public elementary school students were being given stimulants; 750,000 to 1.6 million children were receiving these drugs throughout the United States. Furthermore, some 25% of children in special education classes were receiving stimulant medication. This survey also showed a decrease in the male-to-female ratio from 8:1 to 5:1, an increased use of stimulant medication for adolescents in secondary school, and an increased use of stimulants for children with inattentiveness without hyperactivity.

HISTORY OF STIMULANT USE

Historically, Bradley[17] is given credit for first describing the efficacy of stimulant treatment (amphetamine) in children. He treated children on an inpatient residential ward and noted dramatic improvement in behavior and academic performance. However, his findings were not acted upon until the 1960s, when Eisenberg et al.[26a] reported efficacy of stimulants in decreasing oppositional behavior in boys in a residential school, and Conners et al.[23] reported on the use of standardized parent and teacher rating scales[22] to monitor drug effect. Since then, there have been numerous controlled treatment studies showing the efficacy of stimulant medication over the short term.

EFFECTIVENESS OF STIMULANTS
Short-Term Effectiveness

Wilens and Biederman[99] reviewed 230 studies that addressed the efficacy of stimulant medication in different age groups. They concluded that most (65–75%) children with ADHD respond positively to stimulant treatment. However, they also point out that a very varied placebo response rate has been reported, ranging from 2%[92] to 39%.[5] This would suggest that the proportion of children who truly responded positively to stimulant medication was in fact less than 65–75%. In a recent study, Elia and colleagues[27] showed that if children who were not responsive to one of the stimulant medications were tried on another, 98% were found to be responsive to one of the two (methylphenidate or amphetamine).

EFFECTS ON COGNITION AND ACADEMIC ACHIEVEMENT

Many studies have shown that stimulants improve cognition, vigilance, reaction time, short-term memory, and learning of verbal and nonverbal material (see reviews by Barkley[5] and [Gittelman-]Klein[35]). Stimulants have also been shown to improve measures of inattention and distractibility.

Early reviews by Barkley[5] and Gadow[32] concluded that despite the significant cognitive improvements outlined above, stimulant treatment was associated with only minimal improvement in academic performance. However, studies at that time usually used the Wide Range Achievement Test—a relatively insensitive measure for detecting changes in the short term—to measure academic improvement. More recently, Douglas et al.,[25] Rapport et al.,[71,72] and Famularo and Fenton[28] showed that methylphenidate improved academic productivity and accuracy. One must remember that some ADHD children also have specific learning disabilities, which will not improve with stimulant medication alone. It is thus still unclear whether these short-term academic improvements will result in longer-term scholastic success.

There is significant controversy regarding the effects of different dose levels of stimulants on performance and cognitive tasks. In an important early study, Sprague and Sleator[87] found that short-term memory tests improved most on dose levels of 0.3 mg/kg, whereas greatest improvement in hyperactivity was seen at a higher dosage (i.e., 1 mg/kg). It was therefore suggested that higher dosages may improve behavior but are not optimal cognitively. However, (Gittelman-)Klein[35] reviewed 11 studies that addressed the dose–response issue as it related to cognitive function, and found only two reporting that higher doses impaired cognition. All nine other studies showed improved cognitive functioning with increasing dosages. Similarly, recent studies by Tannock et al.,[91] Rapport et al.,[71] and Kupietz et al.[56a] that have looked at various dosage ranges have all shown improved cognitive functioning at higher dosages.

It has been suggested that higher dosages of stimulants may result in constriction of attention or overfocusing, resulting in reduction of cognitive flexibility. A study by Solanto and Wender[86] of 19 ADHD children aged 6 to 10, which explored cognitive flexibility via the Wallach–Kogen Battery at three different dosages (0.3, 0.6, and 1.0 mg/kg), did not show any negative effect for overfocusing. These findings were replicated by Tannock and colleagues[91] using other tasks. It is therefore reasonable to conclude that cognition generally improves with increasing dosages in the range of 0.3 to 1.0 mg/kg, without negative effects on flexibility or overfocusing. Even so, titration should be individualized, with the optimal cognitive dose determined for each child.

BEHAVIORAL EFFECTS

MOTOR ACTIVITY. Stimulants reduce the excessive motor activity characteristic of ADHD. Early measures to demonstrate this effect were relatively insensitive and could only carry out measurement over short periods of time. These early measures included laboratory observations, counting grid crossings, stabilimetric chairs, and wrist and ankle actometers. There were suggestions that motor activity per se did not differentiate ADHD children from normals as much as purposeless activity did.

Recent technical development of a portable actometer with a solid-state memory enabled researchers to record number of movements over a 10-day period. Using such a device on 12 hyperactive boys, Porrino et al.[67,68] showed that ADHD children had higher activity levels at all times, even during sleep, than did normal controls. These researchers further illustrated that activity levels significantly decreased with the administration of dextroamphetamine and increased beyond the initial level when the drug wore off, thus demonstrating the existence of "rebound."

These findings were elaborated on by Borcherding et al.,[16] who compared dextroamphetamine (0.2 to 0.6 mg/kg twice daily) and methylphenidate (0.45 to 1.25 mg/kg twice daily) on activity levels. The authors found that methylphenidate reduced motor activity more than dextroamphetamine did, and that plasma drug levels did not correlate with activity changes. These studies clearly indicate that stimulants decrease motor activity.

IMPULSIVITY. Rapport and colleagues[73] particularly focused on the effects of different dosages of methylphenidate on impulsivity. Impulsive behavior has a negative effect on academic performance and peer relationships, and may contribute to accident proneness and delinquency. Impulsivity has been measured via latency times and error rates on the Matching Familiar Figures Test and via parent and teacher ratings of self-control. More recently, Tannock et al.[90] assessed inhibitory control at two doses of methylphenidate (0.3 and 1.0 mg/kg/day) and found improvement in this function with increasing dosages.

AGGRESSIVENESS. ADHD children who are aggressive have a more negative long-term outcome.[58] Thus, a number of recent studies by Klorman et al.,[56] Barkley et al.,[8] Gadow et al.,[33] and Kaplan et al.[54] suggesting that methylphenidate can decrease aggressive behavior are encouraging. This improvement in aggressive symptoms appears to be dose-dependent, with greater improvement at higher dosages. However, at similar dosages, Hinshaw et al.[50] found only slight decreases in aggression in 24 school-age boys, while in another study, Hinshaw[49] suggested that methylphenidate may have an effect on covert aggression such as stealing or vandalism. We may conclude that aggressive behavior may be improved by stimulant medication, but that the effect is probably a relatively weak one.

CLASSROOM BEHAVIOR. Abikoff and Gittelman[2] conducted a study in which they evaluated classroom behavior of 28 ADHD children treated for 8 weeks on methylphenidate (mean dose 41.5 mg/day). The evaluations were carried out via direct observations by "blinded" observers using a structured observational scale. The stimulant-treated ADHD children were indistinguishable from controls on measures of gross and fine motor movements, hyperactivity, noncompliance, and interference.

RELATIONSHIPS

FAMILY RELATIONSHIPS. A number of studies have shown that stimulant treatment of the ADHD child has a positive effect on mother–child interactions,[6,7] sibling interactions,[81] and overall family interactions.[81] Generally, stimulant-treated ADHD children are more compliant with maternal commands. Mothers, on the other hand, become less controlling and intrusive, less critical, and warmer. There are fewer negative interactions with siblings, and the family as a whole is more open to other psychosocial interventions.

PEER RELATIONSHIPS. Stimulants have been shown to improve peer relationships in ADHD children. In one early study, Whalen et al.[97] showed that when on methylphenidate at doses of 5 to 40 mg/day, ADHD children were less intense, became more involved in tasks, communicated more effectively, and were generally more socially responsive. Similarly, Swanson et al.[88] found that children on stimulants showed fewer negative social behaviors than when they were off stimulants.

More recently, Whalen et al.[98] showed that the social judgment of ADHD children was improved on stimulants. Whalen[96] also showed that ADHD boys on stimulant medication obtained more peer nominations for being "cooperative," being "fun to be with," and acting like a "best friend" than they obtained in the nonmedicated state. However, these ratings remained below those of children without ADHD.

Generally, the studies mentioned above have indicated that social improvement is better on higher dosages (e.g., 0.3 vs. 0.6 mg/kg). It is clear that with stimulant medication alone, many interpersonal problems of ADHD children persist, and other interventions (such as social skills training and parent training) may also be required. However, stimulants appear to improve the situation, and may make other additional interventions easier to implement and more likely to succeed.

Long-Term Effects

Few well-controlled studies have evaluated the effect of stimulant medication in ADHD children over the long term. In an early study, Weiss et al.[94] compared the adolescent outcome of ADHD children who received stimulant treatment (methylphenidate) for 3–5 years in childhood with that of children who did not receive such medication. Surprisingly, no significant differences were found in adolescence between the treated and untreated hyperactive groups. In a subsequent study, Hechtman et al.[48] compared prospectively followed ADHD children when they were about 19 to 25 years of age. One group had received 3–5 years of stimulant medication during childhood, while the other had not. There were few significant differences between the two groups at 19 to 25 years of age with regard to education completed, job status, psychiatric history, or antisocial behavior (including drug and alcohol abuse). However, the group who had received stimulant treatment in childhood viewed their childhoods more positively and had somewhat better social skills and self-esteem. It thus seems clear that stimulant treatment is very effective in short-term studies, where it has been shown to improve cognitive, behavioral, and social functioning. However, additional interventions may be required to obtain a more positive long-term outcome.

ADVERSE EFFECTS (SIDE EFFECTS) OF STIMULANTS
Short-Term Side Effects

Generally, stimulant side effects are dose-dependent, are mild to moderate in most children, and can be managed either by decreasing the dose or changing the time when medication is given. In an early review, Barkley[5] summarized the findings from 110 studies involving some 4200 patients. More recently, Barkley et al.[9] conducted a systematic study of 83 ADHD children, involving placebo and two doses of methylphenidate (0.6 mg and 1.0 mg/kg/day) for 7–10 days. They carefully recorded adverse short-term effects. These authors discovered a very high (< 50%) and variable rate of side effects reported on placebo. Some of these "placebo" side effects (e.g., staring, lack of interest, sadness, and anxiety) were reduced with methylphenidate treatment. Only 4% of children receiving stimulants had to discontinue treatment because of side effects.

COMMON SIDE EFFECTS

The most commonly reported stimulant side effects include insomnia, decreased appetite, weight loss, abdominal pain, headaches, irritability, and increased crying. Minor increases in heart rate and diastolic and systolic blood pressure have also been reported; these effects are very variable and seem somewhat related to dose.[55] It seems that these cardiovascular effects decrease with long-term treatment.[18] Most side effects can be reduced by decreasing the dose of medication. In addition, insomnia can be treated by giving most of the medication early in the day. If this is ineffective or undesirable (i.e., the child needs medication later in the day), diphenhydramine (Benadryl®) can be used at bedtime. Gastrointestinal symptoms can be alleviated by giving the medication in the middle of the meal or by administering some antacids. Weight loss can be avoided by adding a significant snack at bedtime, when most of the medication has worn off.

INFREQUENT SIDE EFFECTS

TICS. An important, although infrequent, side effect of stimulant medication is the appearance of motor tics. Usually these are facial tics, but repetitive throat clearing or sniffing may also occur. Generally, ADHD children should be screened for tics, as well as for a history of tic disorder or Tourette's syndrome in the family. If any of these is present, stimulants may be contraindicated. If tics develop on stimulant medication, the medication should be discontinued. It is estimated that 1% of ADHD children who are treated with stimulants will develop a tic disorder and that 13% will show exacerbation of pre-existing tics.[23a] Generally, reducing or discontinuing the stimulant medication eliminates the tics. A trial of another class of medication (e.g., clonidine or desipramine) may be considered.

BEHAVIORAL REBOUND. Behavioral rebound is seen when children experience stimulant withdrawal at the end of the school day. Common symptoms include irritability, excitability, motor hyperactivity, overtalkativeness, and insomnia. Among the first investigators to describe behavioral rebound were Rapoport *et al.*[69] This group showed that three-quarters of 14 ADHD boys receiving dextroamphetamine showed rebound, but none of the subjects on placebo showed this behavior. A more recent careful study by Johnston *et al.*[53] found that only one-third of 21 children treated with methylphenidate at two dosages (0.3 mg/kg and 0.6 mg/kg) showed rebound. Furthermore, the magnitude of the rebound varied considerably on different days for the same child. A measure such as reducing the noon dose or adding a small dose later in the afternoon usually deals adequately with the rebound. Medication rarely has to be discontinued because of rebound effects.

OTHER INFREQUENT SYMPTOMS. Loss of spontaneity is a side effect occasionally reported by the parents and is generally easily dealt with by decreasing the dose of stimulant medication.

RARE SIDE EFFECTS

PSYCHOSIS. Stimulant-induced toxic psychosis is rare in children. Only 30 cases have been reported in the literature.[41] Pre-existing psychosis should be a contraindication for stimulant use, as stimulants can exacerbate a psychotic episode. If psychotic symptoms develop, stimulant medication should be discontinued.

Alopecia and leucocytosis are rare side effects not published in treatment studies but listed in the *Physicians' Desk Reference*.[64] A yearly routine blood count coupled with regular clinical monitoring should adequately address this problem.

Hypersensitivity reactions, which can include skin rash, urticaria, fever, arthralgia, dermatitis, erythema multiforme, necrotizing vasculitis, thrombocytopenia purpura, angina, and cardiac arrhythmias, are again mentioned in the *Physicians' Desk Reference*[64] but not reported in clinical therapeutic studies.

SEIZURE DISORDERS. It was generally believed that stimulants lowered seizure thresholds, and so children with pre-existing seizure disorders should not be given stimulants. However, a recent study by Feldman et al.[29] illustrated that children with seizure disorders and ADHD can be given stimulants and anticonvulsants, with no increase in seizure frequency or EEG changes. Plasma levels of anticonvulsants need to be monitored to avoid toxicity resulting from methylphenidate's competitive inhibition of metabolic pathways, boosting the plasma levels of both drugs.

Long-Term Side Effects

TOLERANCE

In a recent review, Greenhill[41] summarized the findings of 17 studies that appeared between 1988 and 1992; most of these were of fairly short duration (4 to 12 weeks). Tolerance may not be detected in short-term studies. Other studies had few subjects, large attrition rates, or no measure of drug compliance. All these factors make assessing the presence or absence of tolerance very difficult. One study by Abikoff et al.[1] followed a medication control group for 40 weeks. Attrition was low, and no tolerance was detected. Generally, to date there has been no well-documented report of drug tolerance effects.

GROWTH EFFECTS

The effect of stimulant treatment on height and weight remains unclear. The initial report by Safer et al.[78] on 29 ADHD children showed that stimulant medication (dextroamphetamine more than methylphenidate) reduced weight and height gain. However, there was "growth rebound"—that is, more than expected growth during summer drug holidays when the drug was discontinued. These findings led to the conclusion that stimulants may suppress growth. However, a number of other studies by Gross,[44] (Gittelman-)Klein et al.,[37] and Vincent et al.[93] all suggested that with relatively short-term use (6 months) of methylphenidate, there was no significant growth suppression. Wilens and Biederman[99] have suggested that a small subset of ADHD children may experience significant growth suppression on methylphenidate. These children need to be detected, carefully assessed, and appropriately treated.

Significant drug holidays (e.g., summer vacations) have been advocated to deal with growth suppression, as growth rebound has been reported[37,77] during such drug holidays. However, Satterfield et al.[80] did not detect any differences in growth between those ADHD children who did and those who did not have summer drug holidays. In contrast, (Gittelman-)Klein and colleagues[37] randomly assessed 58 ADHD children on methylphenidate to on-drug and off-drug conditions during the summer, and found a positive effect for height but not weight after two summer drug holidays.

In summary, it is clear from work by Hechtman et al.[47] that subjects with ADHD who received no stimulant medication in childhood reach expected height in adulthood, so there is no reduction in height resulting from the condition itself. It has also been shown by Gittelman and Mannuzza[38] that 65 ADHD children who received methylphenidate in childhood did show an initial growth velocity loss, but "caught up" during adolescence and reached expected heights at age 18. These results thus confirm the conclusions of Roche et al.[76] in their review of the topic that stimulants have mild and transient effects on weight, and only rarely affect final height levels. It has been shown by Greenhill and colleagues[42,43] that growth suppression does not occur via the effects of stimulants on growth hormone or prolactin, and that it most likely is attributable to the effect of the medication in suppressing appetite. However, this assumption has not been systematically investigated with calorie counts and control groups. Even though decreased height velocity is not likely to be a significant problem for most ADHD children on stimulants, it may be an issue for a small subgroup. Therefore, height and weight should be regularly monitored (at least every 6 months) when an ADHD child is on stimulants, to ensure that he or she stays in his particular growth curve.

OTHER LONG-TERM SIDE EFFECTS

CARDIOVASCULAR EFFECTS. Stimulant medication has been reported to have mild effects in increasing heart rate and blood pressure. However, Hechtman et al. showed that in adulthood, the blood pressure and pulse of hyperactives who did not receive stimulants in childhood did not differ significantly from those of matched normal controls[47] or from those of hyperactives who received 3–5 years of stimulant treatment during childhood.[48] These findings are reassuring, but some concern that ADHD children treated with stimulants in childhood may have increased risk for cardiovascular problems in middle or later life remains. This important issue needs to be addressed more systematically in long-term follow-up studies.

FUTURE DRUG USE OR ABUSE. Parents are often concerned that stimulant treatment in childhood may result in future abuse of stimulants or other drugs by their children. A review of this area[46] has not supported this concern (see also Chapter 8, this volume). Generally, stimulant treatment in childhood had not resulted in greater drug abuse in adolescence or adulthood.

ATTRIBUTION. Another concern raised by parents and clinicians is that ADHD children will attribute their improved behavior and/or cognition to the drug, and will feel that they have no control over or responsibility for their behavior; thus, development of self-control and responsibility will be significantly impaired. No detailed controlled studies have addressed this issue, but this is a complex area. ADHD children generally tend to blame others for their problem while at the same time they have a rather negative self-image and poor self-esteem, suggesting that a great deal of self-blame also exists. Medication is often given with the statement that it will help the child control and improve his or her own behavior and academic performance. Thus, the medication does not rob the child of a sense of control or responsibility. However, detailed studies may be required to address this issue more clearly. This problem can be ameliorated if the child is given a careful explanation of what Ritalin does and does not do, leaving the child with the feeling that he or she can exert considerable control over behavior (the drugs will be a help in this regard), and that he or she is an important partner in a therapeutic enterprise (see Ian Murray's "Postscript").

COMORBIDITY AND SIDE EFFECTS. As described by Bieder-man and colleagues[14] and outlined in Chapter 22 of this volume, the whole area of the presence of comorbid conditions in ADHD children has received increasing attention in recent years. Some authors[66,89] have suggested that these comorbid conditions may affect the ADHD child's reaction to stimulant medication. Specifically, Pliszka[66] found that children with ADHD and Anxiety Disorder were less responsive to stimulant medication than were ADHD children without Anxiety Disorder. In a double-blind, randomized crossover study, Tannock and colleagues[89] found that children with ADHD and anxiety were just as responsive but had significantly more side effects than did the ADHD group without comorbid Anxiety Disorder. Thus, various comorbid conditions, particularly anxiety, may affect stimulant treatment response and side effects in ADHD children.

LONG-ACTING STIMULANTS

Generally, the long-acting stimulants were developed to improve compliance and to decrease any stigma associated with taking medication. They enable the ADHD child to take one long-acting tablet in the morning, avoiding the lunch-time dose at school, which will exert its effect for most of the day; this eliminates the need to take medication at school. Currently, three types of long-acting medications are available. These include Ritalin SR® (methylphenidate in a wax matrix for slow release), a dextroamphetamine "spansule" containing small medication particles, and Cylert® (pemoline). Generally, regular Ritalin is available in 10- and 20-mg dosages, and the Ritalin SR is available in 20-mg slow-release dosage. The daily dose range is between 2.5 and 60 mg/day. Dexedrine (or dextroamphetamine) is available in 5-mg tablets and spansules, and 10- and 15-mg spansules. The daily dose range is between 2.5 and 40 mg/day. Cylert is available in 18.75-, 37.5-, and 75-mg tablets. The daily dose range is between 18.75 and 112.5 mg/day. As described earlier, dosages should be carefully titrated for each child so as to determine the lowest optimal dose with the fewest side effects.

The slow-release stimulants have a more gradually rising peak, and maximum drug effect (behavioral and cognitive) at about 3 hours postingestion, as opposed to 2 hours with short-acting stimulants. Generally, a number of controlled studies that have compared equivalent dose effects of long- and short-term stimulants have shown that the effect of an 8 A.M. dose of 20-mg Ritalin SR is equivalent clinically to two 10-mg doses of regular Ritalin at 8 A.M. and 12 noon.[11,30,61,62] However, other authors[26] have suggested that the long-acting Ritalin SR-20 may not be as effective as the short-acting Ritalin. It has been hypothesized[15] that the steeper absorption curve of the short-acting methylphenidate gives it a more powerful beneficial effect. The steeper absorption curve may also result in more side effects. In addition, some concerns have been raised about unpredictable release of active methylphenidate from the wax matrix of the slow-release preparation. Thus, the question of the clinical efficacy of long-acting versus short-acting stimulants has as yet not been definitively resolved.

The advantages of pemoline include minimal cardiovascular effects and less intense rebound when compared to methylphenidate or dextroamphetamine. The disadvantages include the fact that clinical benefits may be seen only after 3–4 weeks of use and that the effects when seen are not as great as with methylphenidate or dexedrine. Another important concern with pemoline is that of possible hepatotoxic effects. From 1% to 3% of ADHD children treated with pemoline may develop elevated liver enzymes. These effects are usually reversed when the drug is withdrawn. However, regular monitoring (approximately every 2–3 months) with liver function tests is recommended.

MECHANISM OF STIMULANT ACTION

The mechanism of action of stimulants in improving ADHD symptoms has not been completely worked out. However, it has been shown that stimulants block the reuptake of dopamine and norepinephrine at presynaptic neurons and increase the release of these neurotransmitters into the extraneuronal space.[27] They also function as direct agonists at postsynaptic adrenergic receptors.

One proposed model of stimulant action in ADHD[100] suggests that noradrenergic areas of the frontal cortex exerting inhibitory influences act on lower striatal structures (mainly dopaminergic). Serotonin activity does not appear to be greatly involved.

Stimulant effect on neurohormone release remains unclear. Dextroamphetamine was shown to suppress sleep-related prolactin release. Other hormonal responses were not suppressed (e.g., cortisol and sleep-related human growth hormone).[42, 43] Given over the long term, methylphenidate has been shown to suppress prolactin, release human growth hormone, and increase beta-endorphins.[74]

Greenhill[41] has pointed out that stimulants suppress somatomedin *in vitro*. This would limit long bone growth if it occurred *in vivo*. The author reports that in 13 boys given 0.8 mg/kg of dextroamphetamine for 12 months, there was a trend ($p < .07$) for a decrease in somatomedin and a decrease in height and weight velocity. Thus, there is much yet to be learned about the neuroendocrine effects of various stimulants.

STIMULANT ABSORPTION AND METABOLISM

Stimulants are rapidly absorbed from the gastrointestinal tract and thus exert their action quickly, often within 30 minutes after ingestion. Food enhances absorption[20] For methylphenidate, peak behavioral effects generally occur within 1–2 hours postingestion and dissipate within 3 to 5 hours. Peak plasma concentration occurs within 1 to 2 hours, and the half-life of this drug is 2 to 3 hours.[60,83] Generally, little methylphenidate is bound in the plasma; this makes it readily available to cross the blood–brain barrier. There is a six- to eight-fold preferential uptake of methylphenidate into the central nervous system compared to serum. This would partially explain the efficacy of methylphenidate in relatively low doses, as well as the poor correlations between clinical effect and plasma levels.

Dextroamphetamine's peak behavioral effects occur within 1–2 hours and dissipate within 4 to 5 hours postingestion. Peak plasma concentration occurs within 2–3 hours, with a half-life of 4 to 6 hours.

Slow-release methylphenidate has a peak behavioral effect within 2–3 hours and lasts up to 8 hours postingestion. The half-life is 2 to 6 hours, with a peak plasma level from 1 to 4 hours. The corresponding limit for slow-release dextroamphetamine is somewhat longer. The time response behavioral characteristics of pemoline have not been well documented. Pemoline has a half-life of 7 to 8 hours and reaches peak plasma levels 1 to 4 hours postingestion. Seventy-five percent of the dose is excreted in the urine within 24 hours.

Generally, methylphenidate is metabolized quickly, as it is not greatly bound to plasma protein or directed to fat stores. It is almost entirely metabolized within 12 hours. The parent compound is metabolized by hydrolysis; 20% is oxidized as well as conjugated by the liver.[63]

DRUG INTERACTIONS

Generally, mixing stimulants with other medications is not recommended. The addition of a monoamine oxidase inhibitor, often used as an antidepressant, to stimulants may result in extremely high, potentially lethal blood pressure levels. Zametkin and colleagues[101] have even advised against the use of one such drug, tranylcypromine (Parnate), for ADHD children, despite its effectiveness; the fear is that parents may mistakenly use methylphenidate at times if they run out of the Parnate, resulting in a potentially lethal rise in blood pressure.

The addition of stimulants to oral medications used to treat asthma (e.g., theophylline) can result in dizziness, tachycardia, palpitations, weakness, and agitation.

Stimulants may compete with other drugs for the same metabolic pathways, thus increasing plasma levels of both drugs. Thus methylphenidate elevates plasma levels of tricyclic antidepressants, fluoxetine, anticonvulsants, coumarin, anticoagulants, and phenylbutazone.

Stimulants can also interfere with the action of other drugs. Thus, methylphenidate can block the antihypertensive action of guanethidine. Dextroamphetamine can slow the absorption of phenytoin and phenobarbital, and can block the action of some beta-adrenergic antagonists. Generally, drug interactions need to be kept in mind when stimulants are administered, and parents should be made aware of the potential problems of mixing various medications.

NONSTIMULANT DRUGS IN THE TREATMENT OF ADHD

It is generally agreed among clinicians and researchers that stimulants, particularly methylphenidate, are the drugs of choice in the psychopharmacological treatment of children with ADHD. However, close to 25% of patients diagnosed with ADHD do not respond adequately to stimulant medication: There may be little improvement in designated symptoms, or patients may develop serious side effects that cannot be adequately controlled. Patients may also have comorbid conditions (e.g., anxiety, depression, psychosis, tic disorder, or Tourette's syndrome) that make stimulants less effective or contraindicated. Finally, a combination of stimulants and another drug may be used to produce synergistic or augmented effects. Therefore, there are many reasons why second-order medications may need to be considered.

In an excellent review of this topic, Green[40] provides details of studies utilizing various nonstimulant medications in the treatment of ADHD children.

Tricyclic Antidepressants

The tricyclic antidepressants are the second-line drugs most frequently used in treating ADHD children. Most double-blind studies comparing tricyclic antidepressants with stimulants and placebo show that both drugs are superior to placebo and that stimulants are generally superior to the tricyclic antidepressants.[65,95]

Tricyclic antidepressants have been shown to improve mood and decrease hyperactivity, but they are somewhat sedating and do not improve concentration or cognitive tasks.[24] They may also affect motor coordination. These effects are not usually clinically significant.[45] The longer therapeutic effects and the absence of a significant "rebound" effect generally result in better parent ratings. In addition, the longer duration of action enables the drug to be given once a day at home, thus eliminating the need for administering medication at school. Unlike stimulants, plasma levels of tricyclic antidepressants reflect both therapeutic concentrations (i.e., 150–200 mg/ml) and toxic levels (over 250 mg/ml). Thus, the oral dose can be adjusted through the use of blood level concentrations.

Clinicians should be aware of the fact that 5% of individuals in the general population are genetically predisposed to metabolize tricyclic antidepressants more slowly because of deficiencies in desipramine hydroxylators. This results in two to four times the concentration of tricyclics per unit dose.

Generally, desipramine is said to have fewer side effects than imipramine, amitriptyline, and clomipramine; it has thus been the most widely studied tricyclic antidepressant.[12,13]

The most worrisome side effects with tricyclic antidepressants involve cardiovascular effects. These medications have been shown to increase diastolic blood pressure and heart rate. They also affect cardiac conduction by increasing the PR and QRS intervals; cardiac arrhythmias, tachycardia, and heart block can result. Four sudden deaths have been reported among children receiving tricyclic antidepressants.[59] These reports have resulted in guidelines that include starting at 10 to 25 mg (0.5 to 1.0 mg/kg/day) in divided dosages. Some children will respond at 2 mg/kg, while others will require 5 mg/kg/day. This latter dose should be the maximum dose used. It has been recommended that a 2-week period be used to evaluate any particular dose level. Thus, gradual, slow increases are suggested.

Electrocardiographic monitoring should occur at baseline, 1 mg/kg, 3 mg/kg, and 5 mg/kg; it should be repeated every 3 months. Heart rate should remain under 130 beats per minute, PR interval less than 210 milliseconds, QTc interval less than 450 milliseconds, and QRS interval not in excess of 30% over baseline. If these measures are exceeded, the medication needs to be adjusted downward until the electrocardiogram returns to normal.[13,82]

Other reported side effects include dry mouth, decreased appetite, weight loss, headaches, abdominal discomfort, tiredness, dizziness, and insomnia.[12]

If tricyclics need to be discontinued, this should be done slowly over a 10-day period to decrease any symptoms associated with sudden withdrawal. Such symptoms may also be seen when subjects have poor compliance.

Other Antidepressants

MONOAMINE OXIDASE INHIBITORS

Zametkin et al.[101] demonstrated that a monoamine oxidase A inhibitor (clorgyline) and a mixed A and B inhibitor (tranylcypromine sulfate) were effective in treating children with ADHD. However, a inhibitor (L-deprenyl) was not effective. The potential side effect of extreme blood pressure elevation if required dietary restrictions are not followed, or if Ritalin is inadvertently used as well, makes these medications an unlikely choice in the treatment of ADHD children (see above).

BUPROPION HYDROCHLORIDE

Three studies[19,21,85] have looked at bupropion (Wellbutrin®) in ADHD children. Generally, the children receiving bupropion improved. Optimal dosages ranged from 100 to 250 mg/day or 3 to 6 mg/kg/day. Side effects included skin rash, agitation, dry mouth, insomnia, headache, nausea, vomiting, constipation, and tremor. Seizures have been reported in 4 of 1000 patients; these occurred at predominantly high dosages.

FLUOXETINE HYDROCHLORIDE

Few studies have looked at the efficacy of fluoxetine (Prozac®) for children with ADHD; the few that have been conducted give conflicting results. In a 6-week open study of 19 children with ADHD, Barrickman and colleagues[10] reported that 11 showed significant or moderate improvement. In another study, Riddle and colleagues[75] examined the behavior effects of fluoxetine on 24 children and noted that all 3 children with ADHD showed worsening of their symptoms on the drug. Gammon and Brown[34] reported on a study involving 16 children with ADHD and other comorbid conditions (such as dysthymia, Conduct Disorder, and/or Oppositional Defiant Disorder) who did not respond adequately to methylphenidate alone, so fluoxetine was added. The authors reported that the addition of fluoxetine improved depressive, anxious, conduct, and ADHD symptoms. Greatest improvement was seen in the most significantly disturbed children. Much research is still needed to clarify the usefulness of this medication in ADHD, either by itself or as an adjunct to stimulant treatment.

Antipsychotic Agents

Generally, antipsychotic agents are less effective in treating ADHD symptoms than are stimulants.[39] Furthermore, the potential risk of irreversible tardive dyskinesias and their sedating qualities, which can affect cognition and learning, limit their value. However, recent studies by Aman and colleagues[3,4] suggest that thioridazine may be superior to stimulants in treating a subgroup of mentally retarded patients who also have ADHD symptomatology. Furthermore, (Gittelman-)Klein[36] has suggested that cognitive impairment may be minimized with proper dosages of thioridazine.

Generally, this class of drugs should be considered as third-order drugs. However, they may be useful in retarded children with ADHD symptomatology for whom stimulants and other medications are ineffective.

Clonidine

Clonidine is an antihypertensive agent that is thought to be an alpha-noradrenergic agonist acting on presynaptic neurons to inhibit endogenous release of norepinephrine in the brain. It has been shown to decrease rates of firing in the locus coeruleus, an area rich in norepinephrine neuron cell bodies linked to hyperarousal states.[52] Clonidine has been reported to be most effective in children who are "hyperaroused," with high levels of motor activity, impulsivity, and aggression. These children are often comorbid for Conduct Disorder or Oppositional Disorder. Hunt and colleagues[51] reported that clonidine resulted in improved frustration tolerance, compliance, and coopera- tion, which in turn resulted in better learning and achievement. The medication was not useful in treating distractibility in children with ADD without hyperactivity.

The medication should be increased gradually, with careful monitoring of blood pressure. The initial dose is usually 0.05 mg/day orally, with a gradual 0.05-mg/day increase every third day to a maximum total dose range of 3 to 5 mg/kg (about 0.05 mg four times a day). Hunt et al.[51] have also done studies using a transdermal patch that delivers 0.1, 0.2, or 0.3 mg. The efficacy of the patch usually wears off after 5 days; however, the patch may be useful when compliance with pill taking is an issue. Some children treated by Hunt et al.[52] have benefited from the medication for up to 5 years. If clonidine is discontinued, this should be done gradually over 2 to 4 days to prevent hypertension and withdrawal symptoms, such as headache and agitation.

Side effects include sedation, which usually begins 1 hour after ingestion and lasts 30 to 60 minutes. Tolerance to this side effect usually develops after 3 weeks. Orthostatic hypotension and a general decrease in blood pressure by about 10% can occur. Depression develops in about 5% of children treated. This side effect is often seen in patients with pre-existing depression, a history of depression, or a family history of mood disorder. The medication is therefore not recommended in ADHD children with such histories. Other side effects include headaches, dizziness, stomachache, nausea, vomiting, and cardia arrhythmias.

Leckman et al.[57] have reported clonidine to be effective in a single-blind control trial for patients with ADHD and Tourette's syndrome. It may thus be useful in ADHD children who have tic disorders or who develop tic side effects with stimulants.

Hunt et al.[51] have also advocated the combined use of clonidine and methylphenidate for ADHD children who are comorbid for Conduct Disorder or Oppositional Defiant Disorder, or who have significant side effects on stimulants. The addition of clonidine enabled these authors to decrease the stimulant dose by 40%, thus decreasing stimulant side effects.

In summary, clonidine may be useful for children who have tic disorders or other significant stimulant side effects. However, more studies are needed on its safety and efficacy relative to other second-order medications, such as tricyclic antidepressants.

Other Drugs

As Green[40] points out in his review, fenfluramine, benzodiazepines, and lithium have all be shown to be ineffective in treating ADHD.

CONCLUSION

In conclusion, stimulants remain the drug of choice in the treatment of ADHD. Methylphenidate generally has fewer side effects than dextroamphetamine and is therefore the preferred drug. Long-acting stimulants have certain advantages but also some particular limitations. Some combination of long- and short-acting stimulants may circumvent these problems, but controlled studies are required to clarify this.

Second-order nonstimulant medication usually involves tricyclic antidepressants. Clinicians must carefully monitor potential cardiotoxic side effects. Clonidine has been reported to be useful in ADHD children with tic disorders and other significant stimulant side effects; however, more research is needed on the safety and efficacy of this drug in comparison to other medications. There appears to be greater use of combinations of other medications (fluoxetine, clonidine) with stimulants. These combinations also need further studies regarding safety and efficacy.

CHAPTER TWENTY-FOUR

PSYCHOSOCIAL TREATMENT OF ADHD

BEHAVIOR MODIFICATION

The efficacy of stimulant medication has been clearly shown in various short-term, controlled studies. It decreases activity level and inattention,[12] improves rote learning and short-term memory,[45] and ameliorates classroom behavior.[33,39] However, stimulant medication has its limitations. Twenty to thirty percent of children do not respond favorably to stimulant medication. Even in children with ADHD who do respond, this response is not sufficient to bring the children's academic and social behavior into the normal range. The improvement seen with stimulants is only evident when the drug is physiologically active. Because of possible side effects, medication is usually not given in the late afternoon or early evening. Therefore, a child's behavior and functioning are not improved by stimulants throughout the entire day. Finally, stimulant treatment has not resulted in significantly improved long-term outcome.[14] For all these reasons, despite the apparent efficacy of stimulant medication, additional interventions appear to be needed.

Behavior modification has been an important intervention that has received a good deal of study. The efficacy and limitations of behavior modification therapy for ADHD children have been recently addressed by a number of excellent reviews and studies.[6,12,21,34,35] Generally, behavioral interventions with ADHD children can be divided into three types: (1) clinical behavior therapy, (2) direct contingency management, and (3) cognitive–behavioral intervention.

Clinical Behavior Therapy

Clinical behavior therapy was used in early studies; it generally involves training parents and/or teachers to carry out contingency management programs with the child. Parents are given assigned reading material and taught classical behavioral techniques (e.g., a point system, time out, and the importance of contingent attention).

Teachers are taught classroom management strategies, and often a daily report card is instituted to provide parents with a view of the child's school performance, which is then rewarded at home. This daily report card usually defines four to five specific target behaviors (e.g., completing tasks accurately, completing homework, etc.). Appropriate expectations are set for each individual child. The target behaviors are often components of overall goals (e.g., improved academic performance). Expectations and target behaviors need to be broken into small achievable units, and are adjusted as treatment proceeds. Rewards are set with the child and parents.

Frequent monitoring and modification may be required, particularly in the early phases. Most such interventions involve weekly meetings with parents and teachers. Studies examining the outcome in ADHD children receiving this intervention have usually lasted 8 to 20 weeks. Comparison of pre- and posttreatment ratings and direct observations generally show improvement in both school and home settings. Generally, however, behavioral treatment is not as effective as stimulant treatment.[6,12,34] Furthermore, even though ADHD subjects improve, they do not reach normal levels of functioning and do not improve in all areas (e.g., parent ratings, teacher ratings, peer ratings) across the board.[36] These limitations have been thought to be partially attributable to the fact that the intervention is indirect—that is, carried out by parents and teachers who may not always faithfully adhere to or carry out the program. This limitation is addressed by direct contingency management.

Direct Contingency Management

The treatment components of direct contingency management are usually similar to those of clinical behavior therapy described above. However, contingency management usually involves more intensive intervention directly by a professional, and usually takes place in a specialized treatment facility or demonstration classroom, where there is significant control over treatment implementation. Contingency management frequently involves a point or token reward system, time out, and a response-cost program. Rapport et al.[38] clearly demonstrated the efficacy of a direct response-cost program in which a child lost a minute of free time if he or she was not working. These losses were recorded via a flip card system for the teacher and the child, in which each card had a descending number from 20 to 0. When the child was not working, the teacher would flip a card signaling a 1-minute loss of free time. The child had to monitor the teacher's cards and match his or hers to the teachers. Even though this approach was shown to be as effective as stimulant medication, it was only used with two children in a normal classroom. However, Pelham *et al.*[34] combined response cost with rewards and showed the combination to be effective in managing the children's classroom behavior. The importance of negative consequence in improving behavior in children with ADHD has been shown by O'Leary and colleagues in a number of studies.[40,46] These authors showed that negative consequences (verbal reprimand backed up by time out and loss of privileges) were more effective than positive consequences (teacher attention and praise). Negative consequences were more effective when they were used in the classroom at the outset than when they were gradually introduced. Finally, maintenance of appropriate behavior after withdrawing consequences was better for negative consequences in response costs than for rewards.

The ultimate goal of most behavioral intervention programs is for ADHD children to control and monitor their own behavior, as opposed to having it be controlled by positive or negative contingencies. Cognitive–behavioral interventions were designed to develop such self-instruction and monitoring.

Cognitive–Behavioral Interventions

Among the early proponents of cognitive–behavioral therapy were Meichenbaum and Goodman.[25] They suggested training impulsive children to talk to themselves as a means of developing self-control.

Cognitive therapy was designed to promote self-controlled behavior by enhancing mediation and self-controlling strategies. It was hoped that this would provide internal mediators that would facilitate generalization and maintain effects of behavior therapy. Cognitive–behavioral therapy has taken various forms: verbal self-instruction, problem-solving strategies, cognitive modeling, self-evaluation, and self-reinforcement.

Cognitive–behavioral therapy is usually carried out once or twice a week, with the therapist attempting to teach the child cognitive techniques that he or she can use to control problematic behavior in other settings. Thus, the child is taught to stop, think, and identify the problem; to suggest several possible solutions; to evaluate different solutions; and then to act out the best solution. Techniques are explained to the child. Role play and supervised practice are also used. The child is then encouraged to use these approaches in other settings, such as home and school.

Controlled studies that have evaluated cognitive therapy[1,2,4] have shown that cognitive programs focusing primarily on self-instruction produce little clinical improvement in behavior and academic performance, and do not result in lasting or generalized gains.

Even behavioral treatments that have been shown to be effective have their limitations. First, the improvements noted do not bring the children into the normal range of functioning. Second, no studies have shown long-term maintenance of treatment effects; usually, gains are lost once treatment stops. Often parents and teachers cannot maintain a treatment for long periods of time (e.g., months or years), and thus the treatment probably does not affect long-term outcome. Finally, a small proportion of ADHD children do not improve with behavior modification.

Combined Behavior Modification and Stimulant Medication

The limitations described above, coupled with the significant demands and costs of intensive, well-controlled behavioral programs, have led people to explore the combined effect of behavior modification and stimulant medication. A number of studies[6,12,34] have clearly shown the combined treatment to be superior to either intervention alone. In a comprehensive review of this issue, Pelham and Murphy[35] concluded that two-thirds of the studies reviewed showed the combined intervention to be superior for at least one area of functioning to either intervention alone.

The combined treatment is also more cost-effective because with the introduction of stimulant medication, the scope and complexity of the behavioral intervention can be reduced and so it becomes much less expensive. Furthermore, Carlson et al.[6] have shown that when medication is combined with behavioral therapy, one can achieve the same results with half the stimulant dose. Despite the promise of this combined treatment, its maintenance, generalizability, and effect on long-term outcome have yet to be determined.

PARENT TRAINING

A number of parent training manuals originally devised for reducing oppositional and/or aggressive behaviors have been applied to help parents with children diagnosed with ADHD. Many of these children, even when they fall short of a diagnosis of Oppositional Defiant Disorder or Conduct Disorder, have some oppositional, noncompliant, or aggressive features. Barkley's *Defiant Children*,[3] Patterson's approach,[31] and Forehand and McMahon's protocol[9] have all been used. The differences among these parent training manuals have been summarized elsewhere.[29]

We have used Barkley's approach in parent training for our multimodality treatment study, and this approach is the one discussed here in some detail. We follow up the 12 sessions with weekly individual parent therapy for 1 year.

Treatment Objectives

1. To increase parents' knowledge about ADHD through psychoeducation, and to help them use this knowledge to understand and manage their child better.

2. To provide parents with ongoing clinical supervision, within the context of a group, in the use of specialized contingency management techniques. These techniques address motivational deficits as well as the various noncompliant behaviors.

3. To facilitate the parents' adjustment to having a child with ADHD. (This affects the couple's relationship and the parents' relationship with the ADHD child's sibling[s], as well as the total family functioning.)

4. To employ specific cognitive–behavioral strategies to enhance parental compliance. The group process helps the parents to carry out the program. (Perhaps the lack of group support is partly responsible for the gradual fading out of parental compliance in carrying out the contingency management when the group ends.)

Specific Training Steps

The program can be completed in about 12 sessions. Each session builds on what has been learned in a previous session.

Step I: Introduction
1. An overview of the program is given.
2. A didactic review of ADHD is presented:

- History
- Terminology
- Core symptoms
- Clinical criteria for diagnosis
- Prevalence
- Different types of deficits
- Outcome
- Treatments

There is an emphasis, right from the beginning, and on the fact that ADHD is a lifelong condition and that it can be modified but not cured.

Step II: Understanding parent–child relationships and principles of behavior management
　　1. Parents are helped to understand four factors that contribute to or maintain deviant behaviors:

- Child characteristics
- Parent characteristics
- Situational consequences
- Family stressors

The parents are told that while the child may have inborn characteristics, it is the nature of parent–child interactions that can reliably influence the child's behavior. This stresses the importance of the parents' learning to modify their behaviors.
　　2. Parents are now taught the beginning principles of behavior management, which is covered in increasing detail in subsequent sessions. Parents learn to understand the meaning of antecedent variables (which precede a given behavior), consequences (which influence the rate of that behavior), and feedback conditions.

Step III: Enhancing parents' attending skills ("You get what you see"); emphasizing the importance and technique of "special time"
　　Because of the nature of hyperactive chidren's behavior, they usually elicit few positive parental responses. Most of their parents' reactions to them are corrective, critical, and derogatory. Parents are taught special attending skills and ignoring skills in the context of special periods of time. In this "special time" (perhaps 10–20 minutes), the child has a parent to himself or herself, and can choose the activity. During "special time," the parent must remain noncritical and nondirective, and must learn to ignore deviant behavior during this time. Parents learn to become socially reinforcing and are taught that any behavior management technique is ineffective if there is no positive relationship between the parent and child. We have noted that after parent groups end, contingency management tends to fade (unless specifically reinforced), but "special time" continues longer because the children demand its continuation.

Step IV: Paying attention to appropriate independent play and compliance; giving directions more effectively

Parents learn to look for and reinforce compliance and independent play. They learn to "catch their children being good." Parents are also taught to make their demands more effectively:

- They must only demand that which they will follow through on.
- They must make the demand simple.
- They must make sure they have the child's attention (e.g., eye contact) and get the child to repeat the demand.

Step V: Establishing a home token system to increase motivation

For 9- to 11-year olds, points are usually used; for younger children, chips or tiddlywinks can be used. Positive behaviors are now rewarded with tokens, and at this stage negative behaviors are ignored.

Step VI: Reviewing of the home token economy system; introducing response cost

To the concept of gaining tokens for compliance, response cost adds the refinement of losing tokens for noncompliance. Parents may find this step difficult, and they should review together what works and how. Up to this point, parents have not been taught to use punishments, in order to ensure that positive interaction skills are well established. It is, of course, likely that parents will continue to use their old punishments in addition to the token economy. At this point, tokens are lost for one or two particularly troubling behaviors (e.g., breaking important rules). The number of tokens lost is equivalent to the number that could have been gained had compliance taken place.

Step VII: Using time out from reinforcement

The token economy and response cost are discussed to see how well they are working. Parents are asked to pick the most troubling noncompliant behavior. When this occurs, the child is put into a special room for "time out." Time out is not to be used for long periods. It is difficult for parents to carry this out when their child absolutely refuses; these situations are discussed in the group.

Step VIII: Managing children's behavior in public places

The management of behavior in public places is discussed with the child. The same principles of contingency management response cost, and time out are applied. Expected behaviors and consequences while out of the home are all made very clear to the child, who may be asked to repeat what is expected.

Step IX: Handling future behavior problems
The long-term duration of the disorder is once again emphasized. A booster meeting is planned. At the last meeting, parents often bring up new problems that they have not previously dealt with; a fair amount of anxiety and feelings of loss are usually expressed. In our multimodality study, we follow up the initial parent group training with weekly individual parent guidance sessions for 9 more months, and then monthly sessions for another year.

Efficacy of the Program

Parents learn about ADHD and about behavior management skills. The skills will spill over to the ADHD child's sibling(s), and there may also be a lessening of marital tension. The ADHD child may feel better because he or she is more often rewarded and has special time. While parent training has demonstrated efficacy for noncompliant and aggressive children, its efficacy for children with ADHD is not yet established. The technique of following up the brief parent training sessions with weekly individual parent therapy for 1 year has also not been evaluated.

Contraindications

- Severe marital discord
- Psychopathology of a parent that requires prior treatment
- Psychopathology of a child that is comorbid with ADHD (e.g., depression); this may require a specific intervention

Parent Support Groups

Organizations have sprung up in the past 20 years that are led by parents of children with ADHD or by adults who have ADHD. CHADD (Children with ADD[H]) is one example, and AD-IN (ADD Information Service) and ADDA (Attention Deficit Disorder Association) are others. All over the United States, parents can usually find a self-help group run by parents for parents. Professionals may be asked to give talks to the parents who run their own groups. In these self-help parent groups, one of the most beneficial aspects is the parents' feeling that they are not alone; much mutual support takes place. The purpose of the various national organizations is to empower parents to feel competent in disciplining and nurturing their children, and to work together as partners with professionals. These organizations are also very helpful in disseminating information about where parents can receive competent help.

SOCIAL SKILLS INTERVENTIONS

Children with ADHD have significant interpersonal problems. These arise from the fact that their social interactions are often characterized by impulsivity, intrusiveness, bossiness, aggressiveness, uncoopera- tiveness, noncompliance and social insensitivity. Parker and Asher[30] have clearly shown that peer rejection puts children at risk for school dropout, delinquency, and psychiatric maladjustment. Furthermore, the effects of social skills deficits tend to escalate with time as social rejection leads to poor self-esteem, decreased social interaction, and increasing social skill deficits and interpersonal problems. It is thus crucial to develop effective interventions to enable ADHD children to become socially competent and improve their interpersonal function- ing.

Social skills interventions have included a mixture of techniques operant procedures, modeling appropriate peer behavior; shaping of concrete conversational skills; training in social problem solving; instruction in anger control, self-assessment, and self-monitoring, and strategies to enhance moral development. These variations in focus and approach can be attributed to the fact that social deficits in ADHD children have not been specified and clearly defined. These deficits may, in fact, be significantly different in different ADHD children; therefore, social skills deficits that need to be addressed will vary, as will specific approaches.

In an effort to pinpoint the nature of the social difficulties of ADHD children, Whalen and Henker[49] and Hinshaw et al.[19] showed that children with ADHD do not have deficiencies in global *rates* of social interactions and often display prosocial behaviors. However, the nature and quality of many of their interactions are problematic. They have problems in modulating their responses, in modifying behavior to adapt to changing tasks or situations, and in adhering to plans for carrying out smooth social exchanges. Interventions thus need to modify the *nature* of the social interactions of ADHD children. This is particularly true for children who have ADHD and are also aggressive. Hinshaw[15] showed that aggression was the strongest factor predicting early peer rejection in a summer camp setting for normal and ADHD children. He thus advocates that any treatment must directly target aggressive behavior. Milich and Dodge[26] have shown that children with ADHD and aggression display impulsive and distorted processing of social information. Specifically, these children underutilize social information and quickly attribute hostile intent to people involved in ambiguous social provocative situations. Price and Dodge[37] have further elaborated how such deficient and distorted social information processing gives rise to reactive and retaliatory aggressive behavior. Thus, as Lochman et al.[24] have pointed out, behavioral *and* cognitive treatment approaches may be needed for these aggressive children.

It is clear that social deficits in ADHD children are multiple and varied. Therefore, effective social skills interventions may need to help these children decrease negative peer interactions, increase prosocial skills, increase the accuracy of social information processing, improve general social behavior, and improve academic performance. Clearly, focusing on only one of these aspects will not improve social competence, and a multimodal approach that addresses all these areas may be needed.

Some social skills interventions have improved children's sociometric ratings,[8] and some aggressive children have benefited from cognitive–behavioral and anger control interventions.[22,24] However, a number of recent reviews[16,32,50] have indicated that no treatment or treatment combination results in significant lasting improvement of peer disturbances in children with ADHD. A number of studies have shown that behavioral changes seen by parents and teachers or noted in direct observation did not seem to register with peers. Hinshaw and McHale[20] have suggested that changes may not be perceived by peers because of the lasting effects of a negative social reputation. Undoing such a reputation is indeed difficult. Another factor that may limit the effectiveness of social skills interventions is that social interactions often occur in informal settings without adult supervision. Therefore, it is frequently impossible for teachers and/or parents to control environmental contingencies of the children's social interactions.

Therefore, cognitive–behavioral approaches have been used to improve children's problem-solving strategies. However, as has been shown by Hinshaw et al.,[17,18] the cognitive–behavioral approach is most effective if it is combined with behavioral rehearsal to practice newly developed social skills, explicit reinforcement for appropriate social behavior, and accurate self-assessment and self-monitoring.

Stimulant medication has been shown to decrease the aggressive behavior of ADHD children[15,20,28] without increasing social isolation.[19] The effect of stimulants on ADHD children's aggression does not appear to be mediated by any change in their distortion of social information processing. Stimulants also change peers' appraisal of the children, even though it still does not reach normal levels.[51]

Thus, an approach that combines stimulant medication and behavioral and cognitive–behavioral treatments is generally advocated in addressing the significant social problems of ADHD children.[12,17] Furthermore, treatments need to be individualized and carried out for long periods (years as opposed to months) to help children with ADHD deal adequately with the ever-increasing complexity of social situations.

ACADEMIC SKILLS TRAINING AND REMEDIATION

Organizational Skills Training

It has been clear for many years that the cardinal symptoms of ADHD children—inattention, hyperactivity, and impulsivity—often result in very poor organizational skills. These poor organizational skills are often coupled with specific deficits in visual and/or auditory processing and sequencing. All these difficulties impede academic achievement. Thus, a program that specifically addresses the poor organization strategies of many ADHD children is often required, in addition to any specific remediation designed to deal with specific learning disabilities.

One such program used in our multimodal treatment study for ADHD children involves weekly 1-hour sessions for 16 weeks. Each group consists of four to five children with two educational specialists. The program focuses on strategies to help the children pay attention, follow directions (both written and oral), and develop skills in planning and organizing homework assignments and projects. Developing study skills, note taking, and studying for tests are also addressed. Self-monitoring by checking one's work and strategies to avoid careless mistakes are taught as well; self-monitoring and self-evaluation are reinforced via response cost for inaccurate evaluations. (Children begin each session with a "bank" of points. Point deductions are contingent on mismatches between a child's and trainer's evaluations of the quality of the child's work. In this manner, the children learn to assess their own performance more accurately.) Finally, awareness of time and efficient use of time are dealt with.

Some activities involving the areas outlined above are individualized; others require that children work together to organize, plan, and carry out a project. Every attempt is made to make the activities enjoyable, and social praise and recognition are constant and ongoing for appropriate behavior. Skills learned in one session are reinforced in all subsequent sessions. The organizational and self-monitoring skills are also reinforced in weekly academic remediation sessions, which continue for the remainder of the first year of the treatment, and during regular monthly booster sessions, which occur in the second year of treatment.

Remedial Education and Tutoring

The academic problems of hyperactive children have been well documented.[5,27] Stimulant medication does not eliminate academic handicaps. A placebo-controlled study compared the effects of tutoring and amphetamine in various combinations,[7] but many children did not comply, and the results are uninterpretable. The usefulness of remedial tutoring has been documented in reading-disabled nonhyperactive children.[11] Stimulants added little to reading performance, but arithmetic performance improved significantly. These studies suggest that hyperactives, who are often far behind academically and who at times also have specific learning disabilities, could benefit from remedial tutoring.

Academic remediation in our multimodal study is carried out by a special education teacher, usually once or twice a week. The program is individualized according to each child's specific academic skills deficit. Diagnostic evaluation in key academic areas is carried out for each child, and an individualized program is then designed.

INDIVIDUAL PSYCHOTHERAPY

Chapter 18 deals with individual psychotherapy with children, adolescents, and adults who have ADHD. Clinical vignettes are used to illustrate the different presenting problems and different techniques of therapy at different ages. For example, the case of Derrick illustrates the intensity of the therapeutic relationship that can be formed, as well as its enduring quality. Derrick was a child with severe ADHD who received play therapy between the ages of 5 and 7 years; he was not seen again (because he had moved out of town) until he was 24 years old, at which time he was married and his wife was about to give birth to their first child. At the last session of his 2-year play therapy, he gave the therapist a gift—a mink tail, his transitional object, which had always accompanied him even to his play therapy sessions. Seen again at age 24, Derrick asked about his mink tail, and was delighted when the therapist produced it for him. He expressed an interest in taking it home after his child was born. Out of a range of treatments, it was his play therapy that Derrick remembered as most important.

Since Derrick was treated many years ago, we have gained much more experience with this treatment modality, which this section is designed to summarize and to place in context with other treatments. It is an expensive treatment whose short- or long-term benefit has not been demonstrated for children with ADHD.

For more details about individual psychotherapy with children with ADHD, the reader is referred to a chapter written by one of us together with colleagues,[13] all of whom are engaged in carrying out this treatment as part of the controlled multimodality treatment study for children with ADHD, which is described in a later section. Additional information is also available in a manual of supportive-expressive play psychotherapy for children with externalizing disorders.[23] This manual is helpful for those engaged in psychotherapy with children who have ADHD and oppositional behavior or conduct problems.

Individual child psychotherapy is defined as a process set in motion between a child with ADHD and a trained therapist who meet at least once a week for months, for the purpose of ameliorating specific aspects of the child's difficulties. The main therapeutic vehicle is the formation of a therapeutic alliance between the child and therapist; this forms the basis of a variety of interventions, such as interpretation, confrontation, clarification, and sharing and identifying affects. This form of therapy should never be used as the only treatment of a child with ADHD, but it may become important for certain children as part of a global treatment program.

Individual psychotherapy given to children with ADHD, according to the clinical literature, is controversial. Wender,[48] in a classic article, stated, "Individual psychotherapy is definitely of limited value in treating the common symptoms of MBD" (now termed ADHD). He was referring to the core symptoms of the syndrome (hyperactivity, inattention, and impulsivity, which respond best to stimulant medication). He then cautiously recommended psychotherapy for the many indirect consequences of having this syndrome. These consequences have been graphically described more recently by Henry Smith[44]:

For as each stage of development imposes its own tasks on a child who has failed to master the previous stages and their tasks, failure is compounded with failure, development becomes extremely distorted and delayed, and one begins to see how the original neurophysiological blueprint has undermined the entire structure of the building, resulting in a child who cannot work, cannot play, and has no friends (p. 255)

Smith emphasizes the necessity of psychotherapy for some of these problems.

Divergences from Traditional Forms of Psychotherapy

Certain attributes of children with ADHD make them difficult candidates for traditional forms of psychotherapy:

1. The child with ADHD often does not acknowledge that he or she has a problem and would like to do something about it. Instead, he or she may blankly deny any problems or project them onto others (e.g., "a crummy teacher").

2. The child with ADHD may never have had the experience of being soothed by an adult when distressed. This prior experience is the basis for the formation of an alliance with a therapist. The relative lack of a positive internal or external object (a parent) may result in a very negative transference to the therapist at the beginning of therapy. "I don't want to be here, it's boring, I'm missing my hockey game, I want to go home," is a common response to the start of therapy.

3. The child with ADHD often lacks good communication skills, such as the ability to verbally express and identify affects. Instead, he or she will tend to "act," short-circuiting the affect. For example, Jimmy, aged 9, would have a temper tantrum when something did not go his way, but could not say that he was mad or upset. Jimmy, like many others with ADHD, could not confide, did not want to confide, did not want this therapy, and could not at first interact mutually with his therapist. However, he learned to do this to some degree over time.[13]

4. The child with ADHD may not have the cognitive structures, even if he or she is highly intelligent, to symbolize, understand metaphor, internalize, or generalize. This includes the internalization of a corrective emotional experience and the generalization of a new therapeutic relationship with trust to other relationships. The difficulty of fantasizing and free-associating makes these children unable to play at first.

All this having been said, children with ADHD vary a great deal in their skills, personalities, and deficits; some have some or many of the problematic attributes discussed, while others are much better endowed. It has been our aim in doing psychotherapy (in the multimodality treatment study) to help children develop these abilities, with varying success. Some of the children we have treated, but not all, have responded very well to individual psychotherapy. For some children, this modality becomes almost mandatory:

1. Those with disabling associated or reactive disorders (whose core problems are treated by other means, such as medication):

- Low self-esteem, going as far as self-hate at times
- Feelings of hopelessness and helplessness (cognitive–behav-

ioral therapy techniques are valuable here as part of the therapeutic alliance)

- Strong feelings of rejection, which can reach levels of feeling persecuted
- Suicidal thoughts or attempts
- Withdrawal

2. Those with Major Depression, marked dysphoria, or Anxiety Disorders as comorbid disorders.

3. Children with ADHD who have undergone acute trauma. ADHD children have traumatic episodes more frequently than do other children. They get into more accidents, and they may be physically abused by parents or others because of their provocative behavior. One child treated in our program for ADHD ran away from home, was kidnapped, and sexually abused.

Changes need to be made in traditional techniques of dynamic play therapy for these children:

1. The therapist takes a more active role by structuring the sessions. Interactions that hold the child's interest and make him or her into an active play partner are sought. Role playing, story telling,[10] "squiggles,"[52] and the "Ungame"[47] have all been found to accomplish this.

2. Both in terms of theoretical background and in actual techniques of intervention, we have borrowed from many schools of therapy—behavior therapy, cognitive–behavioral therapy, and analytic play therapy. This flexibility is a necessity for children with ADHD. These techniques are used initially to establish the therapeutic alliance and later to promote change.

3. We have found that termination of therapy is very difficult for children with ADHD. In lay terms, one might put it that having learned to relate to someone and confide, the children do not want to relinquish this. Because of the chronicity of the disorder, many psychotherapists, after the intensive phase has ended, make themselves available for crises throughout the children's lives if this is feasible.

Case Vignette

Andy, a 7-year-old with severe ADHD well controlled by methylphenidate, was started in individual psychotherapy for symptoms of extreme jealousy of his younger brother, David, who was 4 years old. He had once injured David and they could not be left alone. Andy had recently refused to go to school, partly because of separation anxiety and partly because he felt "dumb" at school and could not master reading. (Andy also received social skills training and remedial reading, and his parents were in a parent group.)

At initial sessions, the therapist failed to create structure. Andy liked coming (unlike many children), but did not know what to do in a session; instead, he was all over the office touching various toys, but playing with none. The sessions were structured by removing toys from the office and giving Andy a choice of three of five games to play in the session. At first, he chose Legos®, story telling, and "squiggles." Later, Andy made up games to add to the original five, and he was always given a choice among the games at each session. He played out his poor self-esteem by destroying beautiful Legos designs he made, saying, "It's no good." He also played out rivalry situations, drowning his younger brother. In the play story-telling techniques, the therapist suggested different endings to the drowning episodes. These interpretations were made through the play (e.g., "This child is now sorry he drowned the kid because he has no one to play with. He is going to go ahead and save him and the kid will like him for that").

Andy began to want to go to school as his self-esteem improved (he now wanted the therapist to save his Legos designs for him, and he liked them). His reading improved only slowly with his remediation, but this speeded up as his motivation to learn improved. This child is still in therapy.

MULTIMODAL TREATMENT

It is clear that children with ADHD have multiple deficits in academic, social, and emotional spheres. It is also apparent that stimulant medication alone or in combination with any particular type of intervention cannot address the multiple problems most ADHD children have. Thus, early reports by Satterfield and colleagues[41,42,43] that multiple interventions may have far-reaching short- and long-term effects generated a great deal of interest. In Satterfield et al.'s study,[42] children (n = 117) received stimulant treatment; in addition, 41% received individual psychotherapy, 30% group therapy, and 41% education therapy. As for the parents, 57% received individual counseling, 30% group counseling, and 48% family therapy. Children and families received any combination and any number of these. The investigators felt that the outcome of this comprehensively treated group was unusually good, compared to the results of other outcome studies. This view was further supported in a follow-up study,[43] which compared the felony arrests and institutionalization records of hyperactives who received drug treatment only and those who received multimodal treatment. The drug-only group had significantly more arrests and institutionalizations than the multimodal group.

These results do not come from systematic studies (i.e., treatment was not random or controlled), but the results are suggestive of the superiority of multimodal treatment. There is a need for well-controlled studies to assess this approach, which, at this time, is only promising. As noted, hyperactive children have a multiplicity of problems; however, no single treatment has had a satisfactorily broad therapeutic impact. Few studies have used concurrent treatments for an extended time, though a multimodal approach seems optimal. On the basis of the documented deficits of ADHD children and the clinical reports of Satterfield and colleagues, we have embarked on a multimodal treatment study that includes the following interventions in a treatment package: stimulant medication, social skills training, academic skills training, remedial tutoring, parent training and counseling, and individual psychotherapy.

Generally, our inclusion criteria are as follows: Children must be 7–9 years of age, have IQs of 85 or above, and meet DSM-III-R and Diagnostic Interview Schedule for Children diagnoses for ADHD. They also have to have a Conners Teacher Rating Scale score of at least 1.5. Furthermore, all children accepted into the study must be responsive to stimulants as shown by a placebo deterioration, and must be living at home with at least one parent. (Thus, children in institutions or group and foster homes are excluded.) Other exclusion criteria are severe learning disabilities (more than 2 years behind); Conduct Disorder, significant neurological disorders, such as tics, epilepsy, or cerebral palsy; and past or current physical abuse. These exclusion criteria were set up because some make stimulant treatment difficult or dangerous (e.g., tic disorder) and some comorbid diagnoses overshadow the ADHD and require their own particular treatment or cannot be left untreated (e.g., Conduct Disorder, physical abuse, or severe learning disability).

Manuals have been prepared for all interventions, with specific detail outlines for each session. Descriptions of the various treatment modalities have been provided in preceding sections of this chapter.

Once a child has been comprehensively assessed and has met the inclusion criteria, he or she is randomly assigned to one of three groups. Group I, the multimodal treatment group, receives the following:

1. Well-titrated stimulant medication
2. Weekly social skills group, with four children in the group
3. Weekly academic skills training and academic remediation

4. Weekly parent training group for 16 weeks, followed by weekly parental counseling
5. Weekly individual therapy for each child

Group II, the attentional control group, receives the following:

1. Well-titrated stimulant medication
2. Weekly peer activity group
3. Weekly academic homework group
4. Weekly parent support group and parental support
5. Weekly supportive relationship therapy for each child

Group III, the conventionally treated group, receives the following:

1. Well-titrated stimulant medication
2. Monthly meeting for medication monitoring, family support, and counseling
3. Crisis intervention, school consultation, and other interventions to deal with a crisis when necessary (to a maximum of six to eight sessions)

The intensive-treatment groups, Groups I and II, receive weekly interventions in the context of an after-school program twice a week for 1 year, and monthly boosters for a second year. All groups receive a placebo trial after 1 year of treatment, to see whether the children still need medication. If so, they are retitrated to see whether they can function as well on less medication.

The study is ongoing, and the numbers are still too small to present meaningful results. However, we have tried to share, in some considerable detail, a multimodal treatment approach that we are currently testing. We hypothesize that these children, with their multiple and varied social, academic, and emotional problems, will benefit from such a comprehensive treatment approach.

This view has been shared by the U.S. National Institute of Mental Health, which is currently sponsoring a six-site study (our clinic is one of the participating sites) to study multimodal treatment for ADHD. This multisite study is still in the process of synthesizing a mutually acceptable protocol. However, more than 700 ADHD children will be treated in this study, so some answers regarding optimal treatment for this condition should be forthcoming.

CHAPTER TWENTY-FIVE

ASSESSMENT, DIAGNOSIS, AND TREATMENT OF ADULT ADHD

INTRODUCTION: THE EXISTENCE OF ADULT ADHD

Pediatricians up to the 1960s generally considered that the hyperactive syndrome, now termed ADHD, was slowly outgrown during childhood and remitted by adolescence. Among the various reasons for this belief, one reason may have been that during adolescence, many patients stopped seeing their pediatricians and became patients of family physicians. A second reason was probably that the core symptoms of the syndrome (hyperactivity, impulsivity, and attentional deficits) generally diminish in intensity (to varying degrees) as a child enters adolescence, and may no longer be complained about even if still present, while other difficulties or symptoms are now presented as primary problems (e.g., poor school performance and social rejection).[22] Finally, systematic, controlled follow-up studies of hyperactive children had not yet been carried out.

Laufer and Denhoff,[13] clinicians who ably described this syndrome (which they termed "Hyperkinetic Impulse Disorder") and who had had extensive experience with hyperactive children, wrote in 1957, "In later years, this syndrome tends to wane and spontaneously disappear. We have not seen it in those patients we followed to adult life" (p. 464). This became an interesting example of a situation in which widely held clinical folklore could not be substantiated by findings from systematic research once these were available, and clinical beliefs had to be brought into line with new research findings. These same authors decided to send out questionnaires to parents of 100 of their child patients, seen many years previously. Sixty-six percent of the parents contacted returned the questionnaires, which indicated that their now adult children were still having difficulties, sometimes of a serious nature.[12]

In general, the relationship between behavior or emotional disorders of childhood and later adult psychopathology has gained widespread interest for clinicians and researchers, since knowledge in this area of developmental psychopathology is crucial theoretically (for understanding the genesis of adult disorders) and also clinically (for planning adequate services for the different age groups, and, where possible, for preventing continued morbidity). For most conditions of childhood that have been systematically followed into adolescence and adulthood, continuous or intermittent morbidity seems to continue into adult life.

Numerous possibilities exist when a childhood disorder is followed into adulthood, some of which are not mutually exclusive: (1) A varying percentage of children may grow out of the childhood disorder; (2) the disorder may still be present, but some resilient adults may have learned to compensate for their handicaps and have no complaints; (3) for some, the childhood disorder may remit in part, but some aspects will continue to disable them as adults; (4) some adults may still manifest the full childhood syndrome, in a somewhat altered form compatible with their adult status; (5) the childhood disorder may predispose the adults to one or more other mental disorders; or (6) the childhood disorder may predispose the adults to increased psychiatric symptomatology in general, not specifically indicative of a single disorder.

Which of these possibilities constitute the adult outcome of ADHD in childhood? Answers to this questions been provided by three different kinds of studies, all of which have demonstrated first that ADHD is indeed seen in the adulthood of many children with ADHD, and second that all of the possibilities for outcome may be true for different children with this disorder.

The earliest studies that established the existence of the disorder in adulthood were the retrospective follow-up studies carried out in the 1970s, which have been described in detail in the early sections of Chapter 5. "Catch-up retrospective studies" began with reviews of charts from many years previously, followed by tracing the adults whose childhood charts had been reviewed, and determining their adult functioning. "Follow-back" (also retrospective) studies evaluated adults who came for help because they were maladjusted and manifested ADHD-like symptoms, which disabled them. The investigators then elicited the childhood history, which was ascertained from their parents, who had often kept their now adult children's old report cards from school.

A second type of investigation establishing the existence of adult ADHD is genetic research, which for several years has suggested that genetic factors play a role in transmission of ADHD. Recent genetic studies, reviewed in detail in Chapter 22, have clearly demonstrated the fact of genetic transmission (possibly even by a single gene): About 27% of the first-degree relatives of a child with ADHD have the same disorder.[4]

Finally, the third type of study has given us the most direct evidence of the existence of various forms of adult ADHD—namely, controlled, prospective follow-up research, carried out in the late 1970s and still proceeding. In prospective follow-up studies, the diagnosis is clearly established in childhood through interviews and observations at the time; the children are assessed at regular intervals as they are growing up; and thus an impression is gained of continuity or discontinuity of the disorder (partial or complete remission) during the children's development into adult life. These studies have also provided evidence for risk factors for other mental disorders, such as Antisocial Personality Disorder, alcoholism, substance abuse, or depression, which in adult life may be comorbid with continued ADHD.

Denckla has written that the knowledge gained from these prospective follow-up studies (which indicate that 31–66% of adults with the childhood disorder continue to be disabled as adults) is one of the most important findings to come out of the vast research on ADHD.[5] For details of the adult outcome of long-term, prospective, controlled follow-up studies, the reader is referred to Chapter 5. Here we examine the findings from these studies in terms of what they have taught us about the adult disorder.

1. For many children with ADHD, the core symptoms diminished in intensity by adolescence.[22] Many adults outgrew their childhood disorder and became indistinguishable from normal controls.[8,21]

2. At least one disabling residual symptom of the childhood syndrome of ADHD caused impairment of functioning in 66% of the adults followed from childhood.[21]

3. The full syndrome of ADHD was still present in 31% of young adults (mean age = 18 years; range = 16–23 years)[8] and in 8% of older adults (mean age = 26 years; range = 24–33 years).[7]

4. Comorbidity was higher in adults who had been diagnosed as having ADHD in their childhood; that is, they carried more diagnoses of various types than did normal controls.[21] However, the only single diagnosis which clearly distinguished hyperactives and normal controls was Antisocial Personality Disorder, and about 23% of the adults previously hyperactive had this disorder.[8,21] The development of Antisocial Personality Disorder in adolescence and adulthood was highly correlated with continued symptoms of ADHD and with drug and alcohol abuse.[8]

5. Compared to matched normal controls, adults with a childhood history of ADHD had more symptoms of psychopathology, lower self-esteem, and impaired social skills. They had completed less education, and though the majority were working, their work record (according to their employers) and work status were inferior.[21]

6. Two major prospective follow-up studies did not find that childhood ADHD was a risk factor for schizophrenia, Major Depression, or bipolar disorders.[8,21]

These conclusions indicate the variety of possible outcomes of the childhood disorder and suggest variability, including comorbidity, in those adults who continue to be disabled. They also clearly demonstrate the existence of adult ADHD.

DIAGNOSTIC ASSESSMENT

The DSM-III Classification

The older DSM-III classification of 1980[1] recognized that childhood ADD only or ADD(H) may continue into adult life, with hyperactivity itself at times no longer being a main problem in ADD(H). A diagnosis of Attention Deficit Disorder with Hyperactivity, Residual Type (ADD[H]-RT) was defined as characterizing those adults who as children met criteria for ADD(H) and in whom hyperactivity is no longer present, but whose other signs have persisted to the present without remission (e.g., attentional deficits, difficulty in organizing work and completing tasks, and a tendency to make sudden decisions without thinking of consequences). These descriptions indeed accurately reflect the common symptoms of the adult disorder, except that hyperactivity may be manifested not as motor restlessness, but instead as an inner feeling of restlessness, a feeling of being driven.

The DSM-III-R Classification

The DSM-III-R classification of 1987[2] is the current classification, although by the time of publication DSM-IV may be available. DSM-III-R does not have a category for the residual state. Instead, the adult diagnosis is established from the 14 listed childhood problems, some of which tend to refer to the classroom. The task of translating these 14 symptoms to make them truly descriptive of the adult disorder and its unique features is far from easy. In the DSM-III-R classification system in general, both the diagnosis of a childhood disorder from the adult criteria (e.g., Major Depression) and the diagnosis of an adult disorder from the childhood criteria remain problematic, since the adult and child disorders frequently do not have identical manifestations.

Alternative diagnostic procedures refined over time have been used instead of or as well as DSM-III-R for the diagnosis of adult ADHD. Currently, two diagnostic protocols are in use in both research and clinical contexts. These are the Utah criteria and the protocol used by the University of Massachusetts Medical Center (UMMC), both of which are described here. Many researchers and clinicians use both sets of criteria.

The Utah Criteria

The Utah criteria were selected and refined over time by Paul Wender and his colleagues. They were published in 1987 in Wender's book *The Hyperactive Child, Adolescent and Adult: Attention Deficit Disorder through the Life Span*,[23] which was the first publication to clearly describe the various forms of the adult disorder.

The first requirement for diagnosis is the establishment of a history of the childhood disorder, preferably by the subject himself or herself, as well as by his or her parents or old school report cards. Wenders recommends that the Abbreviated Conners Parent Rating Scale be completed by the mother of the adult to be assessed, with a score greater than 12 indicating the presence of childhood ADD(H). Once the childhood disorder is established, the following two characteristics must have been present continuously from childhood to adulthood:

1. Persistent motor activity, as manifested by restlessness, inability to relax, nervousness (meaning inability to settle down rather than anxiety), inability to persist in sedentary activities (e.g., reading), being on the go, and dysphoria when inactive.

2. Attention deficits, as manifested by inability to keep the mind on conversation, distractibility, inability to concentrate on reading materials, difficulty focusing on the job, and frequent forgetfulness (often losing or misplacing things, forgetting plans, mind frequently "somewhere else").

In addition, Wender requires two of the following five:

1. Affective lability (mood shifts from being down, bored, or discontented to excited, lasting usually only hours or a few days).

2. Inability to complete tasks (lack of organization in job or at home; switches from one task to another; difficulty organizing activities, problem solving, or planning time).

3. Hot temper (explosive, short-lived outbursts; transient loss of control; easily provoked; irritable). This may interfere with personal relationships.

4. Impulsivity (decisions made quickly without reflection, often with insufficient information). There is an inability to delay acting without experiencing discomfort. Manifestations may include poor work performance, abrupt initiation or termination of relationships (e.g., multiple marriages), antisocial behaviors, or excessive involve-

ment in pleasurable activities without considering risks (e.g., buying sprees, reckless driving).

5. Stress intolerance. The subject cannot take ordinary stresses in stride and reacts excessively or inappropriately (depression, anxiety, confusion, anger), which interferes with appropriate problem solving.

For the diagnosis of ADD(H)-RT, Wender excludes patients who have the following primary diagnoses:

- Antisocial Personality Disorder
- Major Affective Disorder or Bipolar Disorder
- Schizophrenia, Schizoaffective Personality Disorder, or Schizotypal Personality Disorder
- Borderline Personality Disorder

He notes a number of associated features: marital instability; academic and vocational success less than expected on the basis of intelligence and education; alcohol or drug abuse; atypical responses to psychoactive medications; family history of similar characteristics; ADD(H) in childhood; Antisocial Personality Disorder; and Briquet's syndrome.

Criticisms of the Utah criteria include the use of DSM-III (instead of DSM-III-R) criteria, lack of field trials, and lack of normative data, so that the number of symptoms required for any cutoff is arbitrary. There is also a lack of distinction between learning disabilities and Oppositional Defiant Disorder. Barkley[3] suggests that item 5 above, stress intolerance, should be listed as an associated symptom: It may be secondary rather than primary, it is not always present, and it is not required by DSM-III or DSM-III-R childhood criteria. Furthermore, what is listed under stress intolerance may contaminate the criteria with mood or anxiety disorders.

These difficulties with the Utah criteria are valid, most particularly the lack of field trials and the difficulty of establishing a clear cutoff point. Nevertheless, in our experience, Wender's criteria very accurately describe what one actually sees in adults with ADHD (some of them parents of children we treat), as well as the adult "hyperactives" we followed for 15 years, who continued to be disabled by symptoms of the disorder. A simple translation of the 14 symptoms in DSM-III-R for ADHD in childhood would not cover the variety of adult manifestations, which require probing to make an accurate diagnosis.

The UMMC Protocol

Barkley[3] has described in some detail an assessment protocol for adults with possible ADHD, used by him and his coworkers at UMMC. He stresses, as does Wender, that the patient is asked to bring a significant other to the interview (a parent, a spouse, or a close friend). On arrival, the patient fills out a number of questionnaires: the Symptom Checklist 90—Revised (SCL-90-R[6]); the UMMC Ambulatory Psychiatry Symptom Rating Scale; a checklist of physical complaints to provide a baseline for later side effects; and a checklist of 18 symptoms characteristic of adults with ADHD, 14 translated from DSM-III-R and 4 added from a questionnaire developed by Gittelman. These are rated on a 4-point scale "not at all," "just a little," "pretty much," "very much":

1. Physical restlessness
2. Mental restlessness
3. Easily distracted
4. Impatient
5. Hot or explosive temper
6. Unpredictable behavior
7. Difficulty completing tasks
8. Shifting from one task to another
9. Difficulty sustaining attention
10. Impulsive
11. Talks too much
12. Difficulty doing tasks alone
13. Often interrupts others
14. Doesn't appear to listen to others
15. Loses a lot of things
16. Forgets to do things
17. Engages in physically daring activities
18. Always on the go, as if driven by a motor

This checklist does not tap mood lability, organizational problems, or underachievement in education and/or work, which also characterize adults who have ADHD.

Barkley suggests that the usual time for filling out the questionnaires is about 15 minutes, but that the whole diagnostic interview takes 1 1/2 to 2 hours. The person accompanying the patient also completes the above-listed questionnaires about the patient. A semistructured interview is held to assess current and childhood symptoms, including those associated with ADHD. A psychiatric history (the presence of affective disorders, schizophrenia, Anxiety Disorders, Obsessive Compulsive Disorder, character disorders, substance abuse) and a detailed social, occupational, and legal history are taken. Barkley points out that during the whole assessment, the clinician observes whether the patient is restless, has attentional problems, is coherent, and is able to focus on the task. The patient is informed about the importance of substance abuse for planning future treatment, and is asked for a urine specimen for toxicology.

For those patients whose symptoms indicate ADHD, a neuropsychological assessment is carried out. To test attention, Mirsky's[15] four attentional processes are evaluated:

Focused attention	Trail Making Tests A and B[19]
	Wechsler Adult Intelligence Scale—
	Revised (WAIS-R)
	Digit Symbol test[20]
Encoding/manipulating	WAIS-R Digit Span test[20]
	WAIS-R Arithmetic test[20]
Sustained attention	Adaptive Rate California Psychological
	Inventory (CPI)[11]
Flexibility	Wisconsin Card Sorting Test[10]

For more details of Barkley's neuropsychological assessment, the reader is referred to Chapter 18 of his book.[3] Memory tests are given, intellectual level and academic achievement are evaluated, and observational measures are recommended.

CLINICAL ASSESSMENT OF INDIVIDUAL SYMPTOMS

Attention

Barkley's neuropsychological tests for assessment of the various kinds of attentional difficulties are described above. Only certain other clinical caveats gained from experience are mentioned here.

When the history is taken, attentional problems may range from being predominant among the patient's reasons for seeking evaluation, to being totally denied. Many adults who have ADHD do not complain of attentional problems, because they have found work where little sustained attention is required or where those aspects of work requiring attention are delegated to someone else. For example, in the first case vignette below, Danny Johnson's wife, Diane, did all the bookkeeping and administration of their business. Danny did complain that his attention span had not really improved since childhood, but many other patients do not recognize this, and never read or choose to do sedentary activities. (In childhood, they had no choice!)

We ask whether the patients would prefer different work if they had different abilities to concentrate.

When the patients are being evaluated, we look for attentional problems (and related organizational problems) while they are waiting during their interview and while completing forms.

Motor Restlessness

It has been rare in our experience for a patient to present for diagnosis because of restlessness. The patient's spouse or significant other may describe that this is present, but often the activity has been incorporated into the work or life situation. The patient may have chosen an active, even risky, job or may be holding down two jobs. In the history, one can ask for a description of the activity required during a normal day. Furthermore, some adults with ADHD are no longer physically restless. Instead, they "feel restless" or "feel driven." Wender has suggested that they may feel dysphoric when forced to be sedentary (see the Utah criteria, above).

Restlessness or fidgetiness can be observed during the assessment, and should be looked for. We have not carried out electronic measurements of physical activity, but for research purposes these would be of interest.

Impulsivity

It has already been stressed how important it is for the patient being diagnosed to be accompanied by a significant other. Impulsivity is very stressful to others in the patient's family. The short fuse may not result in violence, but it impairs all relationships and the problem solving that relationships require.

Patients should be asked how they make decisions (impulsively or with reflection and foresight). Do they say things without anticipating the effect on others? Are they easily frustrated by even small things going wrong or not going their way? Do they have a short fuse? Have they had traffic violations? Have they quit work suddenly for obscure reasons? (One patient almost quit a senior insurance job because his company changed the telephone systems and he thought he could not master the new system. Without treatment, he would probably have become and remained unemployed.)

We observe impulsivity when the questionnaires are filled out. The most extreme example of this impulsivity is described in Chapter 13 in the case of Anthony, who at age 20 years attempted to fill out the CPI (with its 500 questions) and got so frustrated, he came to see us from New Zealand to tell us what he thought about us! With respect to

laboratory tests, the errors of commission on the Continuous Performance Test (CPT) have been used.

Social Skills

Deficient social skills may be the most lasting and most disabling
aspect of childhood and adult ADHD. The history of friendships gives
us an idea to what degree this problem is present. We probe whether
the adult has his or her own friends or forms one part of couple
friendships maintained by the spouse. In a case where this problem is
extreme, the adult with ADHD may antagonize the spouse's relatives
and friends.

During the interview, the ability to relate to the examiner is
noted. Some adults with ADHD can relate well; others may show
inappropriate ways of relating. For example, there may be inappropriate familiarity, such as asking the interviewer personal questions or
calling him or her by the first name, in the absence of any psychotic
features.

In our 15-year prospective follow-up study, we used laboratory
measures to evaluate differences in social skills between grown-up
hyperactives and matched controls. Although these measures indicated poorer social skills in the former (see Chapter 10), and may be
useful to assess any improvements resulting from social skills training,
they are not as useful as the clinical history of relationships over time,
as well as observation of the relationship between patient and
interviewer.

TWO CASE VIGNETTES

The patients assessed and treated by us came as parents of children we
were treating, or were referred by other clinicians from all over because
of the paucity of specialized services. Their main reasons for coming
were that they recognized that they had the same difficulties as their
children, or were grossly underachieving at home and at work. Some
came because of impulsive styles that affected their relationships and
prevented intimacy. These presenting problems were outlined by John
Ratey, whose impressions were similar to ours.

Ratey and coworkers[17] systematically studied 60 adults from
three different referral sources (including Harvard University health
services), who had significant childhood and current symptoms of
ADHD. These had not been diagnosed because the patients presented

with atypical symptoms characteristic of other disorders, such as depression, cyclothymia, or dysphoria (47%); anxiety, somatization, sleep disorders, and eating disorders (30%); or antisocial behaviors (5%). These 60 patients shared the following characteristics:

- Physical and mental restlessness
- Disabling distractibility or poor attention
- Low self-esteem, self-loathing
- A gnawing sense of underachievement
- Specific learning problems

They had had numerous unsuccessful psychiatric treatments for their associated symptoms. Traditional dynamic psychotherapy sometimes only aggravated their low self-esteem. Ratey et al.[17] recommend specific treatments, which are described below in the treatment section. We now present two case vignettes of adult patients we ourselves have seen.

Case Vignette I: Danny Johnson, Age 32 Years

This case vignette was chosen because Danny shows the full adult ADHD syndrome, no current comorbidity, an unsuccessful previous treatment history, and a level of poor self-esteem and impaired functioning that was at first hidden by his joviality and sense of humor. In Danny's case, he came to us for treatment because of the diagnosis of his young son, Jamie, with ADHD, and because his work performance (according to his wife) was much lower than his intellectual level. Before the recognition of the severity of Danny's ADHD and the resulting functional impairment, previous parent training, family therapy, and marital counseling had not been fruitful.

HISTORY

When Jamie was first diagnosed as having ADHD, his father volunteered, "I must have had the same problems as him as a child." This was ignored at the time, perhaps because Danny clearly meant it in the past tense, suggesting that he was fine now. Observation of Danny and his wife, Diane, in a parents' group suggested the presence of current ADHD. The following conversation took place in a subsequent evaluation interview:

DANNY: I had the same as a child, but no one ever diagnosed me. Perhaps they didn't know about it then. I failed Grade 5 and I know I had an IQ test at that time, and they told my parents that I was very bright but lazy. My teachers always thought I could do it if I wanted to, and I came to believe that myself; it made me feel I wasn't really dumb. As time went on and I got into high school, my behavior got worse and worse. I was always elsewhere from where the teacher was. I was frequently truant, since school had become intolerable. I became aggressive whenever I was criticized. I knew I was disliked. I was even a pain for my parents, and they weren't patient and could not figure me out. When I think about what you told me about myself and Jamie, it all makes sense. But my parents never got off my back—I was just a bad egg.

DIANE: (*To Danny, smiling*) You still are. (*To the interviewer*) Daniel can't sit still. He always has to be doing something or going somewhere. It's hard on me, since I just want to relax at times. He never finishes what he starts. For example, he has to get more customers for our business and get busy collecting bills. I have to remind him a million times, and then he resents me behaving like his mother.

The therapist then went back to collect more details of Danny's adolescence. He had failed Grade 10 and worked at various menial jobs, which did not last. His poor organization and short fuse ended many jobs. Between the ages of 16 and 24, Danny abused alcohol and hashish, and had a police record for minor crimes (an assault charge while drunk; drunken driving; other traffic violations, including speeding; possession of drugs, and debts). During adolescence, Danny's self-esteem was at the lowest ebb: He had strong self-loathing then, and he felt totally incompetent and hopeless about the future. At this point in his life, Danny would probably (retrospectively) have been diagnosed as having ADHD, Conduct Disorder, and Oppositional Defiant Disorder. His stronger and healthier ego traits began to become apparent when he met and married Diane at the age of 24 years. In Danny's words, "I settled down. Diane helped a lot. I loved her, and she cared about me. She helped to organize me and acted as my bookkeeper at work. Our life settled down and we had two children. Only Jamie is a problem."

Currently, Danny no longer uses street drugs, and drinks heavily on weekends only; he has not had any police involvement for 7 years. The couple own a house and a small business. As a child, Danny was rejected by other children; as an adolescent, he had drinking pals; currently, the couple have friends together. Danny and his wife have a keen sense of humor and high intelligence.

CURRENT PROBLEMS

Danny has major problems at home and at work. At work, he is disorganized, does not complete tasks, blows his fuse at employees, and avoids unpleasant tasks (e.g., bill collecting); as a result, his work output is erratic. Although his business has not failed in a time of recession, and his wife does all the administration for him as well as holding a senior job of her own, Danny dislikes his work, which bores him and which he considers inferior.

Diane talked in the interview about these problems, but also focused on his sense of humor and the fact that his children love him. She reported, "Danny and Jamie together can be like murder—they blow up at each other every two minutes. At other times they get along beautifully, like two peas in a pod." Diane then described that Danny has no ability to plan and no sense of time. He forgets what he is supposed to do next.

INTERVIEWER: Can you give me an example of that?

DIANE: I'll tell you what happened last week. Jamie had his baseball playoffs. He's great at baseball, and Danny promised him he would be there. He really intended to be there because he kept talking about it. He was playing golf with his friend in the morning, and was supposed to meet us at the game. He never showed up. I felt terrible for Jamie, who kept looking for him. When he came home that evening, he was met by our stony faces. Only then did he remember about the game. He had completely forgotten about it while playing golf.

Danny and Diane also have marital problems, which previous treatment did not change. These stem mainly from Danny's ADHD problems, which affect the marriage in quite specific ways. (We have frequently seen exactly these problems in couples in which one partner has ADHD.) Danny's difficulties with organization, lack of planning or reflection (leading to poor problem solving), his failure to finish what he has begun (especially unpleasant tasks), his impatience with others in the family, his short fuse (though he is never physically violent), and his difficulty in listening to Diane (even when she is not "directing" him) all make everyday life difficult. Both partners agree that their main problems are lack of communication and sexual problems, which we have observed as being very common when one in a marriage has ADHD. Diane said, "Of course they are connected." The spouses do not communicate because Danny is too inattentive to listen to Diane; he also feels that he cannot talk about himself. "I'm no good at talking; you must have figured that out," Danny said to the therapist. At the same time, Danny has a high sexual drive; to him, sexual activity is not only a pleasant release, but proof of his virility and a way of being intimate with Diane, since he feels he cannot be intimate in verbal ways.

Diane is rarely sexually aroused by Danny, since she requires verbal intimacy and quiet affection before, during, and after the sexual act. She said, "I want Danny to talk to me and not just grab me. We need to learn to talk to one another at all times, not only when we have sex." The treatment of Danny and of the couple's relationship are described further in the treatment section.

Three things are of special interest about Danny, and typical of many others like him:

1. He was never evaluated or diagnosed as having ADHD as a child, even though he was a poor student with behavior problems. Retrospectively, his mother gave him a score of 18 on the Abbreviated Conners. Had he been treated early, he might have finished high school and completed university because of his high intelligence.

2. Danny's current ADHD diagnosis could easily have been missed. During the first evaluation of the family all together, the couple alone, and each parent alone, all problems were denied except those of Jamie. Gaining the parents' trust and specific, detailed probing were required before they revealed the real problems.

3. Previous attempts at treatment had failed. Danny had had one year of dynamic psychotherapy at age 26 for dysphoria related to his work situation and poor motivation for work. Marital therapy for the couple had not changed their difficulties. Parent training had been effective while it was going on, but most of what was learned stopped being applied when it ended. Treatment would probably have been successful if the real problems had been diagnosed.

Case Vignette II: Claire Leblanc, Age 36 Years

This vignette was chosen to illustrate many patients who have a single symptom that is disabling in some situations but not in others, and who do not meet the criteria for the full adult ADHD syndrome.

Claire is married and the mother of André, age 12, Nicole, age 10, and Marie, age 8. André was recently tested at school, where he has always done poorly, without actually failing a grade. His behavior had for years been characterized by school underachievement, extreme messiness, some oppositional behaviors, and low self-esteem. At age 9, he had a year of dynamic psychotherapy (and his parents were seen as part of family therapy) without improvement. At age 11, André was given a trial of Ritalin®; this had an immediate beneficial effect on his behavior, and his marks at school have improved considerably.

After André was diagnosed as having ADD without hyperactivity and treated successfully, his mother came to the conclusion that she had always had the same disorder as her son. She thought she had been hyperactive as a child, but her mother did not think so. She had failed no grades in school but had never done well. After graduating from high school, she entered social work school, but flunked out after exams in the second year. She was admitted into a general BA program, but again failed out after exams. She then entered a secretarial college, but dropped out after some months because she could not master shorthand. She feels that these failures were attributable to her short attention span.

Subsequently, Claire married, had three children and went back to work, when Marie was 3 years old. She then worked successfully in two consecutive jobs, each of which lasted several years. In these jobs, she was able to advance because she was able to master the level of attention the jobs demanded.

Recently, Claire decided that she wished to return to university to complete her degree in social work. After 6 months, she began having difficulties with her courses and underwent neuropsychological testing. The latter indicated that while she had no specific learning disabilities and high intelligence, she had difficulties concentrating and memorizing. She was subsequently referred for diagnosis and treatment of these difficulties. At the assessment interview, she requested Ritalin, which she felt would make it easier for her to pass her courses. She had matured over the years and had, for example, developed her own strategies for studying. She felt she could probably get her degree without the use of medication, but she would have to put in three times the effort as anyone else.

It is clear that Claire has done relatively well without medication. It is also likely that medication would improve her academic functioning and facilitate her obtaining a professional degree. Her situation is probably similar to that of many other adults with residual symptoms of varying magnitude of the childhood disorder. Careful clinical judgment must be exercised with respect to the degree of the functional impairment caused by these symptoms. On the one hand, if medication allows an individual to function at his or her optimal level and has few side effects, it should not be withheld. On the other hand, one would also foresee a significant increase in the use of medication, such as stimulants, by patients in these kinds of situations.

DIFFERENTIAL DIAGNOSIS

We encounter two main problems in differential diagnosis. One is to rule out other disorders (from Axis I or Axis II of the DSM-III-R diagnostic system) that simulate ADHD. The other is to do a thorough assessment to determine what other disorders a patient has as well as

ADHD. The presence and nature of comorbidity affect the treatment plan as well as the prognosis.

Conditions That Simulate Adult ADHD

Conditions that may simulate adult ADHD include the following:

1. *Normal variations in attention, activity, and organization.* In general, these are not severely disabling, and there is no childhood history of the same disorder.

2. *Learning disabilities.* These may be comorbid with ADHD, but they may also simulate the disorder. The simulation occurs when attentional problems and restlessness are clearly secondary to the learning disabilities. This is true throughout the life span.

3. *Hypomania.* Hypomania and adult ADHD have several symptoms in common: irritability, fast speech, flight of ideas (confused with disorganized speech content), sleep disturbances, and restlessness. In hypomania, however, we see *ongoing* euphoria and inappropriate cheerfulness as compared to lability of mood, which may occur in adult ADHD. The total denial of all problems, even on careful probing, is not seen in adult ADHD as it is in hypomania. We have seen one adolescent with ADHD develop hypomania; the change in mood was dramatic.

4. *Dysthymia, dysphoria, and cyclothymia.* Many ADHD patients have been treated for one of these disorders, with the presence of ADHD not having been diagnosed. In those with adult ADHD, we see at times low-grade depression or marked lack of optimism, specifically related to the perceived handicaps. Mood lability lasts, when present, for a couple of hours or a day but is not sustained.

5. *Borderline Personality Disorder.* Both adult ADHD and Borderline Personality Disorder are characterized by impulsivity and impaired social relationships. However, those with Borderline Personality Disorder tend to have intense love–hate relationships; those with adult ADHD seek relationships, but may be unsuccessful and feel rejected. Alcohol or drug abuse may occur in either condition. Self-mutilation is occasionally seen in adult ADHD, but is different in quality; it is more an obsessional type of scratching of the skin, for example. Suicide attempts may occur in both conditions, but are more common in Borderline Personality Disorder. Borderline patients lack most of the specific symptoms described for adult ADHD.

6. *Generalized Anxiety Disorder.* Patients with Generalized Anxiety Disorder may have some symptoms similar to those of patients with adult ADHD, but generally differ in their presenting complaints. In

both disorders, one may see fidgetiness, restlessness, insomnia, irritability, impatience, and inability to relax. In patients with ADHD, these latter symptoms are more feelings of being driven. For patients with Generalized Anxiety Disorder, the symptoms are usually of shorter duration, and symptoms of autonomic nervous system overactivity (sweating, clammy hands, palpitations or fast heart rate, dizziness, discomfort in the abdomen, frequent urination, etc.) are nearly always found, whereas these are absent in ADHD patients. The chief complaints of patients with Generalized Anxiety Disorder are intense, lasting feelings of anxiety; worry about the future; and rumination that misfortunes will occur.

Comorbidity

Major Depression (and other depressive conditions), anxiety states, drug or alcohol abuse, Antisocial Personality Disorder, and learning disabilities may all co-occur with adult ADHD and must be diagnosed at initial assessment. They are described in more detail in Chapter 22.

TREATMENT OF ADULT ADHD

New aspects of treatment of children with ADHD are reviewed in Chapters 23 and 24. It is generally considered that children respond best to a combination of treatments, including medication and various kinds of behavior therapies, even though this has not been confirmed as yet in a controlled, systematic, multimodal treatment study. In adults, the same principles apply—namely, that treatments aim to ameliorate the adults' main difficulties.

There are five controlled studies evaluating the efficacy of methylphenidate (Ritalin®) and pemoline (Cylert®) with adults. These are briefly described, as are two recent open-ended studies using L-tyrosine and bupropion. No controlled studies exist that have evaluated the effects of psychological therapies for adults with ADHD, but therapies that have been documented are described.

Controlled Drug Studies

In the first of these studies,[27] 11 patients selected from various outpatient clinics in Salt Lake City when they presented with irritability, inattentiveness, restlessness, and emotional lability (patients with schizophrenia, affective disorders, brain syndromes, and mental retardation were excluded) were studied by means of a double-blind crossover technique comparing methylphenidate with placebo. This was followed by an open trial of pemoline and/or tricyclic antidepressants. The maximum dose of methylphenidate used was 60 mg. Methylphenidate was found to be superior to placebo. Of 15 patients in the open trial, 4 responded well to pemoline, and 2 subjects who had not responded to stimulants responded to tricyclic antidepressants. Nine of the 15 patients were female.

Wender, Wood, and Reimherr[25] did a replication study in which they refined their methodology. They devised operational criteria for the diagnosis of adult ADD and broadened the exclusion criteria (Borderline Personality Disorder and Schizotypal Personality Disorder were excluded, as well as the disorders mentioned above). In addition, they developed a more systematic way of establishing the childhood diagnosis, by asking parents of the adults to complete the Abbreviated Conners Parents Rating Scale from memories of their children in school. Sixty patients entered a double-blind study of pemoline, and 26 of these fulfilled childhood criteria for ADD. It was of interest that only the latter subgroup responded to pemoline as compared to placebo.

In a third study,[26] these authors carried out a double-blind crossover study of methylphenidate and placebo in 37 adults who met the Utah criteria (revised) for ADD(H)-RT. A moderate to marked therapeutic response occurred in 57% of the patients on the active drug, and in 11% on placebo—a highly statistically significant difference.

A fourth study was carried out by Gualtieri and colleagues.[9] Twelve male patients with ADD participated in a double-blind crossover study of methylphenidate (0.3 mg/kg b.i.d.). Improvement compared to placebo was found when an actometer was used to measure activity; the overall number of correct responses on the CPI also increased. All subjects described subjective improvement on the active drug. The authors pointed out that all 12 patients guessed correctly whether they were on the active drug or placebo; hence, the study was not blind.

Mattes and coworkers[14] used a double-blind crossover study of methylphenidate with 35 patients with ADD, who had no evidence of childhood ADD or ADHD, and 26 patients who had such a history. No overall benefit from methylphenidate could be found, nor did the group with the childhood history respond more favorably to the active drug. Hence, this study failed to confirm all findings from the previous four controlled studies. Therefore, it is too early to draw definite conclusions that stimulants are efficacious in helping adults with ADHD.

These studies can be criticized as follows:

1. The doses used (particularly in Gualtieri et al.'s study[9]) were low, and similar to doses used in children.

2. The adult diagnoses, particularly in the first study,[27] were probably overinclusive and heterogeneous. The fact that there were so many women compared to men in three studies[25,26,27] is unusual and suggests lack of diagnostic precision.

3. The target symptoms that responded to stimulants were usually subjective, except in Gualtieri *et al.*'s study, and unexpected symptoms (such as the inability to have orgasms) were ameliorated.

4. In none of the studies was the childhood diagnoses made during childhood, it was made retrospectively. We are currently planning a controlled study of methylphenidate with the ADHD patients we diagnosed as children and followed into adulthood who have adult ADHD or disabling continuing symptoms.

Recent Open-Trial Studies

Because of the interest relating to the catecholamine system in ADHD, Reimherr and colleagues, in 1987,[18] studied the efficacy of L-tyrosine in an open trial with 12 adults who fulfilled the Utah criteria for ADD(H)-RT. With a delay of 2 weeks, 8 of the 12 began to show a response; however, by the 8th week they had developed tolerance. The authors concluded that L-tyrosine was not an effective medication. The same group of investigators, in 1989,[24] treated 19 ADHD adults with bupropion in an open trial. These patients had previously received maintenance levels of stimulant medication for an average of 3–7 years. Fourteen of the 19 patients had a moderate to marked response to bupropion, and 10 of them chose to continue the latter in preference to their previous medication with stimulants. The authors concluded that bupropion may be an alternative to stimulant therapy for some adults with ADHD.

Nonpharmacological Treatments

As already mentioned, no controlled studies of nonpharmacological treatments have been done, so we rely on suggestions from experienced clinicians who have treated adults with ADD or ADHD. Attempts at individual psychotherapy and crisis intervention have been described in Chapter 18.

RATEY AND COLLEAGUES' APPROACH

John Ratey and his colleagues[16,17] have described over 100 patients (many of them students or faculty members at Boston-area universities) who were referred to them for diagnostic assessment of adult

ADD, ADHD, or disabling symptoms of the disorder without the full diagnosis. All these patients had had unsuccessful treatment trials with psychotherapy, psychoanalysis, and drug treatment. Of the group of over 100 patients, 74 met criteria for childhood ADD. In their adulthood, some were academic failures, but others, although they felt like failures, were quite successful (two were MacArthur Fellows). Their common characteristics were as follows:

- They had difficulties in their jobs or studies, which they sometimes compensated for (one female pharmacist could not trust herself to take telephone orders for prescriptions so she taped the calls).
- Whether they were successful or not, all felt like underachievers.
- They could not focus their attention or modulate or integrate incoming stimuli, and hence could not organize their internal and external worlds.
- They were disgruntled and discouraged as a result of their cognitive handicaps, which prevented them from realizing their goals.

Psychotherapy for these patients was often characterized by bouncing from topic to topic, thought to thought, in many cases with no center or core and very little feeling attached. Ratey[16] suggests that this was a form of dyslexithymia in which affects were wrongly interpreted. Although the patients were more than willing to share and explore their distress, they were unable to use psychotherapy in traditional ways; for example, their associations were fast and devoid of affect.

Ratey et al.[17] have described five aspects of successful psychological treatment:

1. *Identification.* This involves delineation of the patients' specific cognitive handicaps (related to attentional problems and a sense of being driven) and how these are associated with actual or perceived failures in their work and/or personal relationships. Ratey et al.'s patients often turned to motor activity and sometimes to drugs or alcohol as an escape. Identification alleviated their guilt and resulted in relief at being understood, and elicited further disclosures of a personal nature.

2. *Drug treatment.* The available controlled drug studies have been described above. Ratey and his colleagues usually start off by using desipramine (a tricyclic antidepressant) in low doses. They emphasize that the "therapeutic window" for responsiveness is low (i.e., 10–30 mg daily). When this is unsuccessful, methylphenidate or

dextroamphetamine is tried. These authors have also used fluoxetine and bupropion.

3. *Structuring the environment.* This involves discussions to enhance the patients' organizational skills so that they can keep their affairs in order (e.g., use of appointment books, calendars, writing down what needs to be done, etc.). The choice of "significant others" is discussed—spouses, friends, and mentors. Sometimes the patients require a high level of stimulation in their lives.

4. *Psychoeducation.* This addresses the fact that attentional difficulties and related problems are the main underlying problem, and explores the ramifications of these handicaps on the patients' lives. The biology of the disorder is discussed, and other relatives with the same disorder (if reported on) are assessed. The patients are taught to manage their mood lability; guilt at their perceived failures is reduced, as the condition is understood for what it is and is not related to a failure to try, laziness, or other character flaws.

5. *Character assault.* The patients have usually developed character adaptations that are ego-syntonic but not adaptive and that require confrontation. Examples include procrastination, avoiding difficult tasks, and avoiding the development of intimacy because of a fear of being unable to achieve it in an enduring way. Some are therefore unable to find lasting relationships or are working in unchallenging jobs for which they are overqualified. Many have not been able to set structured career goals. As these maladaptive character adaptations are lessened, new, more productive adaptations can be made.

According to these workers, long-term therapy based on these principles can be very helpful.

OUR OWN APPROACH: THE TREATMENT OF DANNY

Our own experience is similar to that of Ratey and colleagues. The treatment of Danny (the patient described in the first case vignette above) gives some idea of the ramifications of our different treatment approaches.

Danny and his wife, Diane, initially participated in a parents' group run according to Barkley's principles (see Chapter 24). In this group, they enjoyed the companionship of other parents with similar problems in their children and not infrequently in themselves. They mastered principles of behavior therapy, which made them more effective as parents and reduced chaotic child management or aggressive responses. Those parents such as Danny, who had the same disorder as their childrenm developed insight into this.

After 12 parent training sessions were completed, the couples were seen primarily to reinforce what had been learned. However, in many of the couples who had completed the parent training, we noted the following:

1. Parents soon stopped carrying out the specific behavioral interventions learned; they mentioned "being too busy" and the like. Some of the more positive attitudes learned lasted better (e.g., special time with their children or with each other).

2. When each couple was seen alone, problems related to lack of intimacy between the spouses and resultant sexual problems became the choice topics of the treatment, so that treatment centering around these issues had to be combined with reinforcing the skills of behavior management.

One aspect of marital therapy for Danny and Diane was treating Danny with Ritalin®. He took this medication when he got home and in the evening rather than during work, where he learned to succeed by structuring his time better. The Ritalin did not cause him any sleep problems, even when he took it in the evening. The benefits of the medication combined with couples therapy were that he became less explosive with his children and said, "For the first time, I can actually listen when Diane is telling me something." Intimacy was improved, and their sexual relationship became more mutually satisfying. Danny learned that Diane wanted to be listened to, but he also learned that she was interested in listening to his stories. Danny had been so humiliated that his job was less skilled than Diane's that he felt anything he said about it had to be boring. He had also believed that his language skills (written and oral) were so much poorer than his wife's, that he avoided verbal communication. The therapist noticed, however, that he could "talk" competently and pointed this out. The two practiced verbal communication.

More individual therapy along psychoeducational lines is planned to help Danny structure his work performance, stop putting off unpleasant and difficult tasks, and develop higher self-esteem in regard to his real abilities (which he still has trouble believing he has).

For some of these patients, like Danny, writing down or saying what they want from their partners or what they want from themselves to improve their work life is extremely unpleasant. They may refuse because they believe that they "cannot write" or "cannot talk." Often the therapist is astonished at how well they actually write or speak, in view of their failures in school to master language skills.

In summary, it is our clinical belief that adult patients with ADHD can be helped by medication, behavioral therapies, and psychoeducation. When the patients are married or living in couple relationships, marital therapy is likely to be needed. If they are parents, they will also require help in the parental role—for example, parent training. Vocational assessment and guidance may be needed. Self-help groups have been very helpful for many parents. Controlled treatment studies involving medication, psychological therapies, and their combination are sorely lacking and urgently needed.

CONCLUSIONS

Any conclusions drawn from the body of studies reviewed may have to be revised as new studies on adult outcome of the childhood condition are completed. Nevertheless, it is worthwhile to draw some conclusions from the various studies summarized in this book.

1. *Core features of syndrome.* The manifestation of the syndrome differs from infancy through the preschool and school years to adulthood. Certain core features, however, can be identified early in life and generally continue through adolescence and sometimes into adult life. These are inappropriate restlessness, attentional difficulties, and impulsivity, which manifest themselves in different ways at different ages.

2. *Adolescent outcome.* Most studies indicate that the core symptoms are still present in the majority of adolescents who had the childhood condition but have somewhat abated. Frequently they are no longer the presenting complaints, which tend instead to be poor school performance, social deviancy, and difficulties in relationships with peers and adults.

• A significant percentage of subjects, usually about 25% but varying in different studies between 10% and 50%, have a history of antisocial behavior. Not only the number of subjects in any one group but also the severity of these behaviors differ from study to study.

• While hyperactive adolescents may consume more alcohol and use nonmedical drugs (usually hash or marijuana) more frequently, there is no evidence of alcoholism or significant drug addiction when compared to normal controls.

• Hyperactive adolescents have been found to have lower self-esteem, poorer social skills, and impulsive cognitive styles compared to normal controls.

3. *Adult outcome.* While the symptoms of the syndrome may continue into adult life in varying degrees of severity, most studies indicate that a substantial proportion of subjects (perhaps a third to a half of any group studied) become indistinguishable from normal adults, and indeed "outgrow" the childhood condition, as was originally postulated by pediatricians many years earlier. The percentage of hyperactive children who continue to be troubled by symptoms of the syndrome in

adulthood is approximately one-third to one-half in most studies. The variation between studies with respect to continuation of core symptoms is probably related to the age of the subjects at the time of study and also to how the core symptoms are measured and by whom. In a recent controlled follow-up study which unfortunately was completed too late for detailed description in this book, it was found that antisocial behavior and drug use and abuse when present strongly correlated with continuing symptoms of the syndrome, so that the significance of the continuation of the core symptoms requires further study.

• As for adolescence, in adulthood all studies indicated that a higher percentage of hyperactive subjects than normal controls had a history of antisocial behavior and used alcohol and hash or marijuana more frequently and/or more intensively. Again the severity of these problems differed in different studies (approximately 25%), indicating regional and socioeconomic differences, as well as probable differences between studies in the initial degree and extent of conduct disorders in the subjects at intake. There is evidence also that about 20% or more have Antisocial Personality Disorders as measured by DSM-III or modified SADS-L criteria, and acts of physical violence as well as carrying weapons may be more frequent than in normal controls. However only a small minority land up in jail or in psychiatric hospitals.

• In general, studies did not indicate that drug addiction or alcoholism in adulthood was an outcome of the childhood syndrome.

• Using a variety of types of measures of psychopathology, it has been found that hyperactive adults generally have more malaise and nonspecific evidence of psychopathology than normal controls. For example, hyperactive adults score worse on self-rating scales (such as the SCL-90, CPI, self-esteem tests), as well as on indicators of overall level of functioning such as the General Adaptation Scale. In addition, hyperactive subjects were given more DSM-III diagnoses and complained of more symptoms apart from those of the core syndrome.

• Hyperactive adults had impaired social skills compared to normals in studies which measured this.

• In two controlled studies in which this was systematically assessed, hyperactive subjects were generally economically self-sufficient and gainfully employed. Nevertheless, their work status was inferior to that of normal controls. They held jobs for a shorter duration, were laid off or quit more frequently, had lower ratings with respect to the Hollingshead Scale of Work Status, and were inferior to normal controls on employer ratings of work performance.

• In general, EEG's had normalized sometimes during adolescence, and there was no difference on this measure in adulthood. There was no evidence that hyperactive adults differed in height and weight or blood pressure from normals. Treatment with stimulants for at least 3 years in childhood did not significantly affect final adult height. In the study in which this was found, however, dosages were not high, drug holidays were given, children were prepubertal, and the number of subjects was small. It would be advisable for children receiving stimulants to have regular checks of height and weight.

• Family factors may exert their influence via genetic or environmental means or via a combination of the two. Siblings of hyperactive children generally score more deviant on a vareity of measures than do normal controls. Mothers observed interacting with their hyperactive children were generally found to be more punitive and less rewarding than control mothers. Cause and effect are hard to determine with respect to the interaction of the hyperactive child and his or her mother.

In several studies the families of hyperactive children were found to have more psychopathology, particularly antisocial behavior, alcoholism, and hysteria, than normal control families. Family functioning in one study improved when the hyperactive subjects left home.

The genetic influence in the etiology of hyperactivity remains uncertain. However, the family's handling of their hyperactive child, as well as overall family function, undoubtedly affect the eventual outcome of these children.

4. *Treatment of the adolescent and adult hyperactive.* Individual psychotherapy as assessed from clinical experience with a few subjects was ineffective for some problems (e.g., core symptoms) and useful, in varying degrees, for other problems for which medication would be unlikely to be successful.

In well-controlled acute studies, stimulants continued to be efficacious for core symptoms in those adolescents in whom these continued to be present. Short-term efficacy studies of stimulants for adults who continue to have symptoms of the syndrome have given conflicting results, so that definitive conclusions are premature and further studies are required.

5. *Prediction of outcome.* Studies that addressed themselves to predicting outcome indicated that in adolescence, initial measures of aggression predicted antisocial behavior measures, which were correlated both at intake and at follow-up. Intelligence, socioeconomic status, and aspects of family functioning were also important predictors. Multivariate studies on predictors of adult outcome highlighted the importance of the interaction of different initial variables in predicting outcome. Important predictors once again were intelligence, socioeconomic status, and family functioning.

6. *Hyperactive subjects' view of what helped them.* When adult subjects

assessed the treatment they had received as children and what factors had helped them the most, they chose individual persons (a parent, a teacher, a counselor, or a friend) who had been particularly significant for them. While stimulants were viewed as more beneficial than other medications, taking any "pills" was strongly disliked by the majority of hyperactive adults. The main reasons given were "feeling different" and feeling ashamed when other children found out (e.g., when teachers made a comment about medication in front of the class). Reasons for disliking medication seemed relatively unrelated to its efficacy, but were sometimes related to its side effects. Subjects felt that the physicians who prescribed their medication had not adequately discussed with them why this was indicated and what the possible side effects might be. They indicated that they only remembered being told "the pills would be helpful," and wished that they had been given more opportunity to talk to their doctor about taking medication.

In summary, hyperactive syndrome in childhood carries with it some risk for adult psychopathology, as well as the continuation of the core symptoms. For this reason children require early diagnosis and treatment or remediation of the various deficits (social, emotional, and cognitive) which they have. That such a broad-based intervention indeed improves their outcome is suggested by one study, although definitive evidence of the efficacy of multimodal treatment is lacking and is very hard to acquire, since random assignment to different treatment modalities is not ethical. Treatment of continuing symptoms in adulthood continues to be the focus of more investigation. If the strong correlation between antisocial behavior and substance abuse, with the presence of continuing symptoms, is borne out in other studies, it will be of great importance to treat remaining core symptoms with the hope of reducing more serious disorders.

The adult outcome of any one group of hyperactive children studied is not uniform. Some cannot be distinguished from normal controls, while others are in adult jails or psychiatric hospitals. However, most are self-supporting and live in society with continuing symptoms of the syndrome and other social and emotional problems. Factors and interventions which affect this varied outcome are beginning to be identified. It is hoped that future research will point a way for more hyperactive children to achieve positive adult outcomes.

SECOND EDITION: 1993

Research has provided new evidence that genetic factors are important in the etiology of ADHD. The mode of transmission and the specific biological abnormality are yet to be identified, but recent technological advances (e.g., neuroimaging techniques) may enable researchers to unravel the biological underpinnings of ADHD. The clinical importance of possible genetic transmission is already being felt as clinicians actively identify other affected family members, particularly parents and siblings, whose treatment becomes an essential part of a comprehensive treatment program.

Increased awareness of comorbid conditions highlights the necessity of a comprehensive diagnosis to adequately treat the various subgroups.

It is now generally accepted that treatment of ADHD calls for a comprehensive approach that includes medication and psychosocial treatments. Stimulants remain the most widely used group of medications, with methylphenidate the most commonly used drug in this group. Long-acting stimulants have advantages, but also limitations. Combinations of short- and long-acting stimulants are used more frequently, but more research is needed to investigate their efficacy and safety. Other second-order drugs (e.g., tricyclic antidepressants and clonidine) are also used alone or in combination with stimulants. Again, further investigation is needed to clarify the usefulness of these combinations.

Psychosocial treatments include behavior modification, social skills training, parent training, academic skills training and remediation, and individual psychotherapy. Various combinations of these interventions, usually in conjunction with medication, may be useful for particular patients. The efficacy of this multimodal treatment approach is currently receiving more rigorous investigation.

The prospective and retrospective follow-up studies described in this book have established the presence of ADHD in adulthood. Some adults no longer have the full diagnosis but remain disabled by one or more continuing symptoms of the childhood disorder. Structured rating scales are being developed to diagnose the condition in adults, in whom comorbidity is often present as it is in children. Adults with this disorder are often helped by stimulants, desipramine, or other medications, together with various psychological therapies. Treatment outcome in adulthood requires more research to determine optimal treatments for the disorder and for specific remaining symptoms.

In summary, there are exciting new developments in our understanding and treatment of ADHD in children and adults. It is hoped that these will result in a more positive long-term outcome.

REFERENCES

CHAPTER 1

1. Safer, D. J., & Allen, R. P. *Hyperactive Children: Diagnosis and Management.* Baltimore: University Park Press, 1976.

2. Barkley, R. A. *Hyperactive Children: A Handbook for Diagnosis and Treatment.* New York: Guilford Press, 1981.

3. Ross, D. M., & Ross, S. A. *Hyperactivity: Theory, Research and Action* (2nd Ed.). New York: Wiley, 1982.

4. Still, G. F. The Coulstonian Lectures on Some Abnormal Physical Conditions in Children. *Lancet*, 1: 1008–1012, 1077–1082, 1163–1168, 1902.

5. Hohman, L. B. Post-Encephalitic Behavior Disorder in Children. *Johns Hopkins Hospital Bulletin*, 33: 372–375, 1922.

6. Ebaugh, F. G. Neuropsychiatric Sequelae of Acute Epidemic Encephalitis in Children. *American Journal of Diseases in Children*, 25: 89–97, 1923.

7. Kahn, E., & Cohen, L. Organic Driveness: A Brain Stem Syndrome and an Experience. *New England Journal of Medicine*, 210: 748–756, 1934.

8. Bond, E., & Smith, L. H. Post-Encephalitic Behavior Disorders: A 10-Year Review of the Franklin School. *American Journal of Psychiatry*, 92: 17–33, 1935.

9. Bradley, C. The Behavior of Children Receiving Benzedrine. *American Journal of Psychiatry*, 94: 577–585, 1937.

10. Rapoport, J. L., Buchsbaum, M. S., Zahn, T. P., Weingartner, H., Ludlow, C., & Mikkelsen, E. J. Dextroamphetamine: Cognitive and Behavioral Effects in Normal Prepubertal Boys. *Science*, 199: 560–563, 1978.

11. Wender, Paul H. Some Speculations Concerning a Possible Biochemical Basis of Minimal Brain Dysfunction. *Annals of the New York Academy of Sciences*, 205: 18–28, 1973.

12. Strauss, A. A., & Kephart, N. C. *Psychopathology and Education of the Brain-Injured Child* (Vols. 1 & 2). New York: Grune & Stratton, 1955.

13. Hallahan, D. P., & Cruikshank, W. M. *Psychoeducational Foundations of Learning Disabilities.* Englewood Cliffs, NJ: Prentice-Hall, 1973.

14. Clemmens, R. L., & Kenny, T. J. Clinical Correlates of Learning Disabilities, Minimal Brain Dysfunction, and Hyperactivity. *Clinical Pediatrics*, 11: 311–313, 1972.

15. Knobloch, H., & Pasamanick, B. Syndrome of Minimal Cerebral Damage in Infancy. *Journal of the American Medical Association*, 170: 1384–1387, 1959.

16. Pasamanick, B., Rogers, M. E., & Lilienfeld, A. Pregnancy Experience and the Development of Behavior Disorder in Children. *American Journal of Psychiatry*, 112: 613–617, 1956.

17. Clements, S. D., & Peters, J. E. Minimal Brain Dysfunctions in the School Age Child. *Archives of General Psychiatry*, 6: 185–197, 1962.

18. Birch, H. G. *Brain Damage in Children: The Biological and Social Aspects.* Baltimore: Williams & Wilkins, 1964.

19. MacKeith, R. Foreword. Minimal Brain Damage: A Concept Discarded. In *Proceedings of the International Study Group of Minimal Brain Dysfunction* (Little Club Clinics in Developmental Medicine, 10). London: Heinemann, 1963.

20. Bender, L. A Career in Clinical Research in Child Psychiatry. In E. J. Anthony (Ed.), *Explorations in Child Psychiatry*. New York: Plenum Press, 1975.

21. Bakwin, H., & Bakwin, R. M. *Clinical Management of Behavior Disorders in Children*. Philadelphia: Saunders, 1966.

22. Laufer, M. W., & Denhoff, E. Hyperkinetic Behavior Syndrome in Children. *Journal of Pediatrics*, 50: 463-474, 1957.

23. Dykman, R. A., Ackerman, P. T., Clements, S. D., & Peters, J. E. Specific Learning Disabilities: An Attention Deficit Syndrome. In H. R. Myklebust (Ed.), *Progress in Learning Disabilities* (Vol. 2). New York: Grune & Stratton, 1971.

24. Douglas, V. I. Attentional and Cognitive Problems. In M. Rutter (Ed.), *Developmental Neuropsychiatry*. New York: Guilford, 1983.

25. American Psychiatric Association. *Diagnostic and Statistical Manual of Mental Disorders* (3rd Ed.; DSM-III). Washington, D.C.: APA, 1980.

26. Milman, M. Resources and Recourses in the Management of Compound "Intractable" Pain. *Drug Therapy*, 8: 65-80, 1978.

27. Sleator, E. K., Von Neumann, A., & Sprague, R. L. Hyperactive Children: A Continuous Long-Term Placebo Controlled Follow-Up. *Journal of the American Medical Association*, 229: 316-317, 1974.

28. Weiss, G., Kruger, E., Danielson, U., & Elman, M. Effect of Long-Term Treatment of Hyperactive Children with Methylphenidate, *Canadian Medical Association Journal*, 112: 159-165, 1975.

29. Riddle, K. D., & Rapoport, J. L. A Two-Year Follow-Up of 72 Hyperactive Boys. *Journal of Nervous and Mental Disease*, 162: 126-134, 1976.

30. Blouin, A. G. A., Bornstein, R., & Trites, R. Teenage Alcohol Use among Hyperactive Children: A 5-Year Follow-Up Study. *Journal of Pediatric Psychology*, 3: 188-194, 1978.

31. Charles, L., & Schain, R. A Four-Year Follow-Up Study of the Effect of Methylphenidate on the Behavior and Academic Achievement of Hyperactive Children. *Journal of Abnormal Child Psychology*, 9: 495-505, 1981.

32. Weiss, G., Hechtman, L., Perlman, T., Hopkins, J., & Wener, A. Hyperactives as Young Adults. A Controlled Prospective Ten-Year Follow-Up of 75 Children. *Archives of General Psychiatry*, 36: 675-681, 1979.

33. Hechtman, L., Weiss, G., Perlman, T., & Tuck, D. Hyperactives as Young Adults: Various Clinical Outcomes. *Adolescent Psychiatry*, 9: 295-306, 1981.

34. Borland, B. L., & Heckman, H. K. Hyperactive Boys and Their Brothers: A 25-Year Follow-Up Study. *Archives of General Psychiatry*, 33: 669-676, 1976.

35. Milich, R. S., & Loney, J. The Role of Hyperactive and Aggressive Symptomatology in Predicting Adolescent Outcome among Hyperactive Children. *Journal of Pediatric Psychology*, 4: 93-108, 1979.

36. Sprague, R. L. Assessment of Intervention. In R. Trites (Ed.), *Hyperactivity in Children*. Baltimore: University Park Press, 1979.

37. Douglas, V. I. Stop, Look and Listen: The Problem of Sustained Attention and Impulse Control in Hyperactive and Normal Children. *Canadian Journal of Behavioural Science*, 4: 259-282, 1972.

38. Shaffer, D., & Greenhill, L. A Critical Note on the Predictive Validity of the Hyperkinetic Syndrome. *Journal of Child Psychology and Psychiatry*, 20: 61-72, 1979.

39. Rapoport, J. L., Buchsbaum, M. S., Zahn, T. P., Weingartner, H., Ludlow, C., & Mikkelsen, E. J. Dextroamphetamine: Cognitive and Behavioral Effects in Normal Prepubertal Boys. *Science*, 199: 560-563, 1978.

40. Werner, E. E., & Smith, R. S. *Kauai's Children Come of Age*. Honolulu: University of Hawaii Press, 1977.

41. Nichols, P., & Chen, T.-C. *Minimal Brain Dysfunction: A Prospective Study*. Hillsdale, NJ: Erlbaum, 1981.

42. Werry, J. S., Minde, K., Guzman, A., Weiss, G., Dogan, K., & Hoy, E. Studies on the Hyperactive Child VII. Neurological Status Compared with Neurotic and Normal Children. *American Journal of Orthopsychiatry*, 42: 441–451, 1972.

43. Rapoport, J. L., & Quinn, P. O. Minor Physical Anomalies (Stigmata) and Early Developmental Deviation: A Major Biological Subgroup of "Hyperactive Children." *International Journal of Mental Health*, 4: 29–44, 1975.

44. Waldrop, M. F., & Halverson, C. F. Minor Physical Anomalies and Hyperactive Behavior in Young Children. In J. Hellmuth (Ed.), *The Exceptional Infant*. New York: Brunner/Mazel, 1971.

45. Ferguson, H. B., & Pappas, B. A. Evaluation of Psychophysiological, Neurochemical, and Animal Models of Hyperactivity. In R. L. Trites (Ed.), *Hyperactivity in Children*. Baltimore: University Park Press, 1979.

46. Hastings, J. E., & Barkley, R. A. A Review of Psychophysiological Research with Hyperkinetic Children. *Journal of Abnormal Child Psychology*, 6: 413–448, 1978.

47. Cunningham, C. E., & Barkley, R. A. The Interactions of Normal and Hyperactive Children with Their Mothers in Free Play and Structured Tasks. *Child Development*, 50: 217–224, 1979.

48. Shaywitz, S. E., Cohen, D. J., & Shaywitz, B. A. Behavior and Learning Difficulties of Children of Normal Intelligence Born to Alcoholic Mothers. *Journal of Pediatrics*, 96: 978–982, 1980.

49. Morrison, J. R., & Stewart, M. A. The Psychiatric Status of the Legal Families of Adopted Hyperactive Children. *Archives of General Psychiatry*, 23: 888–891, 1973.

50. Cantwell, D. P. Psychiatric Illness in the Families of Hyperactive Children. *Archives of General Psychiatry*, 27: 414–417, 1972.

51. Lopez, R. E. Hyperactivity in Twins. *Canadian Psychiatric Association Journal*, 10: 421–426, 1965.

52. Shaywitz, S. E., Cohen, D. J., & Shaywitz, B. A. The Biochemical Basis of Minimal Brain Dysfunction: Evidence of Alleviation in Brain Dopamine. *Journal of Pediatrics*, 92: 179–187, 1978.

53. Shekim, W. O., Dekirmenjian, H., & Chapel, J. L. Urinary MHPG Excretion in Minimal Brain Dysfunction and Its Modification by D-Amphetamine. *American Journal of Psychiatry*, 136: 667–671, 1979.

54. Gillberg, C., Carlström, G., & Rasmussen, P. Hyperkinetic Disorders in 7-Year-Old Children with Perceptual Motor and Attentional Deficits. *Journal of Child Psychology and Psychiatry*, 24: 233–246, 1983.

55. Schachar, R., Rutter, M., & Smith, A. The Characteristics of Situationally and Pervasively Hyperactive Children: Implications for Syndrome Definition. *Journal of Child Psychology and Psychiatry*, 22: 375–392, 1981.

56. McGee, R., Williams, S., & Silva, P. Behavioral and Developmental Characteristics of Aggressive, Hyperactive, and Aggressive–Hyperactive Boys. *Journal of the American Academy of Child Psychiatry*, 23: 280–284, 1984.

57. Rutter, M. Syndromes Attributed to "Minimal Brain Dysfunction" in Childhood. *American Journal of Psychiatry*, 139: 21–33, 1982.

58. Kenny, T., Clemens, R., & Hudson, B. Characteristics of Children Referred Because of Hyperactivity. *Journal of Pediatrics*, 79: 618–629, 1971.

59. Lambert, N. M., Sandoval, J., & Sassone, D. Prevalence of Hyperactivity in Elementary School Children as a Function of Social System Definers. *American Journal of Orthopsychiatry*, 48: 446–463, 1978.

60. Barkley, R. A. Guidelines for Defining Hyperactivity in Children. In B. B. La-

hey & A. E. Kazdin (Eds.), *Advances in Clinical Child Psychology* (Vol. 5). New York: Plenum Press, 1982.

61. Rutter, M., Graham, P., & Yule, W. *A Neuropsychiatric Study in Childhood*. London: Heinemann, 1970.

62. Miller, R. G., Palkes, H. S., & Stewart, M. A. Hyperactive Children in Suburban Elementary Schools. *Child Psychiatry and Human Development*, 4: 121–127, 1973.

63. Quay, H. C. *Conduct Disorder, ADD and Hyperactivity*. Paper presented at the Annual Meeting of the Canadian Psychological Association, Montreal, September 1980.

64. Achenbach, T. DSM-III in the Light of Empirical Research on the Classification of Childhood Psychopathology. *Journal of the American Academy of Child Psychiatry*, 19: 395–412, 1980.

65. Langhorne, J. E., Loney, J., Paternite, C. E., & Bechtoldt, H. P. Childhood Hyperkinesis: A Return to the Source. *Journal of Abnormal Psychology*, 85: 201–209, 1976.

66. Loney, J. Hyperkinesis Comes of Age: What Do We Know and Where Should We Go? *American Journal of Orthopsychiatry*, 50: 28–42, 1980.

67. Trites, R. L., & Laprade, K. Evidence for an Independent Syndrome of Hyperactivity. *Journal of Child Psychology and Psychiatry*, 24: 573–586, 1983.

68. Stewart, M. A., Cummings, C., Singer, S., & deBlois, C. S. The Overlap between Hyperactive and Unsocialized–Aggressive Children. *Journal of Child Psychology and Psychiatry*, 22: 35–47, 1981.

69. McGee, R., Williams, S., & Silva, P. Background Characteristics of Aggressive, Hyperactive, and Aggressive–Hyperactive Boys. *Journal of the American Academy of Child Psychiatry*, 23: 270–279, 1984.

CHAPTER 2

1. Lambert, N. M., Sandoval, J., & Sassone, D. Prevalence of Hyperactivity in Elementary School Children as a Function of Social System Definers. *American Journal of Orthopsychiatry*, 48: 446–463, 1978.

2. Schachar, R., Rutter, M., & Smith, A. The Characteristics of Situationally and Pervasively Hyperactive Children: Implications for Syndrome Definition. *Journal of Child Psychology and Psychiatry*, 22: 375–392, 1981.

3. Werner, E. E., & Smith, R. S. *Kauai's Children Come of Age*. Honolulu: University of Hawaii Press, 1977.

4. Weiss, G. The Natural History of Hyperactivity in Childhood and Treatment with Stimulant Medication at Different Ages. *International Journal of Mental Health*, 4: 213–226, 1975.

5. Weiss, G., Hechtman, L., Perlman, T., Hopkins, J., & Wener, A. Hyperactives as Young Adults: A Controlled Prospective 10-Year Follow-Up of the Psychiatric Status of 75 Hyperactive Children. *Archives of General Psychiatry*, 36: 675–681, 1979.

6. Nichamin, S. J. Recognizing Minimal Cerebral Dysfunction in the Infant and Toddler: Some Clinical Clues and Thoughts on Management. *Clinical Pediatrics*, 11: 255–257, 1972.

7. Werry, J. S., Weiss, G., & Douglas, V. Studies on the Hyperactive Child: I. Some Preliminary Findings. *Canadian Psychiatric Association Journal*, 9: 120–130, 1964.

8. Campbell, S. B., Szumowski, E. K., Ewing, L. J., Gluck, D. S., & Breaux, A. M. A Multidimensional Assessment of Parent-Identified Behavior Problem Toddlers. *Journal of Abnormal Child Psychology*, 10: 569–592, 1982.

9. Campbell, S. B., Breaux, A. M., Ewing, L. J., & Szumowski, E. K. A One-Year Follow-Up Study of Parent-Referred Hyperactive Preschool Children. *Journal of the American Academy of Child Psychiatry*, 23: 243–249, 1984.

10. Wolff, P. H. The Natural History of Crying and Other Vocalisations in Early Infancy. In B. M. Foss (Ed.), *Determinants of Infant Behaviour* (Vol. 4). London: Methuen, 1969.

11. Barnard, K., & Collar, B. S. Early Diagnosis, Interpretation and Intervention: A Commentary on the Nurse's Role. *Annals of the New York Academy of Sciences*, 205: 373–382, 1933.

12. Fiedler, M. F., Lenneberg, E. H., Rolfe, U. T., & Drorbaugh, J. E. A Speech Screening Procedure with Three-Year-Old Children. *Pediatrics*, 48: 268–276, 1971.

13. Waldrop, M. F., Bell, R. Q., McLaughlin, B., & Halverson, C. F. Newborn Minor Physical Anomalies Predict Short Attention Span, Peer Aggression, and Impulsivity at Age 3. *Science*, 199: 563–565, 1978.

14. Winnicott, D. W. Transitional Objects and Transitional Phenomena. *International Journal of Psycho-Analysis*, 34: 89–97, 1953.

15. Battle, E. S., & Lacey, B. A. A Context for Hyperactivity in Children, Over Time. *Child Development*, 43: 757–773, 1972.

16. Mash, E. J., & Johnston, C. Parental Perceptions of Child Behavior Problems, Parenting, Self-Esteem, and Mothers' Reported Stress in Younger and Older Hyperactive Children. *Journal of Counseling and Clinical Psychology*, 51: 86–99, 1983.

17. Pelham, W. E., & Bender, M. E. Peer Interactions of Hyperactive Children: Assessment and Treatment. In K. D. Gadow & I. Gialer (Eds.), *Advances in Learning and Behavior Difficulties*. Greenwich, CT: JAI Press, 1982.

18. Milich, R., Landau, S., Kilby, G., & Whillen, P. Preschool Peer Perceptions of the Behavior of Hyperactive and Aggressive Children. *Journal of Abnormal Child Psychology*, 10: 497–510, 1982.

19. Schleifer, M., Weiss, G., Cohen, N. J., Elman, M., Cvejic, H., & Kruger, E. Hyperactivity in the Preschooler and the Effect of Methylphenidate. *American Journal of Orthopsychiatry*, 45: 38–50, 1975.

20. Morgenstern, G. Observing the Social Behaviour of Preschool Children. *Laval Medical*, 41: 533–536, 1970.

21. Emerich, W. Continuity and Stability in Early Social Development II: Teachers' Ratings. *Child Development*, 37: 17–28, 1966.

22. Campbell, S., Endman, M., & Bernfeld, G. A Three-Year Follow-Up of Hyperactive Preschoolers into Elementary School. *Journal of Child Psychology and Psychiatry*, 18: 238–249, 1977.

23. Campbell, S. B. *Longitudinal Research on Active and Aggressive Preschoolers: Predictors of Problem Severity at School Entry*. Paper presented at the Fourth Annual Highpoint Hospital Symposium on Attention Deficit and Conduct Disorder, Toronto, Ontario, October 15, 1984.

24. Conners, C. K. Controlled Trial of Methylphenidate in Preschool Children with Minimal Brain Dysfunction. In R. Gittelman (Ed.), *Recent Advances in Child Psychopharmacology*. New York: Human Sciences Press, 1975.

25. Chapel, J. L., Robins, A. J., McGee, R. O., Williams, S. M., & Silva, P. A. A Follow-Up of Inattentive and/or Hyperactive Children from Birth to 7 Years of Age. *Journal of Operational Psychiatry*, 13: 17–26, 1982.

CHAPTER 3

1. Rutter, M. Syndromes Attributed to "Minimal Brain Dysfunction" in Childhood. *American Journal of Psychiatry*, 139: 21–33, 1982.

2. Campbell, S. B., Endman, M. W., Bernfeld, G. A Three-Year Follow-Up of

Hyperactive Preschoolers into Elementary School. *Journal of Child Psychology and Psychiatry,* 18: 239–249, 1977.

3. Klein, A. R., & Young, R. D. Hyperactive Boys in Their Classroom: Assessment of Teacher and Peer Perceptions, Interactions, and Classroom Behavior. *Journal of Abnormal Child Psychology,* 7: 425–442, 1979.

4. Porrino, C. J., Rapoport, J. L., Behar, D., Sceery, W., Ismond, D. R., & Bunney, W. E. A Naturalistic Assessment of the Motor Activity of Hyperactive Boys in Comparison with Normal Boys. *Archives of General Psychiatry,* 40: 681–687, 1983.

5. Douglas, V. I. Stop, Look and Listen: The Problem of Sustained Attention and Impulse Control in Hyperactive and Normal Children. *Canadian Journal of Behavioural Science,* 4: 259–282, 1972.

6. Weiss, G., Minde, K., Werry, J. S., Douglas, V. I., & Nemeth, E. Studies on the Hyperactive Child VIII: Five-Year Follow-Up. *Archives of General Psychiatry,* 24: 409–414, 1971.

7. Douglas, V. I. Attentional and Cognitive Problems. In M. Rutter (Ed.), *Developmental Neuropsychiatry.* New York: Guilford Press, 1983.

8. Sykes, D. H., Douglas, V. I., & Morgenstern, G. The Effect of Methylphenidate (Ritalin) on Sustained Attention in Hyperactive Children. *Psychopharmacologia,* 25: 262–274, 1972.

9. Sykes, D. H., Douglas, V. I., Weiss, G., & Minde, K. Attention in Hyperactive Children and the Effect of Methylphenidate. *Journal of Child Psychology and Psychiatry,* 12: 129–139, 1971.

10. Rosvold, H. E., Mirsky, A. F., Sarason, I., Bransome, E. D., & Beck, L. H. A Continuous Performance Test of Brain Damage. *Journal of Consulting Psychology,* 20: 343–350, 1956.

11. Strauss, A. A., & Lehtinen, L. E. *Psychopathology and Education of the Brain-Injured Child.* New York: Grune & Stratton, 1947.

12. Rosenthal, R. H., & Allen, T. W. Intratask Distractibility in Hyperkinetic and Non-Hyperkinetic Children. *Journal of Abnormal Child Psychology,* 8: 175–187, 1980.

13. Radosh, A., & Gittelman, R. The Effect of Appealing Distractors on the Performance of Hyperactive Children. *Journal of Abnormal Psychology,* 9: 179–189, 1981.

14. Campbell, S. B., Douglas, V. I., & Morgenstern, G. Cognitive Styles in Hyperactive Children and the Effect of Methylphenidate. *Journal of Child Psychology and Psychiatry,* 12: 55–67, 1971.

15. Firestone, P., & Martin, J. E. An Analysis of the Hyperactive Syndrome: A Comparison of Hyperactive Behavior Problem Asthmatic and Normal Children. *Journal of Abnormal Psychology,* 73: 261–274, 1979.

16. Hoy, E., Weiss, G., Minde, K., & Cohen, N. The Hyperactive Child at Adolescence: Emotional, Social, and Cognitive Functioning. *Journal of Abnormal Child Psychology,* 6: 311–324, 1978.

17. Wender, P. *Minimal Brain Dysfunction in Children.* New York: Wiley, 1971.

18. Freibergs, V., & Douglas, V. I. Concept Learning in Hyperactive and Normal Children. *Journal of Abnormal Psychology,* 74: 388–395, 1969.

19. Douglas, V. I., & Peters, K. G. Toward a Clearer Definition of the Attentional Deficit of Hyperactive Children. In G. A. Hale & M. Lewis (Eds.), *Attention and the Development of Cognitive Skills.* New York: Plenum Press, 1979.

20. Douglas, V. I., & Parry, P. Effect of Reward on the Delayed Reaction Time Task Performance of Hyperactive Children. *Journal of Abnormal Psychology,* 11: 313–326, 1983.

21. Cantwell, D. P., & Satterfield, J. H. The Prevalence of Academic Under-Achievement in Hyperactive Children. *Journal of Pediatric Psychology,* 3: 168–171, 1978.

22. Minde, K., Lewin, D., Weiss, G., Lavigueur, H., Douglas, V., & Sykes, D. The Hyperactive Child in Elementary School: A 5-Year Controlled Follow-Up. *Exceptional Children*, 33: 215–221, 1971.

23. Brumback, R. A., & Weinberg, W. A. Relationship of Hyperactivity and Depression in Children. *Perceptual and Motor Skills*, 45: 247–251, 1977.

24. Campbell, S. B., & Cluss, P. Peer Relationships of Young Children with Behavior Problems. In K. H. Rubin & H. S. Ross (Eds.), *Peer Relationships and Social Skills in Childhood*. New York: Springer-Verlag, 1982.

25. Campbell, S. B., & Paulauskas, S. L. Peer Relations in Hyperactive Children. *Journal of Child Psychology and Psychiatry*, 20: 233–246, 1979.

26. Robins, L. *Deviant Children Grown Up*. Baltimore: Williams & Wilkins, 1966.

27. Whalen, C. K., Henker, B., & Dolemoto, S. Teacher Response in the Methylphenidate versus Placebo Status of Hyperactive Boys in the Classroom. *Child Development*, 52: 1005–1014, 1981.

28. Whalen, C. K., Collins, B. E., Henker, B., Alkus, S. R., Adams, D., & Stapp, J. Behavior Observations of Hyperactive Children and Methylphenidate (Ritalin) Effects in Systematically Structured Classroom Environments: Now You See Them, Now You Don't. *Journal of Pediatric Psychology*, 3: 177–187, 1978.

29. Pelham, W. E. *Peer Relations and Hyperactive Children: Description and Treatment Effects*. Paper presented at the meeting of the American Psychological Association, Montreal, September 1980.

30. Bradley, C. The Behavior of Children Receiving Benzedrine. *American Journal of Psychiatry*, 94: 557–585, 1937.

31. Winsberg, B., Bialer, I., Kupietz, S., & Tobias, J. Effects of Imipramine and Dextroamphetamine on Behavior of Neuropsychiatrically Impaired Children. *American Journal of Psychiatry*, 128: 109–115, 1972.

32. Conners, C. K., & Eisenberg, L. The Effects of Methylphenidate on Symptomatology and Learning in Disturbed Children. *American Journal of Psychiatry*, 120: 458–464, 1963.

33. Conners, C. K., Eisenberg, L., & Barcai, A. Effect of Dextroamphetamine on Children: Studies on Subjects with Learning Disabilities and School Behavior Problems. *Archives of General Psychiatry*, 17: 478–485, 1967.

34. Weiss, G., Minde, K., Douglas, V., Werry, J., & Sykes, D. Comparison of the Effect of Chlorpromazine, Dextroamphetamine and Methylphenidate on the Behaviour and Intellectual Functioning of Hyperactive Children. *Canadian Medical Association Journal*, 104: 20–25, 1971.

35. Denhoff, E., Davis, A., & Hawkins, R. Effect of Dextroamphetamine on Hyperkinetic Children: A Controlled Double Blind Study. *Journal of Learning Disabilities*, 4: 491–498, 1971.

36. Conners, C. K., & Rothchild, G. Drugs and Learning in Children. In J. Helmut (Ed.), *Learning Disorders* (Vol. 3). Seattle: Special Child Publications, 1968.

37. Conners, C. K., Eisenberg, L., & Sharpe, L. Effect of Methylphenidate (Ritalin) on Paired Associate Learning and Porteus Maze Performance in Emotionally Disturbed Children. *Journal of Consulting Psychology*, 28: 14–22, 1964.

38. Sprague, R. L., Barnes, K. R., & Werry, J. S. Methylphenidate and Thioridazine: Learning Reaction Time, Activity, and Classroom Behavior in Emotionally Disturbed Children. *American Journal of Orthopsychiatry*, 40: 615–628, 1970.

39. Knights, R. M., & Hinton, G. G. The Effects of Methylphenidate (Ritalin) on the Motor Skills and Behaviour of Children with Learning Problems. *Journal of Nervous and Mental Disease*, 148: 643–653, 1969.

40. Gadow, K. Effects of Stimulant Drugs on Academic Performance in Hyperactive and Learning Disabled Children. *Journal of Learning Disabilities*, 16: 290–299, 1983.

41. Gittelman, R., Klein, D. F., & Feingold, I. Children with Reading Disorders: Effects of Methylphenidate in Combination with Reading Remediation. *Journal of Child Psychology and Psychiatry*, 24: 193–213, 1983.

42. Sprague, R., & Sleator, E. Methylphenidate in Hyperkinetic Children: Differences in Dose Effects on Learning and Social Behavior. *Science*, 198: 1274–1276, 1977.

43. Weiss, G., Kruger, E., Danielson, U., & Elman, M. Effect of Long-Term Treatment of Hyperactive Children with Methylphenidate. *Canadian Medical Association Journal*, 112: 159–165, 1975.

44. Riddle, K. D., & Rapoport, J. L. A 2-Year Follow-Up of 72 Hyperactive Boys. *Journal of Nervous and Mental Disease*, 162: 126–134, 1976.

45. Sleator, E. K., Neumann, A., & Sprague, R. L. Hyperactive Children: A Continuous Long-Term Placebo Controlled Follow-Up. *Journal of the American Medical Association*, 229: 316–317, 1974.

46. Blouin, A. G. A., Bornstein, R., & Trites, R. Teen-Age Alcohol Use among Hyperactive Children: A 5-Year Follow-Up Study. *Journal of Pediatric Psychology*, 3: 188–194, 1978.

47. Stein, R. M., & Reynard, C. L. Observations on Effects of Methylphenidate in Children with Hyperactive Behavior. *Pediatrics*, 55: 709–716, 1955.

48. Charles, L., & Schain, R. A Four-Year Follow-Up Study of the Effects of Methylphenidate on the Behavior and Academic Achievement of Hyperactive Children. *Journal of Abnormal Child Psychology*, 9: 495–505, 1981.

49. Safer, D. J., Allen, R. P., & Barr, L. Depression in Growth in Hyperactive Children on Stimulant Drugs. *New England Journal of Medicine*, 287: 217–220, 1972.

50. Roche, A. F., Lipman, R. S., & Overall, P. E. 76 Effects of Stimulant Medication on the Growth of Hyperactive Children. *Pediatrics*, 63: 847–850, 1979.

51. Ayllon, T., Layman, D., & Kandel, H. J. A Behavioral Educational Alternative to Control of Hyperactive Children. *Journal of Applied Behavior Analysis*, 8: 137–146, 1975.

52. Backman, J. F., Ferguson, H. B., & Trites, R. L. Contingency Contracting with Hyperactive Boy and His Parents. In M. Fine (Ed.), *Intervention with Hyperactive Children: A Case Study Approach*. Jamaica, NY: Spectrum, 1980.

53. Pihl, R. F. Conditioning Procedures with Hyperactive Children. *Neurology*, 17: 421–423, 1967.

54. Allen, K., Henke, L., Harris, F., Baer, D., & Reynolds, N. Control of Hyperactivity by Social Reinforcement of Attending Behavior. *Journal of Educational Psychology*, 58: 231–237, 1967.

55. Safer, D., & Allen, R. *Hyperactive Children: Diagnosis and Management*. Baltimore: University Park Press, 1976.

56. O'Leary, K., Pelham, W., Rosenbaum, A., & Price, G. Behavioral Treatment of Hyperkinetic Children: An Experimental Evaluation of Its Usefulness. *Clinical Pediatrics*, 15: 510–515, 1976.

57. Gittelman-Klein, R., Abikoff, H., Pollack, E., Klein, D., Katz, F., & Mattes, J. A Controlled Trial of Behavior Modification and Methylphenidate in Hyperactive Children. In C. Whalen & B. Henker (Eds.), *Hyperactive Children: The Social Ecology of Identification and Treatment*. New York: Academic Press, 1980.

58. Douglas, V. I., Parry, P., & Morton, P. Assessment of a Cognitive Training Program for Hyperactive Children. *Journal of Abnormal Psychology*, 4: 389–410, 1976.

59. Barkley, R. A., Copeland, A. P., & Sivage, A. C. A Self-Control Classroom for Hyperactive Children. *Journal of Autism and Developmental Disorders*, 10: 75–89, 1980.

60. Satterfield, J. H., Satterfield, B. T., & Cantwell, D. P. Three-Year Multimodality Treatment of 100 Hyperactive Boys. *Journal of Pediatrics*, 98: 650–655, 1981.

CHAPTER 4

1. Hall, G. S. *Adolescence: Its Psychology and Its Relations to Physiology, Anthropology, Sociobiology, Sex, Crime, Religion, and Education* (Vols. 1 & 2). New York: Appleton, 1904.

2. Mead, M. *Coming of Age in Samoa.* New York: Morrow, 1928.

3. Freud, A. Adolescence. *Psychoanalytic Study of the Child*, 13: 255–278, 1958.

4. Offer, D. *The Psychological World of the Teenager.* New York: Basic Books, 1969.

5. Offer, D. Normal Adolescents: Interview Strategy and Selected Results. *Archives of General Psychiatry*, 17: 285–290, 1967.

6. Rutter, M., Graham, P., Chadwick, O. F., & Yule, W. Adolescent Turmoil: Fact or Fiction? *Journal of Child Psychology and Psychiatry*, 17: 35–56, 1976.

7. Erikson, E. Eight Stages of Man. In *Childhood and Society.* New York: Norton, 1950.

8. Huessy, H. R., & Cohen, A. H. Hyperkinetic Behaviors and Learning Disabilities Followed over Seven Years. *Pediatrics*, 57: 4–6, 1976.

9. Bakwin, H., & Bakwin, R. M. *Clinical Management of Behavior Disorders in Children.* Philadelphia: Saunders, 1966.

10. Bradley, C. Characteristics and Management of Children with Behavior Problems Associated with Organic Brain Damage. *Pediatric Clinics of North America*, 4: 1049–1060, 1957.

11. Eisenberg, L. The Management of the Hyperkinetic Child. *Developmental Medicine and Child Neurology*, 8: 593–632, 1966.

12. Laufer, M. W., & Denhoff, E. Hyperkinetic Behavior Syndrome in Children. *Journal of Pediatrics*, 50: 463–474, 1957.

13. Laufer, M. W. Cerebral Dysfunction and Behavior Disorders in Adolescents. *American Journal of Orthopsychiatry*, 32: 501–506, 1962.

14. Anderson, C. M., & Plymate, H. B. Management of the Brain-Damaged Adolescent. *American Journal of Orthopsychiatry*, 32: 492–500, 1962.

15. Mendelson, W. B., Johnson, N. E., & Stewart, M. A. Hyperactive Children as Teenagers: A Follow-Up Study. *Journal of Nervous and Mental Disease*, 153: 273–279, 1971.

16. Stewart, M. A., Mendelson, W. B., & Johnson, N. E. Hyperactive Children as Adolescents: How They Describe Themselves. *Child Psychiatry and Human Development*, 4: 3–11, 1973.

17. Blouin, A. G. A., Bornstein, R., & Trites, R. Teen-Age Alcohol Use among Hyperactive Children: A 5-Year Follow-Up Study. *Journal of Pediatric Psychology*, 3: 188–194, 1978.

18. Feldman, S., Denhoff, E., & Denhoff, J. The Attention Disorders and Related Syndromes: Outcome in Adolescence and Young Adult Life. In E. Denhoff & L. Stern (Eds.), *Minimal Brain Dysfunction: A Developmental Approach.* New York: Masson Publishing (USA), 1979.

19. Weiss, G., Minde, K., Werry, J. S., Douglas, V. I., & Nemeth, E. Studies on the Hyperactive Child VIII: Five Year Follow-Up. *Archives of General Psychiatry*, 24: 409–414, 1971.

20. Minde, K., Weiss, G., & Mendelson, N. A 5-Year Follow-Up of 91 Hyperactive School Children. *Journal of the American Academy of Child Psychiatry*, 11: 595–610, 1972.

21. Werry, J. S., Weiss, G., Douglas, V. I., & Martin, J. Studies on the Hyperactive Child III: The Effect of Chlorpromazine upon Behavior and Learning Ability. *Journal of the American Academy of Child Psychiatry*, 5: 292–312, 1966.

22. Weiss, G., Werry, J. S., Minde, K., Douglas, V., & Sykes, D. Studies on the Hyperactive Child V: The Effects of Dextroamphetamine and Chlorpromazine on

Behavior and Intellectual Functioning. *Journal of Child Psychology and Psychiatry*, 9: 145–156, 1968.

23. Hoy, E., Weiss, G., Minde, K., & Cohen, N. The Hyperactive Child at Adolescence: Emotional, Social, and Cognitive Functioning. *Journal of Abnormal Child Psychology*, 6: 311–324, 1978.

24. Minde, K., Lewin, D., Weiss, G., Lavigueur, H., Douglas, V., & Sykes, E. The Hyperactive Child in Elementary School: A 5-Year Controlled Follow-Up. *Exceptional Children*, 38: 215–221, 1971.

25. Cohen, N. J., Weiss, G., & Minde, K. Cognitive Styles in Adolescents Previously Diagnosed as Hyperactive. *Journal of Child Psychology and Psychiatry*, 13: 203–209, 1972.

26. Ackerman, P. T., Dykman, R. A., & Peters, J. E. Teenage Status of Hyperactive and Nonhyperactive Learning Disabled Boys. *American Journal of Orthopsychiatry*, 47: 577–596, 1977.

27. Satterfield, J. H., Hoppe, C. M., & Schell, A. M. A Prospective Study of Delinquency in 110 Adolescent Boys with Attention Deficit Disorder and 88 Normal Adolescent Boys. *American Journal of Psychiatry*, 139: 797–798, 1982.

28. Cox, A., Rutter, M., Yule, B., & Quinlan, B. Bias Resulting from Missing Information: Some Epidemiological Findings. *British Journal of Preventive Social Medicine*, 31: 131–136, 1977.

29. Langhorne, J. E., Loney, J., Paternite, C. E., & Bechtoldt, H. P. Childhood Hyperkinesis: A Return to the Source. *Journal of Abnormal Psychology*, 85: 201–209, 1976.

30. Loney, J., Langhorne, J. E., & Paternite, C. E. An Empirical Basis for Subgrouping the Hyperkinetic MBD Syndrome. *Journal of Abnormal Psychology*, 87: 431–441, 1978.

CHAPTER 5

1. Weiss, G., Minde, K., Werry, J. S., Douglas, V. I., & Nemeth, E. Studies on the Hyperactive Child VIII: Five Year Follow-Up. *Archives of General Psychiatry*, 24: 409–414, 1971.

2. Mendelson, W. B., Johnson, N. E., & Stewart, M. A. Hyperactive Children as Teenagers: A Follow-Up Study. *Journal of Nervous and Mental Disease*, 153: 273–279, 1971.

3. Menkes, M. M., Rowe, J. S., & Menkes, J. H. A Twenty-Five-Year Follow-Up Study on the Hyperkinetic Child with Minimal Brain Dysfunction. *Pediatrics*, 39: 393–399, 1967.

4. Borland, B. L., & Heckman, H. K. Hyperactive Boys and Their Brothers: A 25-Year Follow-Up Study. *Archives of General Psychiatry*, 33: 669–675, 1976.

5. Feldman, S. A., Denhoff, E., & Denhoff, J. I. The Attention Disorders and Related Syndromes: Outcome in Adolescence and Young Adult Life. In L. Stern & E. Denhoff (Eds.), *Minimal Brain Dysfunction: A Developmental Approach*. New York: Masson Publishing (USA), 1979.

6. Loney, J., Whaley-Klahn, M. A., Kosier, T., & Conboy, J. *Hyperactive Boys and Their Brothers at 21: Predictors of Aggressive and Antisocial Outcomes*. Paper presented at meeting of the Society for Life History Research, Monterey, CA, November 1981.

7. Wood, D. R., Reimherr, F. W., Wender, P. H., & Johnson, G. E. Diagnosis and Treatment of Minimal Brain Dysfunction in Adults. *Archives of General Psychiatry*, 33: 1353–1460, 1976.

8. Shelley, E. M., & Riester, A. A Syndrome of Minimal Brain Damage in Young Adults. *Diseases of the Nervous System*, 33: 335–338, 1972.

9. Goodwin, D. W., Schulsinger, F., & Hermansen, L., Guze, S. B., & Winokur, G. Alcoholism and the Hyperactive Child Syndrome. *Journal of Nervous and Mental Disease*, 160: 349–353, 1975.

10. Gomez, R. L., Janowsky, D., Zeitin, M., Huey, L., & Clopton, P. L. Adult Psychiatric Diagnosis and Symptoms Compatible with the Hyperactive Child Syndrome: A Retrospective Study. *Journal of Clinical Psychiatry*, 42: 389–394, 1981.

11. Weiss, G., Hechtman, L., Perlman, T., Hopkins, J., & Wener, A. Hyperactive Children as Young Adults: A Controlled Prospective 10-Year Follow-Up of the Psychiatric Status of 75 Children. *Archives of General Psychiatry*, 36: 675–681, 1979.

12. Hechtman, L., & Weiss, G. Controlled Prospective Fifteen-Year Follow-Up of Hyperactives as Adults: Non-Medical Drug and Alcohol Use and Antisocial Behavior. Manuscript submitted for publication.

13. Hechtman, L., Weiss, G., & Perlman, T. Hyperactives as Young Adults: Self-Esteem and Social Skills. *Canadian Journal of Psychiatry*, 25: 478–483, 1980.

14. Weiss, G., Hechtman, L., & Perlman, T. Hyperactives as Young Adults: School, Employer and Self-Rating Scales Obtained during Ten-Year Follow-Up Evaluation. *American Journal of Orthopsychiatry*, 48: 438–445, 1978.

15. Hopkins, J., Perlman, T., Hechtman, L., & Weiss, G. Cognitive Style in Adults Originally Diagnosed as Hyperactives. *Journal of Child Psychology and Psychiatry*, 20: 209–216, 1979.

16. Werry, J. S., Weiss, G., Douglas, V. I., & Martin, J. Studies on the Hyperactive Child III: The Effect of Chlorpromazine upon Behavior and Learning Ability. *Journal of the American Academy of Child Psychiatry*, 5: 292–312, 1966.

17. Weiss, G., Werry, J. S., Minde, K., Douglas, V. & Sykes, D. Studies on the Hyperactive Child V: The Effects of Dextroamphetamine and Chlorpromazine on Behavior and Intellectual Functioning. *Journal of Child Psychology and Psychiatry*, 9: 145–156, 1968.

18. Cox, A., Rutter, M., Yule, B., & Quinlan, B. Bias Resulting from Missing Information: Some Epidemiological Findings. *British Journal of Preventive Social Medicine*, 31: 131–136, 1977.

19. Schachar, R., Rutter, M., & Smith, A. The Characteristics of Situationally and Pervasively Hyperactive Children: Implications for Syndrome Definition. *Journal of Child Psychology and Psychiatry*, 22: 375–392, 1981.

20. Overall, J. E., & Gorham, D. R. The Brief Psychiatric Rating Scale. *Psychological Reports*, 10: 799–812, 1962.

21. Gough, H. *California Psychological Inventory* (Rev. Ed.). Palo Alto, CA: Consulting Psychologist Press, 1975.

22. Derogatis, L., Lipman, R., & Covi, L. SCL-90: An Outpatient Psychiatric Rating Scale. *Psychopharmacology Bulletin*, 9: 13–27, 1973.

23. Hechtman, L., Weiss, G., Perlman, T., & Tuck, D. Hyperactives as Young Adults: Various Clinical Outcomes. *Adolescent Psychiatry*, 9: 295–306, 1981.

24. Weiss, G., Hechtman, L., Milroy, T., & Perlman, T. Psychiatric Status of Hyperactives as Adults: A Controlled 15-Year Follow-Up of 63 Hyperactive Children. *Journal of the American Academy of Child Psychiatry*, 24: 211–220, 1985.

25. American Psychiatric Association. *Diagnostic and Statistical Manual of Mental Disorders* (3rd Ed.; DSM-III). Washington, DC: APA, 1980.

26. Endicott, J., & Spitzer, R. L. A Diagnostic Interview: The Schedule for Affective Disorders and Schizophrenia. *Archives of General Psychiatry*, 35: 837–844, 1978.

27. Dykman, R. A., & Ackerman, P. Long-Term Follow-Up Studies of Hyperactive Children. In *Advances in Behavioral Paediatrics* (Vol. 1). Greenwich, CT: JAI Press, 1980.

28. Blouin, A. G. A., Bornstein, R., & Trites, R. Teenage Alcohol Use among

Hyperactive Children: A 5-Year Follow-Up Study. *Journal of Pediatric Psychology*, 3: 188–194, 1978.

29. Satterfield, J. H., Hoppe, C. M., & Schell, A. M. A Prospective Study of Delinquency in 110 Adolescent Boys with Attention Deficit Disorder and 88 Normal Adolescent Boys. *American Journal of Psychiatry*, 139: 797–798, 1982.

30. Gittelman, R., Mannuzza, S., Shenker, R., & Bonagura, N. Hyperactive Boys Almost Grown Up: Psychiatric Status. *Archives of General Psychiatry*, in press.

CHAPTER 6

1. Mendelson, W. B., Johnson, N. E., & Stewart, M. A. Hyperactive Children as Teenagers: A Follow-Up Study. *Journal of Nervous and Mental Disease*, 153: 273–279, 1971.

2. Stewart, M. A., Mendelson, W. B., & Johnson, N. E. Hyperactive Children as Adolescents: How They Describe Themselves. *Child Psychiatry and Human Development*, 4: 3–11, 1973.

3. Weiss, G., Minde, K., Werry, J. S., Douglas, V. I., & Nemeth, E. Studies on the Hyperactive Child VIII: Five-Year Follow-Up. *Archives of General Psychiatry*, 24: 409–414, 1971.

4. Minde, K., Lewin, D., Weiss, G., Lavigueur, H., Douglas, V., & Sykes, E. The Hyperactive Child in Elementary School: A 5-Year Controlled Follow-Up. *Exceptional Children*, 38: 215–221, 1971.

5. Minde, K., Weiss, G., & Mendelson, N. A 5-Year Follow-Up of 91 Hyperactive School Children. *Journal of the American Academy of Child Psychiatry*, 11: 595–610, 1972.

6. Ackerman, P. T., Dykman, R. A., & Peters, J. E. Teenage Status of Hyperactive and Nonhyperactive Learning Disabled Boys. *American Journal of Orthopsychiatry*, 47: 577–596, 1977.

7. Satterfield, J., Hoppe, C. M., & Schell, A. M. A Prospective Study of Delinquency in 110 Adolescent Boys with Attention Deficit Disorder and 88 Normal Adolescent Boys. *American Journal of Psychiatry*, 139: 797–798, 1982.

8. Robins, L. N. *Deviant Children Grown Up*. Baltimore: Williams & Wilkins, 1966.

9. Glueck, S., & Glueck, E. *Juvenile Delinquents Grown Up*. New York: Commonwealth Fund, 1940.

10. Kramer, J., & Loney, J. *Predicting Adolescent Antisocial Behavior among Hyperactive Boys*. Paper presented at Annual Meeting of the American Psychological Association, Toronto, 1978.

11. Loney, J., Kramer, J., & Milich, R. The Hyperkinetic Child Grows Up: Predictors of Symptoms, Delinquency, and Achievement at Follow-Up. In K. D. Gadow & J. Loney (Eds.), *Psychosocial Aspects of Drug Treatment for Hyperactivity*. Boulder, CO: Westview Press, 1981.

12. Rivera, R., Rafferty, F., & Krause, M. *Juvenile Delinquency in Illinois: Highlights of the 1972 Adolescent Survey*. Chicago: Chicago Institute for Juvenile Research, 1972.

13. Hays, M. *Report of the Iowa Study of Drug Attitudes and Behavior among Youth*. Des Moines: State of Iowa Department of Public Instruction, 1976.

14. Chambers, C. *The Incidence and Prevalence of Substance Use and Misuse, Attitudes and Problems within Two Study Populations in the State of Iowa*. Washington, DC: Resource Planning Corporation, 1976.

15. Blouin, A. G. A., Bornstein, R., & Trites, R. Teen-Age Alcohol Use among Hyperactive Children: A 5-Year Follow-Up Study. *Journal of Pediatric Psychology*, 3: 188–194, 1978.

16. Feldman, S., Denhoff, E., & Denhoff, J. The Attention Disorders and Related Syndromes: Outcome in Adolescence and Young Adult Life. In L. Stern & E. Denhoff (Eds.), *Minimal Brain Dysfunction: A Developmental Approach.* New York: Masson Publishing (USA), 1979.

17. Morrison, J. R., & Stewart, M. A. A Family Study of the Hyperactive Child Syndrome. *Biological Psychiatry,* 3: 189–195, 1971.

18. Cantwell, D. P. Psychiatric Illness in the Families of Hyperactive Children. *Archives of General Psychiatry,* 27: 414–417, 1972.

19. Morrison, J. R., & Stewart, M. A. The Psychiatric Status of Legal Families of Adopted Hyperactive Children. *Archives of General Psychiatry,* 28: 888–891, 1973.

20. Stewart, M. A., de Blois, C. S., & Cummings, C. Psychiatric Disorder in Parents of Hyperactive Boys and Those With Conduct Disorder. *Journal of Child Psychology and Psychiatry,* 21: 283–292, 1980.

21. Morrison, J. R. Adult Psychiatric Disorders in Parents of Hyperactive Children. *American Journal of Psychiatry,* 137: 825–827, 1980.

22. Morrison, J. R. Diagnosis of Adult Psychiatric Patients with Childhood Hyperactivity. *American Journal of Psychiatry,* 136: 955–958, 1979.

23. Morrison, J. R. Childhood Hyperactivity in an Adult Psychiatric Population: Social Factors. *Journal of Clinical Psychiatry,* 41: 40–43, 1980.

24. Wender, P. H., Reimherr, F. W., & Wood, D. R. Attention Deficit Disorder ("Minimal Brain Dysfunction") in Adults: A Replication Study of Diagnosis and Drug Treatment. *Archives of General Psychiatry,* 38: 449–456, 1981.

25. Wood, D. R., Reimherr, F. W., Wender, P. H., and Johnson, G. E. Diagnosis and Treatment of Minimal Brain Dysfunction in Adults. *Archives of General Psychiatry,* 33: 1453–1460, 1976.

26. Shelley, E. M., & Riester, A. Syndrome of Minimal Brain Damage in Young Adults. *Diseases of the Nervous System,* 33: 335–338, 1972.

27. Morrison, J. R., & Minkoff, K. Explosive Personality as a Sequel to the Hyperactive-Child Syndrome. *Comprehensive Psychiatry,* 16: 343–348, 1975.

28. Gomez, R. L., Janowsky, D., Zeitin, M., Huey, L., & Clopton, P. L. Adult Psychiatric Diagnosis and Symptoms Compatible with the Hyperactive Child Syndrome: A Retrospective Study. *Journal of Clinical Psychiatry,* 42: 389–394, 1981.

29. Mann, H. B., & Greenspan, S. I. The Identification and Treatment of Adult Brain Dysfunction. *American Journal of Psychiatry,* 133: 1013–1017, 1976.

30. Mattes, J., Boswell, L., & Oliver, H. *Methylphenidate Effects on Symptoms of Attention Deficit Disorders in Adults. Archives of General Psychiatry,* 41: 1059–1067, 1984.

31. Menkes, M. M., Rowe, J. S., & Menkes, J. H. A Twenty-Five-Year Follow-Up Study on the Hyperkinetic Child with Minimal Brain Dysfunction. *Pediatrics,* 39: 393–399, 1967.

32. Laufer, M. W. Long-Term Management and Some Follow-Up Findings on the Use of Drugs with Minimal Cerebral Syndromes. *Journal of Learning Disabilities,* 4: 55–58, 1971.

33. Borland, B. L., & Heckman, H. K. Hyperactive Boys and Their Brothers: A 25-Year Follow-Up Study. *Archives of General Psychiatry,* 33: 669–675, 1976.

34. Loney, J., Whaley-Klahn, M. A., Kosier, T., & Conboy, J. *Hyperactive Boys and Their Brothers at 21: Predictors of Aggressive and Antisocial Outcomes.* Paper presented at meeting of the Society for Life History Research, Monterey, CA, November 1981.

35. Endicott, J., & Spitzer, R. L. A Diagnostic Interview: The Schedule for Affective Disorders and Schizophrenia. *Archives of General Psychiatry,* 35: 837–844, 1978.

36. Kramer, J., Loney, J., & Whaley-Klahn, M. A. *The Iowa Crime and Punishment Survey (CAPS).* Unpublished survey, University of Iowa, 1978.

37. Huessy, H., Metoyer, M., & Townsend, M., 8-10 Year Follow-Up of Children Treated in Rural Vermont for Behavioral Disorder. *American Journal of Orthopsychiatry*, 43: 236–238, 1973.

38. Milman, D. H. Minimal Brain Dysfunction in Childhood: Outcome in Late Adolescence and Early Adult Years. *Journal of Clinical Psychiatry*, 9: 371–380, 1979.

39. Gittelman, R., Mannuzza, S., Shenker, R., & Bonagura, N. Hyperactive Boys Almost Grown Up: Psychiatric Status. *Archives of General Psychiatry*, in press.

40. Hechtman, L., Weiss, G., & Perlman, T. Hyperactives as Young Adults: Past and Current Antisocial Behavior (Stealing, Drug–Alcohol Abuse) and Moral Development. *American Journal of Orthopsychiatry*, 54: 415–425, 1984.

41. Weiss, G., Hechtman, L., Perlman, T., Hopkins, J., & Wener, A. Hyperactives as Young Adults: A Controlled Prospective Ten-Year Follow-Up of 75 Children. *Archives of General Psychiatry*, 36: 675–681, 1979.

42. Hechtman, L., Weiss, G., & Perlman, T. Growth and Cardiovascular Measures in Hyperactive Individuals as Young Adults and in Matched Normal Controls. *Canadian Medical Association Journal*, 118: 1247–1250, 1978.

43. Hopkins, J., Perlman, T., Hechtman, L., & Weiss, G. Cognitive Style in Adults Originally Diagnosed as Hyperactives. *Journal of Child Psychology and Psychiatry*, 20: 209–216, 1979.

44. Hechtman, L., Weiss, G., & Metrakos, K. Hyperactive Individuals as Young Adults: Current and Longitudinal Electroencephalographic Evaluation and Its Relation to Outcome. *Canadian Medical Association Journal*, 118: 919–923, 1978.

45. Hechtman, L. Families of Hyperactives. In R. Simmons (Ed.), *Research in Community and Mental Health* (Vol. 2). Greenwich, CT: JAI Press, 1981.

46. Hollingshead, A. B., & Redlich, F. C. *Social Class and Mental Illness: A Community Study*. New York: Wiley, 1958.

47. Kohlberg, L. *Stages in the Development of Moral Thought and Action*. New York: Holt, Rinehart & Winston, 1969.

48. Weiss, G., Hechtman, L., Milroy, T., & Perlman, T. Psychiatric Status of Hyperactives as Adults: A Controlled Prospective 15-Year Follow-Up of 63 Hyperactive Children. *Journal of the American Academy of Child Psychiatry*, 24: 221–227, 1985.

49. Hechtman, L., & Weiss, G. Controlled Prospective Fifteen-Year Follow-Up of Hyperactives as Adults: Non-Medical Drug and Alcohol Use and Antisocial Behavior. Manuscript submitted for publication.

50. Derogatis, L. R., Lipman, R. S., & Covi, L. SCL-90: An Outpatient Psychiatric Rating Scale—Preliminary Report. *Psychopharmacology Bulletin*, 9: 13–28, 1973.

51. Cox, A., Rutter, M., Yule, B., & Quinlan, B. Bias Resulting from Missing Information: Some Epidemiological Findings. *British Journal of Preventive Social Medicine*, 31: 131–136, 1977.

52. Hechtman, L., Weiss, G., Perlman, T., & Tuck, D. Hyperactives as Young Adults: Various Clinical Outcomes. *Adolescent Psychiatry*, 14: 295–306, 1981.

53. Hechtman, L., Weiss, G., Perlman, T., & Amsel, R. Hyperactives as Young Adults: Initial Predictions of Adult Outcome. *Journal of the American Academy of Child Psychiatry*, 24: 250–261, 1984.

CHAPTER 7

1. Endicott, J., & Spitzer, R. L. A Diagnostic Interview: The Schedule for Affective Disorder and Schizophrenia. *Archives of General Psychiatry*, 35: 837–844, 1978.

2. American Psychiatric Association. *Diagnostic and Statistical Manual of Mental Disorders* (3rd Ed.; DSM-III). Washington, DC: APA, 1980.

3. Lampl-de-Groot, J. Ego Ideal and Super-Ego. *Psychoanalytic Study of the Child,* 17: 94–106, 1962.

4. Murray, J. M. Narcissim and the Ego Ideal. *Journal of the American Psychoanalytic Association,* 12: 477–511, 1964.

5. Freud, A. *Normality and Pathology in Childhood: Assessments of Development.* New York: International Press, 1965.

6. Cantwell, D. P. Psychiatric Illness in the Families of Hyperactive Children. *Archives of General Psychiatry,* 27: 414–417, 1972.

7. Stewart, M. A., & Morrison, J. R. Affective Disorder among the Relatives of Hyperactive Children. *Journal of Child Psychology and Psychiatry,* 14: 209–212, 1973.

CHAPTER 8

1. Weiss, G., Minde, K., Werry, J. S., Douglas, V. I., & Nemeth, E. The Hyperactive Child VIII: Five-Year Follow-Up. *Archives of General Psychiatry,* 24: 409–414, 1971.

2. Satterfield, J., Hoppe, C. M., & Schell, A. M. A Prospective Study of Delinquency in 110 Adolescent Boys with Attention Deficit Disorder and 88 Normal Adolescent Boys. *American Journal of Psychiatry,* 139: 797–798, 1982.

3. Blouin, A. G. A., Bornstein, R., Trite, R. Teen-Age Alcohol Use among Hyperactive Children: A 5-Year Follow-Up Study. *Journal of Pediatric Psychology,* 3: 188–194, 1978.

4. Mendelson, W. B., Johnson, N. E., & Stewart, M. A. Hyperactive Children as Teenagers: A Follow-Up Study. *Journal of Nervous and Mental Disease,* 153: 273–279, 1971.

5. Feldman, S., Denhoff, E., & Denhoff, J. The Attention Disorders and Related Syndromes: Outcome in Adolescence and Young Adult Life. In L. Stern & E. Denhoff (Eds.), *Minimal Brain Dysfunction: A Developmental Approach.* New York: Masson Publishing (USA), 1979.

6. Beck, L., Langford, W. S., MacKay, M., & Sum, G. Childhood Chemotherapy and Later Drug Abuse and Growth Curve: A Follow-Up Study of 30 Adolescents. *American Journal of Psychiatry,* 132: 4, 436–438, 1975.

7. Kramer, J., & Loney, J. *Predicting Adolescent Antisocial Behavior among Hyperactive Boys.* Paper presented at the Annual Meeting of the American Psychological Association, Toronto, August 1978.

8. Loney, J., Kramer, J., & Milich, R. The Hyperkinetic Child Grows Up: Predictors of Symptoms, Delinquency and Achievement at Follow-Up. In K. Gadow & J. Loney (Eds.), *Psychosocial Aspects of Drug Treatment for Hyperactivity.* Boulder, CO: Westview Press, 1981.

9. Hays, M. *Report of the Iowa Study of Drug Attitudes and Behavior among Youth.* Des Moines: State of Iowa Department of Public Instruction, 1976.

10. Chambers, C. *The Incidence and Prevalence of Substance Use and Misuse: Attitudes and Problems within Two Study Populations in the State of Iowa.* Washington, DC: Resource Planning Corporation, 1976.

11. Henker, B., Whalen, C., Bugental, D. B., & Barker, C. Licit and Illicit Substance Use Patterns in Stimulant-Treated Children and Their Peers. In K. Gadow & J. Loney (Eds.), *Psychosocial Aspects of Drug Treatment for Hyperactivity.* Boulder, CO: Westview Press, 1981.

12. Goodwin, D. W., Schulsinger, F., Hermansen, L., Guze, S. B., & Winokur, G. Alcoholism and Hyperactive Child Syndrome. *Journal of Nervous and Mental Disease,* 160: 349–353, 1975.

13. Wood, D., Wender, P. H., & Reimherr, F. W. The Prevalence of Attention Deficit Disorder Residual Type or Minimal Brain Dysfunction in a Population of Male Alcoholic Patients. *American Journal of Psychiatry*, 140: 95–98, 1983.

14. Morrison, J. R. Diagnosis of Adult Psychiatric Patients with Childhood Hyperactivity. *American Journal of Psychiatry*, 136: 955–958, 1979.

15. Tarter, R. E., McBride, N., Baonpane, N., & Schneider, D. U. Differentiation of Alcoholics: Children History of Minimal Brain Dysfunction, Family History, and Drinking Pattern. *Archives of General Psychiatry*, 34: 761–768, 1977.

16. Wood, D. R., Reimherr, F. W., Wender, P. H., & Johnson, G. E. Diagnosis and Treatment of Minimal Brain Dysfunction in Adults. *Archives of General Psychiatry*, 33: 1453–1460, 1976.

17. Mattes, J., Boswell, L., & Oliver, H. Methylphenidate Effects on Symptoms of Attention Deficit Disorder in Adults. *Archives of General Psychiatry*, 41: 1059–1067, 1984.

18. Morrison, J. R., and Stewart, M. A. A Family Study of the Hyperactive Child Syndrome. *Biological Psychiatry*, 3: 189–195, 1971.

19. Cantwell, D. P. Psychiatric Illness in the Families of Hyperactive Children. *Archives of General Psychiatry*, 27: 414–417, 1972.

20. Morrison, J. R., & Stewart, M. A. The Psychiatric Status of Legal Families of Adopted Hyperactive Children. *Archives of General Psychiatry*, 3: 888–891, 1973.

21. Stewart, M. A., de Blois, C. S., & Singer, S. Alcoholism and Hyperactivity Revisited: A Preliminary Report. In M. Gallanter (Ed.), *Biomedical Issues and Clinical Effects of Alcoholism* (Vol 5). New York: Grune & Stratton, 1979.

22. Morrison, J. R. Adult Psychiatric Disorders in Parents of Hyperactive Children. *American Journal of Psychiatry*, 137: 825–827, 1980.

23. Offord, D. R., Sullivan, N., Allen, N., & Abrams, N. Delinquency and Hyperactivity. *Journal of Nervous and Mental Disease*, 167: 734–741, 1979.

24. Laufer, M. W. Long-Term Management and Some Follow-Up Findings on the Use of Drugs with Minimal Cerebral Syndrome. *Journal of Learning Disabilities*, 4: 55–58, 1971.

25. Borland, B. L., & Heckman, H. K. Hyperactive Boys and Their Brothers: A 25-Year Follow-Up Study. *Archives of General Psychiatry*, 33: 669–675, 1976.

26. Milman, D. H. Minimal Brain Dysfunction in Childhood: Outcome in Late Adolescence and Early Adult Years. *Journal of Clinical Psychiatry*, 40: 371–380, 1979.

27. Loney, J., Whaley-Klahn, M. A., Kosier, T., and Conboy, J. *Hyperactive Boys and Their Brothers at 21: Predictors of Aggressive and Antisocial Outcomes.* Paper presented at a meeting of the Society for Life History Research, Monterey, CA, November 1981.

28. Abelson, H., & Fishburne, P. *National Survey on Drug Abuse, 1977* (Vol. 2, *Methodology*). Rockville, MD: National Institute on Drug Abuse, 1977.

29. Endicott, J., & Spitzer, R. L. A Diagnostic Interview: The Schedule for Affective Disorders and Schizophrenia. *Archives of General Psychiatry*, 35: 837–844, 1978.

30. Gittelman, R., Mannuzza, S., Shenker, R., & Bonagura, N. Hyperactive Boys Almost Grown Up: Psychiatric Status. *Archives of General Psychiatry*, in press.

31. Lambert, M. *Overview of the Data Base for the Berkeley Hyperactivity Studies and Some Preliminary Findings Related to Substance Use and Mental Health Outcomes.* Personal communication, January 1985.

32. Hechtman, L., Weiss, G., & Perlman, T. Hyperactives as Young Adults: Past and Current Antisocial Behavior (Stealing, Drug and Alcohol Abuse) and Moral Development. *American Journal of Orthopsychiatry*, 54: 415–425, 1984.

33. Robins, L. N. Sturdy Childhood Predictors of Adult Outcomes: Replications form Longitudinal Studies. *Psychological Medicine*, 8: 611–622, 1978.

34. Hechtman, L., & Weiss, G. Controlled Prospective Fifteen-Year Follow-Up of

Hyperactives as Adults: Non-Medical Drug and Alcohol Use and Antisocial Behavior. Manuscript submitted for publication.

CHAPTER 9

1. Menkes, M. M., Rowe, J. S., & Menkes, J. H. A Twenty-Five-Year Follow-Up Study on the Hyperactive Child with Minimal Brain Dysfunction. *Pediatrics*, 39: 393–399, 1967.
2. Feldman, S., Denhoff, E., & Denhoff, J. The Attention Disorders and Related Syndromes: Outcome in Adolescence and Young Adult Life. In L. Stern & E. Denhoff (Eds.), *Minimal Brain Dysfunction: A Developmental Approach*. New York: Masson Publishing (USA), 1979.
3. Borland, B. L., & Heckman, H. K. Hyperactive Boys and Their Brothers: A 25-Year Follow-Up Study. *Archives of General Psychiatry*, 33: 669–675, 1976.
4. Mendelson, W. B., Johnson, N. E., & Stewart, M. A. Hyperactive Children as Teenagers: A Follow-Up Study. *Journal of Nervous and Mental Disease*, 153: 273–279, 1971.
5. Weiss, G., Hechtman, L., & Perlman, T. Hyperactives as Young Adults: School, Employer and Self-Rating Scales Obtained During Ten-Year Follow-Up Evaluation. *American Journal of Orthopsychiatry*, 48: 438–445, 1978.
6. Weiss, G., Perlman, T., Tuck, D., & Hechtman, L. *Hyperactives as Young Adults: Work Record*. Paper presented at the meeting of the Canadian Psychiatric Association, September 1979.
7. Weiss, G., Hechtman, L., Perlman, T., Tuck, D. *Hyperactive Adults: Work Record*. Paper presented at poster session of the meeting of the American and Canadian Academy of Child Psychiatry, September 1984.

CHAPTER 10

1. Weiss, G., Minde, K., Werry, J. S., Douglas, V. I., & Nemeth, E. Studies on the Hyperactive Child VIII: Five-Year Follow-Up. *Archives of General Psychiatry*, 24: 409–414, 1971.
2. Hoy, E., Weiss, G., Minde, K., & Cohen, N. The Hyperactive Child at Adolescence: Emotional, Social, and Cognitive Functioning. *Journal of Abnormal Child Psychology*, 6: 311–324, 1978.
3. Hollingshead, A., & Redlich, F. C. *Social Class and Mental Illness: A Community Study*. New York: 1958.
4. Davidson, H., & Lang, G. Children's Perceptions of Their Teachers' Feelings Toward Them Related to Self-Perception, School Achievement and Behavior. *Journal of Experimental Education*, 29: 107–116, 1960.
5. Ziller, R. C., Hagen, J., & Smith, M. Self-Esteem: A Self-Social Construct. *Journal of Consulting and Clinical Psychology*, 33: 84–95, 1969.
6. Mendelson, W. B., Johnson, N. E., & Stewart, M. A. Hyperactive Children as Teenagers: A Follow-Up Study. *Journal of Nervous and Mental Disease*, 153: 273–279, 1971.
7. Stewart, M. A., Mendelson, W. B., & Johnson, N. E. Hyperactive Children as Adolescents: How They Describe Themselves. *Child Psychiatry and Human Development*, 4: 3–11, 1973.
8. Ackerman, P. T., Dykman, R. A., & Peters, J. E. Teenage Status of Hyperactive and Non-Hyperactive Learning-Disabled Boys. *American Journal of Orthopsychiatry*, 47: 577–596, 1977.

9. Werner, E. E., & Smith, R. S. *Kauai's Children Come of Age.* Honolulu: University of Hawaii Press, 1977.

10. Feldman, S., Denhoff, E., Denhoff, J. The Attention Disorders and Related Syndromes: Outcome in Adolescence and Young Adult Life. In L. Stern & E. Denhoff (Eds.), *Minimal Brain Dysfunction: A Developmental Approach.* New York: Masson Publishing (USA), 1979.

11. Langhorne, J. E., & Loney, J. A Four-Fold Model for Subgrouping the Hyper-kinetic/MBD Syndrome. *Child Psychiatry and Human Development* 9: 153–159, 1979.

12. Paternite, C. E., Loney, J., & Langhorne, J. E. Relationships Between Sympto-matology and SES Related Factors in Hyperkinetic/MBD Boys. *American Journal of Ortho-psychiatry,* 46: 291–301, 1976.

13. Satterfield, J. H., Satterfield, B. T., & Cantwell, D. P. Three-Year Multimodal-ity Treatment Study of 100 Hyperactive Boys. *Journal of Pediatrics,* 98: 650–655, 1981.

14. Borland, B. L., & Heckman, H. K. Hyperactive Boys and Their Brothers: A 25-Year Follow-Up Study. *Archives of General Psychiatry,* 33: 669–675, 1976.

15. Milman, D. H. Minimal Brain Dysfunction in Childhood: Outcome in Late Adolescence and Early Adult Years. *Journal of Clinical Psychiatry,* 40: 371–380, 1979.

16. Weiss, G., Hechtman, L., Perlman, T., Hopkins, J., & Wener, A. Hyperactives as Young Adults: A Controlled Prospective 10 Year Follow-Up of the Psychiatric Status of 75 Hyperactive Children. *Archives of General Psychiatry,* 36: 675–681, 1979.

17. Weiss, G., Hechtman, L., & Perlman, T. Hyperactives as Young Adults: School, Employer, and Self-Rating Scales Obtained during Ten-Year Follow-Up Evaluation. *American Journal of Orthopsychiatry,* 48: 438–445, 1978.

18. Clark, K. W. *Evaluation of a Group Social Skills Training Program with Psychiatric Inpatients: Training Vietnam Veterans in Assertion, Heterosocial and Job Interview Skills.* Unpub-lished doctoral dissertation, University of Wisconsin, 1974.

19. Platt, J. J., Spivack, G., & Bloom, N. *Means–End Problem Solving Procedure (MEPS) Manual and Tentative Norms.* Philadelphia: Department of Mental Health Sciences, Hahne-mann Medical College and Hospital, 1971.

20. Weiss, G., Hechtman, L., Milroy, T., & Perlman, T. Psychiatric Status of Hyperactives as Adults: A Controlled Prospective 15-Year Follow-Up of 63 Hyperactive Children. *Journal of the American Academy of Child Psychiatry,* 24: 211–221, 1985.

21. Hechtman, L., & and Weiss, G. Controlled Prospective Fifteen-Year Follow-Up of Hyperactives as Adults: Non-Medical Drug and Alcohol Use and Antisocial Behavior. Manuscript submitted for publication.

CHAPTER 11

1. Laufer, M. W., Denhoff, E., & Solomons, S. Hyperkinetic Impulse Disorder in Children's Behavior Problems. *Psychosomatic Medicine,* 19: 38–49, 1957.

2. Freibergs, V., & Douglas, V. I. Concept Learning in Hyperactive and Normal Children. *Journal of Abnormal Psychology,* 74: 388–395, 1969.

3. Buckley, R. E. A Neurophysiological Proposal for the Amphetamine Response in Hyperkinetic Children. *Psychosomatics,* 13: 93–99, 1972.

4. Wender, P. H. *Minimal Brain Dysfunction in Children.* New York: Wiley–Inter-science, 1971.

5. Dykman, R. A., Ackerman, P. T., Clements, S. D., & Peters, J. E. Specific Learning Disabilities: An Attention Deficit Syndrome. In H. R. Myklebust (Ed.), *Progress in Learning Disabilities* (Vol. 2). New York: Grune & Stratton, 1972.

6. Werry, J. S. Some Clinical and Laboratory Studies of Psychotropic Drugs in Children: An Overview. In M. K. Smith (Ed.), *Drugs and Cerebral Function*. Springfield, IL: C. C. Thomas, 1970.

7. Satterfield, J. H., & Dawson, M. E. Electrodermal Correlates of Hyperactivity in Children. *Psychophysiology*, 8: 191–197, 1971.

8. Wender, P. H. Some Speculations Concerning a Possible Biochemical Basis of Minimal Brain Dysfunction. *Annals of New York Academy of Sciences*, 205: 18–28, 1973.

9. Zentall, S. S. Optimal Stimulation as a Theoretical Basis of Hyperactivity. *American Journal of Orthopsychiatry*, 45: 549–563, 1975.

10. Rapoport, J. L., & Ferguson, H. B. Biological Validation of the Hyperkinetic Syndrome. *Developmental Medicine and Child Neurology*, 23: 667–682, 1981.

11. Cohen, M., & Douglas, V. Characteristics of the Orienting Response in Hyperactive and Normal Children. *Psychophysiology*, 9: 238–245, 1972.

12. Satterfield, J. H., Cantwell, D. P., Lesser, L. I., & Pososim, R. L. Physiological Studies of the Hyperkinetic Child: I: *American Journal of Psychiatry*, 128: 1418–1424, 1972.

13. Spring, C., Greenberg, L., Scott, J., & Hopwood, J. Electrodermal Activity in Hyperactive Boys Who Are Methlyphenidate Responders. *Psychophysiology*, 11: 436–442, 1974.

14. Montagu, J. D. The Hyperkinetic Child: A Behavioural Electrodermal and EEG Investigation. *Developmental Medicine and Child Neurology*, 17: 299–305, 1975.

15. Zahn, T. P., Abate, F., Little, B. C., & Wender, P. H. Minimal Brain Dysfunction, Stimulant Drugs and Autonomic Nervous System Activity. *Archives of General Psychiatry*, 32: 381–387, 1975.

16. Ferguson, H. B., Simpson, S., & Trites, R. L. Psychophysiological Study of Methlyphenidate Responders and Nonresponders. In R. K. Knights & D. J. Bakker (Eds.), *Neuropsychology of Learning Disorders*. Baltimore: University Park Press, 1976.

17. Barkley, R. A., & Jackson, T. L., Jr. Hyperkinesis, Autonomic Nervous System Activity and Stimulant Drug Effects. *Journal of Child Psychology and Psychiatry*, 18: 347–357, 1977.

18. Porges, S. W., Walter, G. F., Korb, R. J., Sprague, R. L. The Influence of Methlyphenidate on Heart Rate and Behavioral Measures of Attention in Hyperactive Children. *Child Development*, 46: 727–733, 1975.

19. Douglas, V. Attentional and Cognitive Problems. In M. Rutter (Ed.), *Developmental Neuropsychiatry*. New York: Guilford Press, 1983.

20. Sroufe, L. A., Sonies, B. C., West, W. D., & Wright, F. S. Anticipatory Heart Rate Deceleration and Reaction Time in Children with and without Referral for Learning Disability. *Child Development*, 44: 267–273, 1973.

21. Porges, S. W., Gohrer, R. E., Keren, G., Cheuns, M. N., Franks, G. J., & Drasgow, F. The Influence of Methlyphenidate on Spontaneous Autonomic Activity and Behavior in Children Diagnosed as Hyperactive. *Psychophysiology*, 18: 42–48, 1981.

22. Ballard, J. E., Boileau, R. A., Sleator, E. K., Massey, B. H., & Sprague, R. L. Cardiovascular Responses of Hyperactive Children to Methlyphenidate. *Journal of the American Medical Association*, 236: 2870–2874, 1976.

23. Capute, A. J., Niedermeyer, E. F., & Richardson, F. The Electroencephalogram in Children with Minimal Cerebral Dysfunction. *Pediatrics*, 41: 1104–1114, 1968.

24. Klinderfuss, G. H., Lange, P. H., Weinberg, W. A., & O'Leary, J. Electroencephalographic Abnormalities of Children with Hyperkinetic Behavior. *Neurology*, 15: 883–891, 1965.

25. Wikler, A., Dixon, J. R., & Parker, J. B., Jr. Brain Function in Problem Children and Controls: Psychometric, Neurological, and Electroencephalographic Comparison. *American Journal of Psychiatry*, 127: 634–645, 1970.

26. Werry, J. S., Minde, K., Guzman, A., Weiss, G., Dogan, K., & Hoy, E. Studies on the Hyperactive Child VII: Neurological Status Compared with Neurotic and Normal Children. *American Journal of Orthopsychiatry*, 42: 441–451, 1972.

27. Eeg-Olofsson, O. The Development of the Electroencephalogram in Normal Children and Adolescents from the Age of 1 through 21 Years. *Acta Paediatrica Scandinavica*. 208 (Suppl.): 1–46, 1970.

28. Cantwell, D. P. Drugs and Medical Intervention. In H. E. Rie & E. D. Rie (Eds.), *Handbook of Minimal Brain Dysfunction: A Critical Review*. New York: Wiley, 1980.

29. Knights, R. M., & Hinton, G. The Effects of Methylphenidate (Ritalin) on the Motor Skills and Behavior of Children with Learning Problems. *Journal of Nervous and Mental Disease*, 148: 643–653, 1969.

30. Satterfield, J. H., Cantwell, D. P., Saul, R. E., & Usin, A. Intelligence, Academic Achievement, and EEG Abnormalities in Hyperactive Children. *American Journal of Psychiatry*, 133: 391–395, 1974.

31. Grünewald-Zuberbier, E., Grünewald, G., & Rasche, A. Hyperactive Behaviour and EEG Arousal Reactions in Children. *Electroencephalography and Clinical Neurophysiology*, 38: 149–159, 1975.

32. Shetty, T. Some Neurologic Electrophysiologic and Biochemical Correlates of the Hyperkinetic Syndrome. *Pediatric Annals*, 29: 29–38, 1973.

33. Satterfield, J. H. EEG Issues in Children with Minimal Brain Dysfunction. *Seminars in Psychiatry*, 5: 35–46, 1973.

34. Buchsbaum, M., & Wender, P. H. Average Evoked Response in Normal and Minimally Brain Dysfunctioned Children Treated with Amphetamine: A Preliminary Report. *Archives of General Psychiatry*, 29: 764–770, 1973.

35. Hall, R. A., Griffin, R. B., Moyer, D. L., Hopkins, K. H., & Rapoport, J. L. Evoked Potential, Stimulus Intensity, and Drug Treatment in Hyperkinesis. *Psychophysiology*, 13: 405–418, 1976.

36. Milstein, V., Stevens, J., & Sachdev, K. Habituation of the Alpha Attenuation Response in Children and Adults with Psychiatric Disorders. *Electroencephalography, and Clinical Neurophysiology*, 26: 12–18, 1969.

37. Fuller, P. W. Computer Estimated Alpha Attenuation during Problem Solving in Children with Learning Disabilities. *Electroencephalography and Clinical Neurophysiology*, 42: 148–156, 1977.

38. Quinn, P., & Rapoport, J. Minor Physical Anomalies and Neurologic Status in Hyperactive Boys. *Pediatrics*, 53: 742–747, 1974.

39. Shetty, T. Alpha Rhythms in the Hyperkinetic Child. *Nature*, 234: 476, 1971.

40. Greenhill, L. L., Puig-Antich, J., Sassin, J., & Sachar, E. J. Hormone and Growth Response in Hyperkinetic Children on Stimulant Medication. *Psychopharmacology Bulletin*, 13: 33–36, 1977.

41. Nahas, A. D., & Krynicki, V. Effect of Methylphenidate on Sleep Stages and Ultradiam Rhythms in Hyperactive Children. *Journal of Nervous and Mental Disease*, 164: 66–69, 1977.

42. Oettinger, L., Majovski, L. V., Limbeck, G. A., & Gouch, R. Bone Age in Children with Minimal Brain Dysfunction. *Perceptual and Motor Skills*, 39: 1127–1131, 1974.

43. Roche, A. F., Lipman, R. S., Overall, J. E., & Hung, W. The Effects of Stimulant Medication on the Growth of Hyperkinetic Children. *Pediatrics*, 63: 847–851, 1979.

44. Safer, D. J., Allen, R. P., & Barr, E. Depression of Growth in Hyperactive Children on Stimulant Drugs. *New England Journal of Medicine*, 287: 217–220, 1972.

45. Safer, D. J., & Allen, R. P. Factors Influencing the Suppressant Effects of Two Stimulant Drugs on the Growth of Hyperactive Children. *Pediatrics*, 51: 660–667, 1973.

46. Safer, D. J., Allen, R. P., & Barr, E. Growth Rebound after Termination of Stimulant Drugs. *Journal of Pediatrics*, 86: 113–116, 1975.

47. Weiss, G., Kruger, E., Danielson, U., & Elman, M. Effects of Long-Term Treatment of Hyperactive Children with Methylphenidate. *Canadian Medical Association Journal*, 112: 159–165, 1975.

48. Quinn, P. O., & Rapoport, J. L. One-Year Follow-Up of Hyperactive Boys Treated with Imipramine or Methylphenidate. *American Journal of Psychiatry*, 132: 241–245, 1975.

49. Puig-Antich, J., Greenhill, L. L., Sassin, J., & Sachar, E. J. Growth Hormone, Prolactin, and Cortisol Responses and Growth Patterns in Hyperkinetic Children Treated with Dextroamphetamine. *Journal of the American Academy of Child Psychiatry*, 17: 457–475, 1978.

50. Mattes, J. M., & Gittelman, R. Growth of Hyperactive Children on Maintenance Regimen of Methylphenidate. *Archives of General Psychiatry*, 40: 317–321, 1983.

51. McNutt, B. A., Boileau, R. A., & Cohen, M. The Effects of Long-Term Stimulant Medication on the Growth and Body Composition of Hyperactive Children. *Psychopharmacology Bulletin*, 13: 36–38, 1977.

52. Eisenberg, L. The Hyperkinetic Child and Stimulant Drugs. *New England Journal of Medicine*, 287: 249–250, 1972.

53. Gross, M. D. Growth of Hyperkinetic Children Taking Methylphenidate, Dextroamphetamine, or Imipramine/Desipramine. *Pediatrics*, 58: 423–431, 1976.

54. Millichap, J. G., & Millichap, M. Growth of Hyperactive Children [Letter to the editor]. *New England Journal of Medicine*, 292: 1300, 1975.

55. Satterfield, J. H., Cantwell, D. P., Schell, A., & Blaschke, T. Growth of Hyperactive Children Treated with Methylphenidate. *Archives of General Psychiatry*, 36: 212–217, 1979.

56. Friedmann, N., Thomas, J., Carr, R., Elders, J., Ringdahl, I., & Roche, A. Effect on Growth in Pemoline-Treated Children with Attention Deficit Disorder. *American Journal of Diseases of Children*, 135: 329–332, 1981.

57. Beck, L., Langford, W. S., MacKay, M., & Sum, G. Childhood Chemotherapy and Later Drug Abuse and Growth Curve: A Follow-Up Study of 30 Adolescents. *American Journal of Psychiatry*, 132: 436–438, 1975.

58. Loney, J., Whaley-Klahn, M. A., Boles Ponto, L., & Adney, K. Predictions of Adolescent Height and Weight in Hyperkinetic Boys Treated with Methlyphenidate. *Psychopharmacology Bulletin*, 17: 132–134, 1981.

59. Shaywitz, S. E., Hunt, R. D., Jatlow, P., Cohen, D., Young, J. G., Pierce, R., Andersen, G. M., Bennett, A., & Shaywitz, B. A. Psychopharmacology of Attention Deficit Disorder: Pharmacokinetic, Neuroendocrine and Behavioral Measures Following Acute and Chronic Treatment with Methylphenidate. *Pediatrics*, 69: 688–694, 1982.

60. Aarskog, D., Fevang, F. O., Kløve, H., Stda, K. F., & Thorsen, T. The Effect of the Stimulant Drugs Dextroamphetimine and Methylphenidate on Secretion of Growth Hormone in Hyperactive Children. *Journal of Pediatrics*, 90: 136–139, 1977.

61. Hechtman, L., Weiss, G., & Perlman, T. Growth and Cardiovascular Measures in Hyperactive Individuals as Young Adults and in Matched Normal Controls. *Canadian Medical Association Journal*, 118: 1247–1250, 1978.

62. Hechtman, L., Weiss, G., & Perlman, T. Young Adult Outcome of Hyperactive Children Who Received Long-Term Stimulant Treatment. *Journal of the American Academy of Child Psychiatry*, 23: 261–270, 1984.

63. Hechtman, L., Weiss, G., & Metrakos, K. Hyperactive Individuals as Young Adults: Current and Longitudinal Electroencephalographic Evaluation and Its Relationship to Outcome. *Canadian Medical Association Journal*, 118: 919–923, 1978.

64. Stevens, J. R., Sachdev, K., & Milstein, V. Behavior Disorders of Childhood and the Electroencephalogram. *Archives of Neurology,* 18: 160–177, 1968.

65. Hughes, J. R. Electroencephalography and Learning Disabilities. In H. R. Myklebust (Ed.), *Progress in Learning Disabilities* (Vol. 2). New York: Grune & Stratton, 1971.

CHAPTER 12

1. Borland, B. L., & Heckman, H. K. Hyperactive Boys and Their Brothers: A 25-Year Follow-Up Study. *Archives of General Psychiatry,* 33: 669–675, 1976.

2. Feldman, S., Denhoff, E., & Denhoff, J. The Attention Disorders and Related Syndromes: Outcome in Adolescence and Young Adult Life. In L. Stern & E. Denhoff (Eds.), *Minimal Brain Dysfunction: A Developmental Approach.* New York: Masson Publishing (USA), 1979.

3. Loney, J., Whaley-Klahn, M. A., Kosier, T., & Conboy, J. *Hyperactive Boys and Their Brothers at 21: Predictions of Aggressive and Antisocial Outcomes.* Paper presented at a meeting of the Society for Life History Research, Monterey, CA, November 1981.

4. Abelson, H., & Fishburne, P. *National Survey on Drug Abuse* (Vol. 2, Methodology). Rockville, MD: National Institute on Drug Abuse, 1977.

5. Welner, Z., Welner, A., Stewart, M. A., Palkes, H., & Wish, E. A Controlled Study of Siblings of Hyperactive Children. *Journal of Nervous and Mental Disease,* 165: 110–117, 1977.

6. Lopez, R. E. Hyperactivity in Twins. *Canadian Psychiatric Association Journal,* 10: 421–426, 1965.

7. Safer, D. J. A Familial Factor in Minimal Brain Dysfunction. *Behavior Genetics,* 3: 175–186, 1973.

8. Battle, E. S., & Lacey, B. A Context For Hyperactivity in Children, Over Time. *Child Development,* 43: 757–773, 1972.

9. Bettelheim, B. Bringing Up Children. *Ladies' Home Journal,* p. 28, 1973.

10. Bell, R. Q., & Harper, L. V. *Child Effects on Adults.* Hillsdale, NJ: Erlbaum, 1977.

11. Campbell, S. B. Mother–Child Interaction in Reflective, Impulsive, and Hyperactive Children. *Developmental Psychology,* 8: 341–349, 1973.

12. Campbell, S. B. Mother–Child Interaction: A Comparison of Hyperactive, Learning Disabled, and Normal Boys. *American Journal of Orthopsychiatry,* 45: 51–57, 1975.

13. Humphries, T., Kinsbourne, M., & Swanson, J. Stimulant Effects on Cooperation and Social Interaction between Hyperactive Children and Their Mothers. *Journal of Child Psychology and Psychiatry,* 19: 13–22, 1978.

14. Cunningham, C. E., & Barkley, R. A. The Interactions of Normal and Hyperactive Children and Their Mothers in Free Play and Structured Tasks. *Child Development,* 50: 217–224, 1979.

15. Mash, E. J., & Johnston, C. A Comparison of The Mother–Child Interactions of Younger and Older Hyperactive and Normal Children. *Child Development,* 53: 1371–1381, 1982.

16. Barkley, R. A., & Cunningham, C. E. The Parent–Child Interactions of Hyperactive Children and Their Modification by Stimulant Drugs. In R. Knights & D. Bakker (Eds.), *Treatment of Hyperactive and Learning Disabled Children.* Baltimore: University Park Press, 1980.

17. Mash, E. J., & Johnston, C. A Behavioral Assessment of Sibling Interactions in Hyperactive and Normal Children. Unpublished manuscript, University of Calgary (Canada), 1981.

18. Tallmadge, J., & Barkley, R. A. The Interactions of Hyperactive and Normal Boys with Their Fathers and Mothers. *Journal of Abnormal Child Psychology*, 11: 565–579, 1983.

19. Mash, E. J., & Johnston, C. Parental Perceptions of Child Behavior Problems, Parenting, Self-esteem and Mothers' Reported Stress in Younger and Older Hyperactives and Normal Children. *Journal of Consulting and Clinical Psychology*, 51: 86–99, 1983.

20. Morrison, J. R., & Stewart, M. A. A Family Study of the Hyperactive Child Syndrome. *Biological Psychiatry*, 3: 189–195, 1971.

21. Cantwell, D. P. Psychiatric Illness in the Families of Hyperactive Children. *Archives of General Psychiatry*, 27: 414–417, 1972.

22. Cantwell, D. P. Genetics of Hyperactivity. *Journal of Child Psychology and Psychiatry*, 16: 261–264, 1975.

23. Morrison, J. R., & Stewart, M. A. The Psychiatric Status of the Legal Families of Adopted Hyperactives. *Archives of General Psychiatry*, 3: 888–891, 1973.

24. Morrison, J. R., & Stewart, M. A. Evidence for Polygenetic Inheritance in the Hyperactive Child Syndrome. *American Journal of Psychiatry*, 130: 791–792, 1973.

25. Morrison, J. R., & Stewart, M. A. Bilateral Inheritance as Evidence for Polygenicity in the Hyperactive Child Syndrome. *Journal of Nervous and Mental Disease*, 158: 226–228, 1974.

26. Goodwin, D. W., Schulsinger, F., Hermansen, L., Guze, S. B., & Winokur, G. Alcoholism and the Hyperactive Child Syndrome. *Journal of Nervous and Mental Disease*, 160: 349–353, 1975.

27. Stewart, M. A., & Morrison, J. R. Affective Disorder among the Relatives of Hyperactive Children. *Journal of Child Psychology and Psychiatry*, 14: 209–212, 1973.

28. Stewart, M. A., de Blois, C. S., & Cummings, C. Psychiatric Disorder in the Parents of Hyperactive Boys and Those with Conduct Disorder. *Journal of Child Psychology and Psychiatry*, 21: 283–292, 1980.

29. Stewart, M. A., & Leone, L. A Family Study of Unsocialized–Aggressive Boys. *Biological Psychiatry*, 13: 10-7–118, 1978.

30. Stewart, M. A., de Blois, C. S., & Singer, S. Alcoholism and Hyperactivity Revisited In M. Gallanter (Ed.), *Biomedical Issues and Clinical Effects of Alcoholism* (Vol. 5). New York: Grune & Stratton, 1979.

31. Morrison, J. R. Adult Psychiatric Disorders in Parents of Hyperactive Children. *American Journal of Psychiatry*, 137: 825–827, 1980.

32. McMahon, R. F. Genetic Etiology in the Hyperactive Child Syndrome: A Critical Review. *American Journal of Orthopsychiatry*. 50: 145–149, 1980.

33. Hechtman, L. Families of Hyperactives. In J. Greenley (Ed.), *Research in Community and Mental Health* (Vol. 2). Greenwich, CT: JAI Press, 1981.

34. Hechtman, L., Weiss, G., Finkelstein, J., Wener, A., & Benn, R. Hyperactives as Young Adults: Preliminary Report. *Canadian Medical Association Journal*, 115: 625–630, 1976.

35. Menkes, M. M., Rowe, J., & Menkes, J. A Twenty-Five-Year Follow-Up Study on the Hyperactive Child with Minimal Brain Dysfunction. *Pediatrics*, 29: 393–399, 1967.

36. Hogarty, G. E., & Katz, M. M. Norms of Adjustment and Social Behavior. *Archives of General Psychiatry*, 25: 470–480, 1971.

37. Kelman, H. R. The Effect of the Brain-Damaged Child on the Family. In H. C. Birch (Ed.), *Brain Damage in Children: The Biological and Social Aspect*. Baltimore: William and Wilkins, 1964.

38. Delamater, A. M., Lahey, B. B., & Drake, L. Toward an Empirical Subclassification of "Learning Disabilities": A Psychophysiological Comparison of "Hyperactive" and "Non-Hyperactive" Subgroups. *Journal of Abnormal Child Psychology*, 9: 65–77, 1981.

39. Ackerman, P. T., Elardo, P. T., & Dykman, R. A. A Psychosocial Study of Hyperactive and Learning Disabled Boys. *Journal of Abnormal Child Psychology,* 7: 91–100, 1979.

40. Cohen, N. J., & Minde, K. The "Hyperactive Syndrome" in Kindergarten Children: Comparison of Children with Pervasive and Situational Syndromes. *Journal of Child Psychology and Psychiatry,* 24: 443–456, 1983.

41. Langhorne, J. E., Loney, J., Paternite, C. E., & Bechtoldt, H. P. Childhood Hyperkinesis: A Return to Source. *Journal of Abnormal Psychology,* 85: 201–209, 1976.

CHAPTER 13

1. Hechtman, L., Weiss, G., Perlman, T., & Tuck, D. Hyperactives as Young Adults: Various Clinical Outcomes. *Adolescent Psychiatry,* 9: 295–306, 1981.

CHAPTER 14

1. Loney, J., Kramer, J., & Milich, R. The Hyperactive Child Grows Up: Predictors of Symptoms, Delinquency and Achievement at Follow-Up. In K. Gadow & J. Loney (Eds.), *Psychosocial Aspects of Drug Treatment for Hyperactivity.* Boulder, CO: Westview Press, 1981.

2. Hechtman, L., Weiss, G., Perlman, T., & Amsel, R. Hyperactives as Young Adults: Initial Predictors of Adult Outcome. *Journal of the American Academy of Child Psychiatry,* 23: 250–261, 1984.

3. Riddle, K. D., & Rapoport, J. L. A 2-Year Follow-Up of 72 Hyperactive Boys. *Journal of Nervous and Mental Disease,* 162: 126–134, 1976.

4. Ackerman, P. T., Dykman, R. A., & Peters, J. E. Teenage Status of Hyperactive and Non-Hyperactive Learning Disabled Boys. *American Journal of Orthopsychiatry,* 47: 577–596, 1977.

5. Milman, D. H. Minimal Brain Dysfunction in Childhood: Outcome in Late Adolescence and Early Adult Years. *Journal of Clinical Psychiatry,* 40: 371–380, 1979.

6. Menkes, M. M., Rowe, J. S., & Menkes, J. H. A Twenty-Five-Year Follow-Up Study on the Hyperkinetic Child with Minimal Brain Dysfunction. *Pediatrics,* 39: 393–399, 1967.

7. Satterfield, J. The Hyperactive Child Syndrome: A Precursor of Adult Psychopathy. In R. Hare & D. Schalling (Eds.), *Psychopathic Behavior Approaches to Research.* Chichester, England: Wiley, 1976.

8. Weiss, G., Minde, K., Werry, J. S., Douglas, V. I., & Nemeth, E. Studies on the Hyperactive Child VIII: Five-Year Follow-Up. *Archives of General Psychiatry,* 24: 409–414, 1971.

9. Zambelli, A. J., Stamm, J. S., Maitinsky, S., & Loiselle, D. L. Auditory Evoked Potentials and Selective Attention in Formerly Hyperactive Adolescent Boys. *American Journal of Psychiatry,* 134: 742–747, 1977.

10. White, J., Barratt, E., & Adams, P. The Hyperactive Child in Adolescence: A Comparative Study of Physiological and Behavioral Patterns. *Journal of the American Academy of Child Psychiatry,* 18: 154–169, 1979.

11. Hechtman, L., Weiss, G., & Metrakos, K. Hyperactive Individuals as Young Adults: Current and Longitudinal Electroencephalographic Evaluation and Its Relation to Outcome. *Canadian Medical Association Journal,* 118: 919–923, 1978.

12. Mendelson, W. B., Johnson, N. E., & Stewart, M. A. Hyperactive Children as Teenagers: A Follow-Up Study. *Journal of Nervous and Mental Disease,* 153: 273–279, 1971.

13. Minde, K. K., Lewin, D., Weiss, G., Lavigueur, H., Douglas, V., & Sykes, E. The Hyperactive Child in Elementary School: A 5-Year Controlled Follow-Up. *Exceptional Children,* 38: 215–221, 1971.

14. Minde, K. K., Weiss, G., & Mendelson, N. A Five-Year Follow-Up of 91 Hyperactive School Children. *Journal of the American Academy of Child Psychiatry,* 11: 595–610, 1972.

15. Loney, J., Whaley-Klahn, M. A., Kosier, T., & Conboy, J. *Hyperactive Boys and Their Brothers at 21: Predictors of Aggressive and Antisocial Outcomes.* Paper presented at a meeting of the Society for Life History Research, Monterey, CA, November 1981.

16. Endicott, J., & Spitzer, R. L. A Diagnostic Interview: The Schedule for Affective Disorders and Schizophrenia. *Archives of General Psychiatry,* 35: 837–844, 1978.

17. Langhorne, J. E., & Loney, J. A Four-Fold Model For Subgrouping the Hyperkinetic/MBD Syndrome. *Child Psychiatry and Human Development,* 9: 153–159, 1979.

18. Kramer, J., & Loney, J. *Predicting Adolescent Antisocial Behavior among Hyperactive Boys.* Paper presented at the Annual Meeting of the American Psychological Association, Toronto, August 1978.

19. Robins, L. N. Sturdy Childhood Predictors of Adult Outcomes: Replications from Longitudinal Studies. *Psychological Medicine,* 8: 611–622, 1978.

20. Kramer, J., Loney, J., & Whaley-Klahn, M. A. *The Iowa Crime and Punishment Survey (CAPS).* Unpublished survey, University of Iowa, 1978.

21. Abelson, H., & Fishburne, P. *National Survey on Drug Abuse,* 1977 (Vol. 2, *Methodology*). Rockville, MD: National Institute on Drug Abuse, 1977.

CHAPTER 15

1. Morrison, J. R., & Stewart, M. A. A Family Study of the Hyperactive Child Syndrome. *Biological Psychiatry,* 3: 189–195, 1971.

2. Cantwell, D. P. Psychiatric Illness in the Families of Hyperactive Children. *Archives of General Psychiatry,* 27: 414–417, 1972.

3. Stewart, M. A., de Blois, C. S., & Singer, S. Alcoholism and Hyperactivity Revisited. In M. Gallanter (Ed.), *Biomedical Issues and Clinical Effects of Alcoholism* (Vol. 5). New York: Grune & Stratton, 1979.

4. Mendelson, W. B., Johnson, N. E., & Stewart, M. A. Hyperactive Children as Teenagers: A Follow-Up Study. *Journal of Nervous and Mental Disease,* 153: 273–279, 1971.

5. Weiss, G., Minde, K., Werry, J. S., Douglas, V. I., & Nemeth, E. Studies on the Hyperactive Child VIII: Five-Year Follow-Up. *Archives of General Psychiatry,* 24: 409–414, 1971.

6. Minde, K. K., Weiss, G., & Mendelson, N. A 5-Year Follow-Up Study of 91 Hyperactive School Children. *Journal of the American Academy of Child Psychiatry,* 11: 595–610, 1972.

7. Loney, J., Whaley-Klahn, M. A., Kosier, T., & Conboy, J. *Hyperactive Boys and Their Brothers at 21: Predictors of Aggressive and Antisocial Outcomes.* Paper presented at a meeting of the Society for Life History Research, Monterey, CA, November 1981.

8. Endicott, J., & Spitzer, R. L. A Diagnostic Interview: The Schedule for Affective Disorders and Schizophrenia. *Archives of General Psychiatry,* 35: 847–844, 1978.

9. Kramer, J., Loney, J., & Whaley-Klahn, M. A. *The Iowa Crime and Punishment Survey (CAPS).* Unpublished survey, University of Iowa, 1978.

10. Abelson, H., & Fishburne, P. *National Survey on Drug Abuse,* 1977 (Vol. 2, *Methodology*). Rockville, MD: National Institute on Drug Abuse, 1977.

11. Battle, E. S., & Lacey, B. A Context For Hyperactivity in Children, Over Time. *Child Development,* 43: 757–773, 1972.

12. Campbell, S. B. Mother–Child Interaction in Reflective, Impulsive, and Hyperactive Children. *Developmental Psychology,* 8: 341–349, 1973.

13. Campbell, S. B. Mother–Child Interaction: A Comparison of Hyperactive, Learning Disabled, and Normal Boys. *American Journal of Orthopsychiatry,* 45: 51–57, 1975.

14. Humphries, T., Kinsbourne, M., & Swanson, J. Stimulant Effects on Cooperation and Social Interaction between Hyperactive Children and Their Mothers. *Journal of Child Psychology and Psychiatry,* 19: 13–22, 1978.

15. Barkley, R. A., & Cunningham, C. E. The Parent–Child Interactions of Hyperactive Children and Their Modification by Stimulant Drugs. In R. Knights & D. Bakker (Eds.), *Treatment of Hyperactive and Learning Disabled Children.* Baltimore: University Park Press, 1980.

16. Loney, J., Kramer, J., & Milich, R. The Hyperkinetic Child Grows Up: Predictors of Symptoms, Delinquency, and Achievement at Follow-Up. In K. D. Gadow & J. Loney (Eds.), *Psychosocial Aspects of Drug Treatment for Hyperactivity.* Boulder, CO: Westview Press, 1981.

17. Loney, J., Langhorne, J. E., Paternite, C. E., Whaley-Klahn, M. A., Blair-Broeker, C. T., & Hacker, M. *The Iowa HABIT: Hyperactive/Aggressive Boys in Treatment.* Paper presented at a meeting of the Society for Life History Research in Psychopathology, Fort Worth, TX, October 1976.

18. Werner, E. E., & Smith, R. S. *Kauai's Children Come of Age.* Honolulu: University of Hawaii Press, 1977.

19. Paternite, C. E., Loney, J., & Langhorne, J. E. Relationships between Symptomatology and SES-Related Factors in Hyperkinetic/MBD Boys. *American Journal of Orthopsychiatry,* 46: 291–301, 1976.

20. Milman, D. H. Minimal Brain Dysfunction in Childhood: Outcome in Late Adolescence and Early Adult Years. *Journal of Clinical Psychiatry,* 40: 371–380, 1979.

21. Huessy, H. R., Metoyer, M., & Townsend, M. 8–10 Year Follow-Up of 84 Children Treated for Behavioral Disorder in Rural Vermont. *Acta Paedopsychiatrica,* 40: 230–235, 1974.

22. Mellsop, G. W. Psychiatric Patients Seen as Children and Adults: Childhood Predictors of Adult Illness. *Journal of Child Psychology and Psychiatry,* 13: 91–101, 1972.

23. Robins, L. N. Sturdy Childhood Predictors of Adult Outcomes: Replications from Longitudinal Studies. *Psychological Medicine,* 8: 611–622, 1978.

24. Satterfield, J. H., Hoppe, C. M., & Schell, A. M. A Prospective Study of Delinquency in 110 Adolescent Boys with Attention Deficit Disorder and 88 Normal Adolescent Boys. *American Journal of Psychiatry,* 139: 795–798, 1982.

25. Weiss, G., Kruger, E., Danielson, U., & Elman, M. Effects of Long-Term Treatment of Hyperactive Children with Methylphenidate. *Canadian Medical Association Journal,* 112: 159–165, 1975.

26. Conrad, W. G., & Insel, J. Anticipating the Response to Amphetamine Therapy in the Treatment of Hyperkinetic Children. *Pediatrics,* 40: 9–98, 1967.

27. Loney, J., Comly, H. H., & Simon, B. Parental Management, Self-Concept, and Drug Response in Minimal Brain Dysfunction. *Journal of Learning Disabilities,* 8: 187–190, 1975.

28. Menkes, M., Rowe, J. S., & Menkes, J. H. A Twenty-Five-Year Follow-Up Study on the Hyperkinetic Child with Minimal Brain Dysfunction. *Pediatrics,* 39: 393–399, 1967.

29. Chess, S., Thomas, A., Korn, S., Mittelman, M., & Cohen, J. Early Parental

Attitudes, Divorce and Separation, and Young Adult Outcome: Findings of a Longitudinal Study. *Journal of the American Academy of Child Psychiatry,* 22: 47–51, 1983.

CHAPTER 16

1. Mendelson, W. B., Johnson, N. E., & Stewart, M. A. Hyperactive Children as Teenagers: A Follow-Up Study. *Journal of Nervous and Mental Disease,* 153: 273–279, 1971.

2. Minde, K. K., Weiss, G., & Mendelson, N. A 5-Year Follow-Up Study of 91 Hyperactive School Children. *Journal of the American Academy of Child Psychiatry,* 11: 595–610, 1972.

3. Peterson, D. R., & Quay, H. C. *Factor Analyzed Problem Checklist.* Urbana: University of Illinois, Children's Research Center, 1967.

4. Ackerman, P. T., Dykman, R. A., & Peters, J. E. Teenage Status of Hyperactive and Non-Hyperactive Learning Disabled Boys. *American Journal of Orthopsychiatry,* 47: 577–596, 1977.

5. Helper, M. M. Follow-Up of Children with Minimal Brain Dysfunctions: Outcomes and Predictors. In H. E. Rie & E. D. Rie (Eds.), *Handbook of Minimal Brain Dysfunction: A Critical Review.* New York: Wiley, 1980.

6. Menkes, M. M., Rowe, J. S., & Menkes, J. H. A Twenty-Five-Year Follow-Up Study on the Hyperactive Child with Minimal Brain Dysfunction. *Pediatrics,* 39: 393–399, 1967.

7. Weiss, G., Kruger, E., Danielson, U., & Elman, M. Effects of Long-Term Treatment of Hyperactive Children with Methylphenidate. *Canadian Medical Association Journal,* 112: 159–165, 1975.

8. Garfinkle, B. D., Wender, P. H., Sloman, L., & O'Neill, I. Tricyclic Antidepressant and Methylphenidate Treatment of Attention Deficit Disorder in Children. *Journal of the American Academy of Child Psychiatry,* 22: 343–348, 1983.

9. Conrad, W. G., & Insel, J. Anticipating the Response to Amphetamine Therapy in the Treatment of Hyperkinetic Children. *Pediatrics,* 40: 96–98, 1967.

10. Loney, J., Comly, H. H., & Simon, B. Parental Management, Self-Concept, and Drug Response in Minimal Brain Dysfunction. *Journal of Learning Disabilities,* 8: 187–190, 1975.

11. Loney, J., Kramer, J., & Milich, R. The Hyperkinetic Child Grows Up: Predictors of Symptoms, Delinquency, and Achievement at Follow-Up. In K. D. Gadow & J. Loney (Eds.), *Psychosocial Aspects of Drug Treatment for Hyperactivity.* Boulder, CO: Westview Press, 1981.

12. Riddle, K. D., & Rapoport, J. L. A 2-Year Follow-Up of 72 Hyperactive Boys. *Journal of Nervous and Mental Disease,* 162: 126–134, 1976.

13. Blouin, A. G. A., Bornstein, R., & Trites, R. Teen-Age Alcohol Use among Hyperactive Children: A 5-Year Follow-Up Study. *Journal of Pediatric Psychology,* 3: 188–194, 1978.

14. Charles, L., & Stein, R. A Four-Year Follow-Up Study of the Effects of Methylphenidate on the Behavior and Academic Achievement of Hyperactive Children. *Journal of Abnormal Child Psychology,* 9: 495–505, 1981.

15. Satterfield, J., Hoppe, C. M., & Schell, A. M. A Prospective Study of Delinquency in 110 Adolescent Boys with Attention Deficit Disorder and 88 Normal Adolescent Boys. *American Journal of Psychiatry,* 139: 797–798, 1982.

16. Satterfield, J. H., Satterfield, B. T., & Cantwell, D. P. Three-Year Multimodal Treatment Study of 100 Hyperactive Boys. *Journal of Pediatrics,* 98: 650–655, 1981.

17. Feldman, S., Denhoff, E., & Denhoff, J. The Attention Disorders and Related Syndromes: Outcome in Adolescence and Young Adult Life. In L. Stern & E. Denhoff (Eds.), *Minimal Brain Dysfunction: A Developmental Approach.* New York: Masson Publishing (USA), 1979.

18. Loney, J., Whaley-Klahn, M. A., Kosier, T., & Conboy, J. *Hyperactive Boys and Their Brothers at 21: Predictors of Aggressive and Antisocial Outcomes.* Paper presented at a meeting of the Society for Life History Research, Monterey, CA, November 1981.

19. Kagan, J., Rosman, B. L., Day, D., Albert, J., & Phillips, W. Information Processing in the Child: Significance of Analytic and Reflective Attitudes. *Psychological Monographs,* 78 (1, Whole No. 578), 1964.

20. Wilkin, H. A., Dyk, R. B., Goodenough, D. R., & Karp, S. A. *Psychological Differentiation.* New York: Wiley, 1962.

21. Stroop, J. R. Studies of Interference in Serial Verbal Reactions. *Journal of Experimental Psychology,* 18: 643–661, 1965.

22. Endicott, J., & Spitzer, R. L. A Diagnostic Interview: The Schedule for Affective Disorder and Schizophrenia. *Archives of General Psychiatry,* 35: 837–844, 1978.

23. Derogatis, L., Lipman, R., & Covi, L. SCL-90: An Outpatient Psychiatric Rating Scale. *Psychopharmacology Bulletin,* 9: 13–27, 1973.

24. Davidson, H., & Lang, G. Children's Perceptions of Their Teachers' Feelings Towards Them Related to Self-Perception, School Achievement and Behavior. *Journal of Experimental Education,* 29: 107–116, 1960.

25. Ziller, R. C., Hagey, J., Smith, M. D., & Long, B. Self-Esteem: A Self-Social Construct. *Journal of Consulting and Clinical Psychology,* 33: 84–95, 1969.

26. Hoy, E., Weiss, G., Minde, K., & Cohen, N. The Hyperactive Child at Adolescence: Emotional, Social and Cognitive Functioning. *Journal of Abnormal Child Psychology,* 6: 311–324, 1978.

27. Clark, K. W. *Evaluation of a Group Social Skills Training Program with Psychiatric Inpatients: Training Vietnam Veterans in Assertion, Heterosocial and Job Interview Skills.* Unpublished doctoral dissertation, University of Wisconsin, 1974.

28. Lord, I. M. Statistical Adjustment When Comparing Pre-Existing Groups. *Psychological Bulletin,* 72: 336–337, 1969.

29. Henker, B., Whalen, C. K., Bugental, D. B., & Barker, C. Licit and Illicit Drug Use Patterns in Stimulant Treated Children and Their Peers. In K. D. Gadow & J. Loney (Eds.), *Psychosocial Aspects of Drug Treatment for Hyperactivity.* Boulder, CO: Westview Press, 1981.

CHAPTER 17

1. Hechtman, L., Weiss, G., Perlman, T., & Amsel, R. Hyperactives as Young Adults: Initial Predictors of Adult Outcome. *Journal of the American Academy of Child Psychiatry,* 23: 250–261, 1984.

2. Cohen, J., & Cohen, P. *Applied Multiple Regression/Correlation Analysis for the Behavioral Sciences.* Hillsdale, NJ: Elbaum, 1975.

3. Overall, J. E., & Gorham, D. R. The Brief Psychiatric Rating Scale. *Psychological Reports,* 10: 799–812, 1962.

4. Milman, D. H. Minimal Brain Dysfunction in Childhood: Outcome in Late Adolescence and Early Adult Years. *Journal of Clinical Psychiatry,* 40: 371–380, 1979.

5. Loney, J., Kramer, J., & Milich, R. The Hyperkinetic Child Grows Up: Predictors of Symptoms, Delinquency and Achievement at Follow-Up. In K. D. Gadow &

J. Loney (Eds.), *Psychosocial Aspects of Drug Treatment for Hyperactivity.* Boulder, CO: Westview Press, 1981.

CHAPTER 18

1. Eisenberg, L., Conners, C. K., & Sharpe, L. A Controlled Study of the Differential Application of Outpatient Psychiatry Treatment for Children. *Japanese Journal of Child Psychiatry,* 6: 125–132, 1965.
2. Winnicott, D. W. Transitional Objects and Transitional Phenomena. *International Journal of Psycho-Analysis,* 34: 89–97, 1953.

CHAPTER 19

1. Gittelman, R. Hyperkinetic Syndrome: Treatment Issues and Principles. In M. Rutter (Ed.), *Developmental Neuropsychiatry.* New York: Guilford Press, 1983.
2. Weiss, G. Controversial Issues on the Pharmacotherapy of the Hyperactive Child. *Canadian Journal of Psychiatry,* 26: 385–392, 1981.
3. Rapoport, J. L., Buchsbaum, M. S., Zahn, T. P., Weingartner, H., Ludlow, C., & Mikkelsen, E. J. Dextroamphetamine: Cognitive and Behavioral Effects in Normal Prepubertal Boys. *Science,* 199: 560–563, 1978.
4. MacKay, M. C., Beck, L., & Taylor, R. Methylphenidate for Adolescents with Minimal Brain Dysfunction. *New York State Journal of Medicine,* 73: 550–554, 1973.
5. Safer, D. J., & Allen, R. P. Stimulant Drug Treatment of Hyperactive Adolescents. *Diseases of the Nervous System,* 36: 454–457, 1975.
6. Oettinger, L. General Discussion. *Annals of the New York Academy of Science,* 205: 345–348, 1973.
7. Gross, M. B., & Wilson, W. C. *Minimal Brain Dysfunction.* New York: Brunner/Mazel, 1974.
8. Varley, C. Effects of Methylphenidate in Adolescents with Attention Deficit Disorder. *Journal of the American Academy of Child Psychiatry,* 22: 351–354, 1983.
9. Coons, H. W., Klovman, R., & Borgstedt, A. D. Enhancing Effects of Methylphenidate on Sustained Attention and Event Related Potentials of Adolescents with Attention Deficit Disorders. *Psychophysiology,* 21(5): 573–574, 1984.
10. Gastfriend, D. R., Biederman, J., & Jellineck, M. S. Desipramine in the Treatment of Adolescents with Attention Deficit Disorder. *American Journal of Psychiatry,* 141: 906–908, 1984.
11. Arnold, L. E., Strobl, D., & Weisenberg, A. Hyperkinetic Adult: Study of the "Paradoxical" Amphetamine Response. *Journal of the American Medical Association,* 222: 693–694, 1972.
12. Huessy, H. R. The Adult Hyperkinetic [Letter to the editor]. *American Journal of Psychiatry,* 131: 724–725, 1974.
13. Huessy, H. R., Cohen, S. M., Blair, C. L., & Rood, P. Clinical Explorations in Adult Minimal Brain Dysfunction. In L. Bellak (Ed.), *Psychiatric Aspects of Minimal Brain Dysfunction in Adults.* New York: Grune & Stratton, 1979.
14. Gauthier, M. Stimulant Medications in Adults with Attention Deficit Disorder: A Review. *Canadian Journal of Psychiatry,* 29: 435–439, 1984.
15. Mann, H. B., & Greenspan, S. I. The Identification and Treatment of Adult Brain Dysfunction. *American Journal of Psychiatry,* 133: 1013–1017, 1976.

16. DeVeaugh-Geiss, J., & Joseph, A. Paradoxical Response to Amphetamine in a Hyperkinetic Adult. *Psychosomatics*, 21: 247, 251–252, 1980.

17. Wood, D. R., Reimherr, F. W., Wender, P. H., & Johnson, G. E. Diagnosis and Treatment of Minimal Brain Dysfunction in Adults. *Archives of General Psychiatry*, 33: 1453–1460, 1976.

18. Wender, P. H., Reimherr, F. W., & Wood, D. R. Attention Deficit Disorder (Minimal Brain Dysfunction) in Adults: A Replication Study of Diagnosis and Drug Treatment. *Archives of General Psychiatry*, 38: 449–456, 1980.

19. Spitzer, R., Endicott, J., & Robins, E. *Research Diagnostic Criteria for a Selected Group of Functional Disorders*. New York: Biometric Research, 1975.

20. Sprague, R. L., Cohen, M., & Werry, S. *Normative Data on the Conners Teacher Rating Scale and Abbreviated Scale* (Tech. Rep.). Urbana: University of Illinois, Children's Research Center, November 1974.

21. Mattes, J., Boswell, L., & Oliver, H. Methylphenidate Effects on Symptoms of Attention Deficit Disorder in Adults. *Archives of General Psychiatry*, 41: 1059–1067, 1984.

22. Mattes, J. Personal communication, 1984.

CHAPTER 22

1. Alberts-Corush, J., Firestone, P., & Goodman, J. T. Attention and Impulsivity Characteristics of the Biological and Adoptive Parents of Hyperactive and Normal Control Children. *American Journal of Orthopsychiatry*, 56: 413–423, 1986.

2. Anderson, J. C., Williams, S., McGee, R., *et al.* DSM-III Disorders in Pre-Adolescent Children: Prevalence in a Large Sample from the General Population. *Archives of General Psychiatry*, 44: 69, 1987.

3. August, G., & Garfinkel, B. D. Behavioral and Cognitive Subtypes of ADHD. *Journal of the American Academy of Child and Adolescent Psychiatry*, 28: 739–748, 1989.

4. Barkley, R. A., DuPaul, G. J., & McMurray, M. B. Comprehensive Evaluation of Attention Deficit Disorder with and without Hyperactivity as Defined by Research Criteria. *Journal of Consulting and Clinical Psychology*, 58: 775–789, 1990.

5. Barkley, R. A., DuPaul, G. J., & McMurray, M. B. Attention Deficit Disorder with and without Hyperactivity: Clinic Response to Three Dose Levels of Methylphenidate. *Pediatrics*, 87: 519–531, 1991.

6. Barkley, R. A., Fischer, M., Edelbrock, C. S., *et al.* The Adolescent Outcome of Hyperactive Children Diagnosed by Research Criteria: III. Mother–Child Interactions, Family Conflicts and Maternal Psychopathology. *Journal of Child Psychology and Psychiatry*, 32: 233–255, 1991.

7. Benson, F. Role of Frontal Dysfunction in Attention Deficit Hyperactivity Disorder. *Journal of Child Neurology*, 6(Supplement): S9–S12, 1991.

8. Biederman, J., Baldessarini, R. J., Wright, V., *et al.* A Double-Blind Placebo Controlled Study of Desipramine in the Treatment of Attention Deficit Disorder: I. Efficacy. *Journal of the American Academy of Child and Adolescent Psychiatry*, 28: 777, 1989.

9. Biederman, J., Baldessarini, R. J., Wright, V., *et al.* A Double-Blind Placebo Controlled Study of Desipramine in the Treatment of Attention Deficit Disorder: III. Lack of Impact of Comorbidity and Family History Factors on Clinical Response. *Journal of the American Academy of Child and Adolescent Psychiatry*, 32(1): 199–204, 1993.

10. Biederman, J., Faraone, S., Keenan, K., *et al.* Family Genetic and Psychosocial Risk Factors in DSM-III Attention Deficit Disorder. *Journal of the American Academy of Child and Adolescent Psychiatry*, 29: 526–533, 1990.

11. Biederman, J., Faraone, S. V., Keenan, K., *et al.* Further Evidence for

Family–Genetic Risk Factors in Attention Deficit Hyperactivity Disorders: Patterns of Comorbidity in Probands and Relatives in Psychiatrically and Pediatrically Referred Samples. *Archives of General Psychiatry*, 49(9): 728–738, 1992.

12. Biederman, J., Faraone, S. V., & Lapey, K. Comorbidity of Diagnosis in Attention Deficit Hyperactive Disorder, Attention Deficit Disorder. *Child and Adolescent Psychiatric Clinics of North America*, 2: 335–361, 1992.

13. Biederman, J., Munir, K., & Knee, B. A. Conduct and Oppositional Disorder in Clinically Referred Children with Attention Deficit Disorder: A Controlled Family Study. *Journal of the American Academy of Child and Adolescent Psychiatry*, 26: 724–727, 1987.

14. Biederman, J., Newcorn, J., & Sprich, S. E. Comorbidity of Attention Deficit Hyperactive Disorder (ADHD). *American Journal of Psychiatry*, 48: 567–577, 1991.

15. Bird, H. R., Camino, G., Rubic Stipic, M., *et al.* Estimates of Prevalence of Childhood Maladjustment in a Community Survey in Puerto Rico. *Archives of General Psychiatry*, 45: 1120, 1988.

16. Brown, G. L., Ebert, M. H., & Minichiello, M. D. Biochemical and Pharmacological Aspects of Attention Deficit Disorder. In L. M. Bloomingdale (Ed.), *Attention Deficit Disorder: Identification, Course and Treatment Rationale*. New York: Spectrum, 1985.

17. Cadoret, R. J., & Stewart, M. A. An Adoption Study of Attention Deficit Hyperactivity/Aggression and Their Relationship to Adult Antisocial Personality. *Comprehensive Psychiatry*, 32: 73–82, 1991.

18. Cantwell, D. Psychiatric Illness in Families of Hyperactive Children. *Archives of General Psychiatry*, 27: 414–423, 1972.

19. Carlson, C. L., Lahey, B. B., & Neeper, R. Direct Assessment of the Cognitive Correlates of Attention Deficit Disorder With and Without Hyperactivity. *Journal of Behavior Assessment and Psychopathology*, 8: 69–86, 1986.

20. Chelune, G. J., Ferguson, W., Koon, R., & Dickey, T. O. Frontal Lobe Disinhibition in Attention Deficit Disorder. *Child Psychiatry and Human Development*, 16: 221–234, 1986.

21. Comings, D. E., Comings, B. G., Mitleman, D., *et al.* The Dopamine D_2 Receptor Locus as a Modifying Gene in Neuropsychiatric Disorders. *Journal of the American Medical Association*, 266: 1793–1800, 1991.

22. Deutsch, C. K., Matthysse, S., Swanson, J. M., & Farkas, L. G. Genetic Latent Structure Analysis of Dysmorphology in Attention Deficit Disorder. *Journal of the American Academy of Child and Adolescent Psychiatry*, 29: 189–194, 1990.

23. Donnelly, M., Zametkin, A. J., Rapoport, J. L., *et al.* Treatment of Hyperactivity with Desipramine: Plasma Drug Concentration, Cardiovascular Effects, Plasma and Urinary Catecholamine Levels and Clinical Response. *Clinical Pharmacology and Therapeutics*, 39: 72–81, 1986.

24. Edelbrock, C., Costello, A., & Kessler, M. D. Empirical Corroboration of Attention Deficit Disorder. *Journal of the American Academy of Child Psychiatry*, 23: 285–290, 1984.

25. Edelbrock, C., Rende, R., Plomin, R., & Thompson, L. A. Genetic and Environmental Effects on Competence and Problem Behavior in Childhood and Early Adolescence. Manuscript submitted for publication.

26. Elia, J, Borcherding, B. G., Potter, W. Z., *et al.* Stimulant Drug Treatment of Hyperactivity: Biochemical Correlates. *Clinical Pharmacology and Therapeutics*, 48: 57–66, 1990.

27. Everett, J., Thomas, J., Cote, F., *et al.* Cognitive Effects of Psychostimulant Medication in Hyperactive Children. *Child Psychiatry and Human Development*, 22: 79–87, 1991.

28. Faraone, S. V., Biederman, J., Chen, W. J., *et al.* Segregation Analysis of

Attention Deficit Hyperactivity Disorder: Evidence for Single Gene Transmission. Manuscript submitted for publication.

29. Frank, G., & Ben Yun, Y. Toward a Clinical Subgrouping of Hyperactive and Non-Hyperactive Attention Deficit Disorder: Results of a Comprehensive Neurological and Neuropsychological Assessment. *Journal of Disabled Children*, 142: 153–155, 1988.

30. Garfinkel, B. D., Wender, P. H., Sloman, L., et al. Tricyclic Antidepressant and Methylphenidate Treatment of Attention Deficit Disordered Children. *Journal of the American Academy of Child and Adolescent Psychiatry*, 22: 343, 1983.

31. Gilger, J. W., Pennington, B. F., & DeFries, J. C. A Twin Study of the Etiology of Comorbidity: Attention Deficit Hyperactivity Disorder and Dyslexia. *Journal of the American Academy of Child and Adolescent Psychiatry*, 31(2): 343–348, 1992.

32. Gillis, J. J., Gilger, J. W., Pennington, B. F., & DeFries, J. C. Attention Deficit Disorder in Reading-Disabled Twins: Evidence for a Genetic Etiology. *Journal of Abnormal Child Psychology*, 20(3):303–315, 1992.

33. Gittelman, R., Mannuzza, S., Shenkar, R., & Bonagura, N. Hyperactive Boys Almost Grown Up: I. Psychiatric Status. *Archives of General Psychiatry*, 42: 937–947, 1985.

34. Goodman, R., & Stevenson, J. A Twin Study of Hyperactivity: II. The Aetiological Role of Genes, Family Relationship and Perinatal Adversity. *Journal of Child Psychology and Psychiatry*, 30: 691–709, 1989.

35. Gorenstein, E. E., Mammato, C. A., & Sandy, J. M. Performance of Inattentive–Overactive Children on Selected Measures of Prefrontal-Type Function. *Journal of Clinical Psychology*, 45: 619–632, 1989.

36. Hauser, P., Zametkin, A. J., Vitiello, B., et al. Attention Deficit Hyperactivity Disorder in 18 Kindreds with Generalized Resistance to Thyroid Hormone (Abstract). *American Society of Clinical Investigation Proceedings*, 1992.

37. Hechtman, L. T. Developmental Neurobiological and Psychosocial Aspects of Hyperactivity, Impulsivity and Attention. In M. Lewis (Ed.), *Child and Adolescent Psychiatry: A Comprehensive Textbook*. Baltimore: Williams & Wilkins, 1991.

38. Heffron, W. A., Martin, C. A., & Welsh, R. J. Attention Deficit Disorders in Three Pairs of Monozygotic Twins: A Case Report. *Journal of the American Academy of Child Psychiatry*, 23: 299–301, 1984.

39. Heilman, K. M., Voeller, K. S., & Nadeau, S. E. A Possible Pathophysiologic Substrate of Attention Deficit Hyperactivity Disorder. *Journal of Child Neurology*, 6(Supplement): S76–S81, 1991.

40. Herjanic, B., Campbell, J., & Reich, W. Development of a Structural Psychiatric Interview for Children: Agreement Between Child and Parent on Individual Symptoms. *Journal of Abnormal Child Psychology*, 10: 307–324, 1982.

41. Hunt, R. D., Cohen, D. J., Anderson, G., et al. Possible Changes in Noradrenergic Receptor Sensitivity Following Methylphenidate Treatment: Growth Hormone and MHPG Response to Clonidine Challenge in Children with Attention Deficit Disorder and Hyperactivity. *Life Sciences*, 35: 885–879, 1984.

42. Jensen, J. B., & Garfinkel, B. D. Neuroendocrine Aspects of Attention Deficit Hyperactivity Disorder. *Endocrinology and Metabolism Clinics of North America*, 17: 111–129, 1988.

43. King, C., & Young, R. Attention Deficit with and without Hyperactivity: Teacher and Peer Perceptions. *Journal of Abnormal Child Psychology*, 10: 463–496, 1982.

44. Lahey, B. B., Piacentini, J., McBurnett, M., et al. Psychopathology in the Parents of Children with Conduct Disorder and Hyperactivity. *Journal of the American Academy of Child and Adolescent Psychiatry*, 27: 163–170, 1988.

45. Lahey, B. B., Shaughnecy, E. A., Hynd, G. W., et al. Attention Deficit Disorder with and without Hyperactivity: Comparison of Behavior Characteristics of Clinic

Referred Children. *Journal of the American Academy of Child and Adolescent Psychiatry*, 26: 718–723, 1987.

46. Lahey, B. B., Shaughnecy, E. A., Strauss, C., & Frame, C. Are Attention Deficit Disorders with and without Hyperactivity Similar or Dissimilar Disorders? *Journal of the American Academy of Child Psychiatry*, 23: 302–309, 1984.

47. Levy, F., & Hay, D. *ADHD in Twins and Their Siblings*. Paper presented at the Society for Research in Child and Adolescent Psychopathology, Sarasota, FL, February 1992.

48. Lopez, R. E. Hyperactivity in Twins. *Canadian Psychiatric Association Journal*, 10: 421–426, 1965.

49. Lou, H. C., Henricksen, L., Bruhn, P., *et al*. Focal Cerebral Hypoperfusion in Children with Dysphasia and/or Attention Deficit Disorder. *Archives of Neurology*, 41: 825–829, 1984.

50. Lou, H. C., Henriksen, L., Bruhn, P., *et al*. Striatal Dysfunction in Attention Deficit and Hyperkinetic Disorder. *Archives of Neurology*, 46: 48–52, 1989.

51. Mauer, R. G., & Stewart, M. Attention Deficit Disorder Without Hyperactivity in a Child Psychiatry Clinic. *Journal of Clinical Psychiatry*, 41: 232–233, 1980.

52. McCraken, J. A Two Part Model of Stimulant Action on Attention Deficit Hyperactivity Disorder in Children. *Journal of Neuropsychiatry*, 3: 201–209, 1991.

53. Mirsky, A. Behavioral and Psychophysiological Markers of Disordered Attention. *Environmental Health Perspectives*, 74: 191–199, 1987.

54. Morrison, J. L. Adult Psychiatric Disorders in Parents of Hyperactive Children. *American Journal of Psychiatry*, 137: 825–827, 1980.

55. Morrison, J. L., & Stewart, M. A Family Study of the Hyperactive Child Syndrome. *Biological Psychiatry*, 3: 189–195, 1971.

56. Morrison, J. L., & Stewart, M. The Psychiatric Status of Legal Families of Adopted Hyperactives. *Archives of General Psychiatry*, 28: 888–891, 1973.

57. Morrison, J. L., & Stewart, M. Bilateral Inheritance as Evidence of Polygenicity in the Hyperactive Child Syndrome. *Journal of Nervous and Mental Disease*, 158: 226–228, 1974.

58. Munir, K., Biederman, J., & Knee, B. A. Psychiatric Comorbidity in Patients with Attention Deficit Disorder: A Controlled Study. *Journal of the American Academy of Child and Adolescent Psychiatry*, 26: 866–846, 1987.

59. Nasrallah, H. A., Loney, J., Olsen, S. C., *et al*. Cortical Atrophy in Young Adults with a History of Hyperactivity in Childhood. *Psychiatry Research*, 17: 241–246, 1986.

60. Nemzer, E. D., Arnold, L. E., Votolato, N. A., *et al*. Amino Acid Supplementation as Therapy for Attention Deficit Disorder. *Journal of the American Academy of Child and Adolescent Psychiatry*, 25: 509–513, 1986.

61. Omenn, G. S. Genetic Issues in the Syndrome of Minimal Brain Dysfunctions. *Seminars in Psychiatry*, 5: 5–17, 1973.

62. Pauls, D. L. Genetic Factors in the Expression of Attention-Deficit Hyperactivity Disorder. *Journal of Child and Adolescent Psychopharmacology*, 1: 353–360, 1991.

63. Pliszka, S. R. Effect of Anxiety on Cognition, Behavior and Stimulant Response in ADHD. *Journal of the American Academy of Child and Adolescent Psychiatry*, 28: 882–887, 1989.

64. Roeltgen, D., & Schneider, J. S. Chronic Low-Dose MPTP in Non-Human Primates: A Possible Model for Attention Deficit Disorder. *Journal of Child Neurology*, 6(Supplement): S82–S89, 1991.

65. Rubenstein, R. A., & Brown, R. T. An Evaluation of the Validity of the Diagnostic Category of Attention Deficit Disorder. *American Journal of Orthopsychiatry*, 54: 398–414, 1984.

66. Rutter, M., Korn, S., & Birch, H. G. Genetic and Environmental Factors in the Development of "Primary Reaction Patterns." *British Journal of Social and Clinical Psychology*, 2: 162–173, 1963.

67. Safer, D. J. A Familial Factor in Minimal Brain Dysfunction. *Behavior Genetics*, 3: 175–186, 1973.

68. Schneider, J. S., & Kovelowski, C. J. Chronic Exposure to Low Doses of MPTP: Cognitive Deficits in Motor Asymptomatic Monkeys. *Brain Research*, 519: 122–128, 1990.

69. Shaywitz, B. A., Cohen, D. J., & Bower, M. B. CSF Monoamine Metabolites in Children with Minimal Brain Dysfunction: Evidence for Alteration of Brain Dopamine. A Preliminary Report. *Journal of Pediatrics*, 90: 671–677, 1977.

70. Shaywitz, B. A., Shaywitz, S. E., Bryne, T., et al. Attention Deficit Disorder: Quantitative Analysis of CT. *Neurology*, 33: 1500–1503, 1983.

71. Shaywitz, B. A., Yager, R. D., & Klopper, J. H. Selective Brain Dopamine Depletion in Developing Rats. *Science*, 191: 305–308, 1976.

72. Stevenson, J. Evidence for a Genetic Etiology in Hyperactivity in Children. *Behavior Genetics*, 22(3): 337–343, 1992.

73. Szatmari, P., Offord, D. R., & Boyle, M. H. Ontario Child Health Study: Prevalence of Attention Deficit Disorder with Hyperactivity. *Journal of Child Psychology and Psychiatry*, 30: 219–230, 1989.

74. Tannock, R., Schachar, R. J., Carr, R. P., et al. Effects of Methylphenidate on Inhibitory Control in Hyperactive Children. *Journal of Abnormal Child Psychology*, 17: 473–491, 1989.

75. Torgensen, A. M., & Kringlen, E. Genetic Aspects of Temperamental Differences in Infants. *Journal of the American Academy of Child Psychiatry*, 17: 433–444, 1978.

76. Voeller, K. S. Toward a Neurobiologic Nosology of Attention Deficit Hyperactive Disorder. *Journal of Child Neurology*, 6(Supplement): S2–S8, 1991.

77. Weiss, G., Hechtman, L. T., Milroy, T., et al. Psychiatric Studies of Hyperactives as Adults: A Controlled Prospective 15 Year Follow-Up of 63 Hyperactive Children. *Journal of the American Academy of Child Psychiatry*, 24: 211, 1985.

78. Welner, Z., Welner, H., Stewart, M., et al. A Controlled Study of Siblings of Hyperactive Children. *Journal of Nervous and Mental Disease*, 165: 110–117, 1977.

79. Willerman, L. Activity Level and Hyperactivity in Twins. *Child Development*, 44: 286–293, 1973.

80. Zametkin, A. J., Nordahl, T. E., Gross, M., et al. Cerebral Glucose Metabolism in Adults with Hyperactivity of Childhood Onset. *New England Journal of Medicine*, 323: 1361–1366, 1990.

81. Zametkin, A. J., & Rapoport, J. L. The Pathophysiology of Attention Deficit Disorder with Hyperactivity: A Review. In B. B. Lahey & A. E. Kazdin (Eds.), *Advances in Clinical Child Psychology* (Vol. 9). New York: Plenum Press, 1986.

82. Zametkin, A. J., & Rapoport, J. L. Neurobiology of Attention Deficit Disorder with Hyperactivity: Where Have We Come in 50 Years? *Journal of the American Academy of Child and Adolescent Psychiatry*, 26: 676–686, 1987.

CHAPTER 23

1. Abikoff, H., Ganeles, D., Reiter, G., et al. Cognitive Training in Academically Deficient ADDH Boys Receiving Stimulant Medication. *Journal of Abnormal Child Psychology*, 16: 411–432, 1988.

2. Abikoff, H., & Gittelman, R. The Normalizing Effects of Methylphenidate on the Classroom Behavior of ADHD Children. *Journal of Abnormal Child Psychology*, 13: 33–44, 1985.

3. Aman, M. G., Marks, R. E., Turbott, S. H., *et al.* Clinical Effects of Methylphenidate and Thioridazine in Intellectually Subaverage Children. *Journal of the American Academy of Child and Adolescent Psychiatry*, 30: 246–256, 1991.

4. Aman, M. G., Marks, R. E., Turbott, S. H., *et al.* Methylphenidate and Thioridazine in the Treatment of Intellectually Subaverage Children: Effects on Cognitive–Motor Performance. *Journal of the American Academy of Child and Adolescent Psychiatry*, 30: 816–824, 1991.

5. Barkley, R. A. A Review of Stimulant Drug Research with Hyperactive Children. *Journal of Child Psychology and Psychiatry*, 18: 137–165, 1977.

6. Barkley, R. A., & Cunningham, C. E. The Effects of Methylphenidate on the Mother–Child Interactions of Hyperactive Children. *Archives of General Psychiatry*, 36: 201–208, 1979.

7. Barkley, R. A., Karlsson, J., Strzelecki, E., *et al.* Effects of Age and Ritalin Dosage on Mother–Child Interactions of Hyperactive Children. *Journal of Consulting and Clinical Psychology*, 52: 750–758, 1984.

8. Barkley, R. A., McMurray, M. B., Edelbrock, C. S., *et al.* The Response of Aggressive and Nonaggressive ADHD Children to Two Doses of Methylphenidate. *Journal of the American Academy of Child and Adolescent Psychiatry*, 28: 873–881, 1989.

9. Barkley, R. A., McMurray, M. B., Edelbrock, C. S., *et al.* Side Effects of Methylphenidate in Children with Attention Deficit Hyperactivity Disorder: A Systemic, Placebo-Controlled Evaluation. *Pediatrics*, 86: 184–192, 1990.

10. Barrickman, L., Noyes, R., Kuperman, S., *et al.* Treatment of ADHD with Fluoxetine: A Preliminary Trial. *Journal of the American Academy of Child and Adolescent Psychiatry*, 30: 762–767, 1991.

11. Bergman, A., Winters, L., & Cornblatt, B. Methylphenidate: Effects on Sustained Attention. In L. L. Greenhill & B. Osman (Eds.), *Ritalin: Theory and Patient Management.* New York: Mary Ann Leibert, 1991.

12. Biederman, J., Baldessarini, R. J., Wright, V., *et al.* A Double-Blind Placebo Controlled Study of Desipramine in the Treatment of ADD: I. Efficacy. *Journal of the American Academy of Child and Adolescent Psychiatry*, 28: 777–784, 1989.

13. Biederman, J., Baldessarini, R. J., Wright, V., *et al.* A Double-Blind Placebo Controlled Study of Desipramine in the Treatment of ADD: II. Serum Drug Levels and Cardiovascular Findings. *Journal of the American Academy of Child and Adolescent Psychiatry*, 28: 903–911, 1989.

14. Biederman, J., Newcorn, J., & Sprich, S. Comorbidity of Attention Deficit Hyperactivity Disorder with Conduct, Depressive, Anxiety and Other Disorders. *American Journal of Psychiatry*, 148: 564–577, 1991.

15. Birmaher, B. B., Greenhill, L. L., Cooper, M. A., *et al.* Sustained Release Methylphenidate: Pharmacokinetic Studies in ADDH Males. *Journal of the American Academy of Child and Adolescent Psychiatry*, 28: 768–772, 1989.

16. Borcherding, B. G., Keysor, C. S., Cooper, T. B., *et al.* Differential Effects of Methylphenidate and Dextroamphetamine on the Motor Activity Level of Hyperactive Children. *Neuropsychopharmacology*, 2: 255–263, 1989.

17. Bradley, C. The Behavior of Children Receiving Benzedrine. *American Journal of Psychiatry*, 94: 577–585, 1937.

18. Brown, R. T., Wynne, M. E., & Slimmer, L. W. Attention Deficit Disorder and the Effect of Methylphenidate on Attention, Behavioral, and Cardiovascular Functioning. *Journal of Clinical Psychiatry*, 45: 473–476, 1984.

19. Casat, C. D., Pleasants, D. Z., Schroeder, D. H., *et al.* Bupropion in Children with Attention Deficit Disorder. *Psychopharmacology Bulletin*, 25: 198–201, 1989.

20. Chan, Y. P., Swanson, J. M., Soldin, S. S., *et al.* Methylphenidate Hydrochloride

Given with or before Breakfast: II. Effects on Plasma Concentration of Methylphenidate and Ritalinic Acid. *Pediatrics*, 72: 56–59, 1983.

21. Clay, T. H., Gualtieri, C. T., Evans, R. W., *et al*. Clinical and Neuropsychological Effects of the Novel Antidepressant Bupropion. *Psychopharmacology Bulletin*, 24: 143–148, 1988.

22. Conners, C. K. A Teacher Rating Scale for Use in Drug Studies with Children. *American Journal of Psychiatry*, 126: 152–156, 1969.

23. Conners, C. K., Eisenberg, L., & Barcai, A. Effect of Dextroamphetamine on Children: Studies on Subjects with Learning Disabilities and School Behavior Problems. *Archives of General Psychiatry*, 17: 478–485, 1967.

23a. Denckla, M. B. Revised Physical and Neurological Examination for Subtle Signs. *Psychopharmacology Bulletin*, 21: 733–779, 1985.

24. Donnelly, M., Zametkin, A. J., Rapoport, J. L., *et al*. Treatment of Childhood Hyperactivity with Desipramine: Plasma Drug Concentration, Cardiovascular Effects, Plasma and Urinary Catecholamine Levels, and Clinical Response. *Clinical Pharmacology and Therapeutics*, 39: 72–81, 1986.

25. Douglas, V. I., Barr, R. G., O'Neill, M. E., *et al*. Short Term Effects of Methylphenidate on the Cognitive Learning and Academic Performance of Children with Attention Deficit Disorder in the Laboratory and Classroom. *Journal of Child Psychology and Psychiatry*, 27: 191–211, 1986.

26. Dulcan, M. Using Psychostimulants to Treat Behavior Disorders of Children and Adolescents. *Journal of Child and Adolescent Psychopharmacology*, 1: 7–20, 1990.

26a. Eisenberg, L., Lachman, R., Molling, P., *et al*. A Psychopharmacologic Experiment in a Training School for Deliquent Boys: Methods, Problems, and Findings. *American Journal of Orthopsychiatry*, 33: 431–447.

27. Elia, J., Borcherding, B. G., Rapoport, J. L., *et al*. Methylphenidate and Dextroamphetamine Treatment of Hyperactives: Are There True Nonresponders. *Psychiatry Research*, 36: 141–155, 1991.

28. Famularo, R., & Fenton, T. The Effect of Methylphenidate on School Grades in Children with Attention Deficit Disorder without Hyperactivity: A Preliminary Study. *Journal of Clinical Psychiatry*, 48: 112–114, 1987.

29. Feldman, H., Crumrine, P., & Handen, B. L. Methylphenidate in Children with Seizures and Attention-Deficit Disorder. *American Journal of Diseases of Children*, 143: 1081–1086, 1989.

30. Fried, J., Greenhill, L. L., Torres, D., *et al*. Sustained-Release Methylphenidate: Long-Term Clinical Efficacy in ADDH Males. *American Academy of Child and Adolescent Psychiatry: Scientific Proceedings of the Annual Meeting*, 3: 47, 1987.

31. Gadow, K. D. Prevalence of Drug Treatment for Hyperactivity and Other Childhood Behavior Disorders. In K. D. Gadow & J. Loney (Eds.), *Psychosocial Aspects of Drug Treatment for Hyperactivity*. Boulder, CO: Westview Press, 1981.

32. Gadow, K. D. Effects of Stimulant Drugs on Academic Performance in Hyperactive and Learning Disabled Children. *Journal of Learning Disabilities*, 16: 290–299, 1983.

33. Gadow, K. D., Nolan, E. E., Sverd, J., *et al*. Methylphenidate in Aggressive-Hyperactive Boys: I. Effects on Peer Aggression in Public School Settings. *Journal of the American Academy of Child and Adolescent Psychiatry*, 29: 710–718, 1990.

34. Gammon, G. D., & Brown, T. E. Fluoxetine Augmentation of Methylphenidate for Attention Deficit and Comorbid Disorders. *Journal of Child and Adolescent Psychopharmacology*, in press.

35. (Gittelman-)Klein, R. Pharmacotherapy of Childhood Hyperactivity: An Update. In H. Y. Meltzer (Ed.), *Psychopharmacology: The Third Generation of Progress*. New York: Raven Press, 1987.

36. (Gittelman-)Klein, R. Thioridazine Effects on the Cognitive Performance of Children with Attention-Deficit Hyperactivity Disorder. *Journal of Child and Adolescent Psychopharmacology*, 1: 263–270, 1990–1991.

37. (Gittelman-)Klein, R., Landa, B., Mattes, J. A., *et al.* Methylphenidate and Growth in Hyperactive Children. *Archives of General Psychiatry*, 45: 1127–1130, 1988.

38. (Gittelman-)Klein, R., & Mannuzza, S. Hyperactive Boys Almost Grown Up: III. Methylphenidate Effects on Ultimate Height. *Archives of General Psychiatry*, 45: 1131–1134, 1988.

39. Gittelman-Klein, R., Klein, D. F., Katz, S., *et al.* Comparative Effects of Methylphenidate and Thioridazine in Hyperkinetic Children: I. Clinical Results. *Archives of General Psychiatry*, 33: 1217–1237, 1976.

40. Green, W. H. Non-Stimulant Drugs in the Treatment of Attention Deficit Hyperactive Disorder. *Child and Adolescent Psychiatric Clinics of North America*, 2: 449–465, 1992.

41. Greenhill, L. L. Pharmacotherapy Stimulants. *Child and Adolescent Psychiatric Clinics of North America*, 2: 411–447, 1992.

42. Greenhill, L. L., Puig-Antich, J., Chambers, W., *et al.* Growth Hormone, Prolactin, and Growth Responses in Hyperkinetic Males Treated with D-Amphetamine. *Journal of the American Academy of Child and Adolescent Psychiatry*, 20: 84–103, 1981.

43. Greenhill, L. L., Puig-Antich, J., Novacenko, H., *et al.* Prolactin, Growth Hormone and Growth Responses in Boys with Attention Deficit Disorder and Hyperactivity Treated with Methylphenidate. *Journal of the American Academy of Child and Adolescent Psychiatry*, 23: 58–67, 1984.

44. Gross, M. Growth of Hyperkinetic Children Taking Methylphenidate, Dextroamphetamine, or Imipramine/Desipramine. *Pediatrics*, 58: 423–431, 1976.

45. Gualtieri, C. T., Keenan, P. A., & Chandler, M. Clinical and Neuropsychological Effect on Desipramine in Children with Attention Deficit Hyperactivity Disorder. *Journal of Clinical Psychopharmacology*, 11: 155–159, 1991.

46. Hechtman, L. T. Adolescent Outcome of Hyperactive Children Treated with Stimulants in Childhood: A Review. *Psychopharmacology Bulletin*, 21: 178–191, 1985.

47. Hechtman, L. T., Weiss, G., & Perlman, T. Growth and Cardiovascular Measures in Hyperactive Individuals as Young Adults and in Matched Normal Controls. *Canadian Medical Association Journal*, 118: 1247–1250, 1978.

48. Hechtman, L. T., Weiss, G., & Perlman, T. Young Adult Outcome of Hyperactive Children who Received Long-Term Stimulant Treatment. *Journal of the American Academy of Child and Adolescent Psychiatry*, 23: 261–269, 1984.

49. Hinshaw, S. Effects of Methylphenidate on Aggressive and Antisocial Behavior (Abstract). *American Academy of Child and Adolescent Psychiatry: Scientific Proceedings of the Annual Meeting*, 7: 31–32, 1991.

50. Hinshaw, S., Henker, B., Whalen, C., *et al.* Aggressive, Prosocial and Nonsocial Behavior in Hyperactive Boys: Dose Effects of MPH in Naturalistic Settings. *Journal of Consulting and Clinical Psychology*, 57: 636–643, 1989.

51. Hunt, R. D., Capper, L., & O'Connell, P. Clonidine in Child and Adolescent Psychiatry. *Journal of Child and Adolescent Psychopharmacology*, 1: 87–102, 1990.

52. Hunt, R. D., Lau, S., & Ryu, J. Alternative Therapies for ADHD. In L. L. Greenhill & B. B. Osman (Eds.), *Ritalin: Theory and Patient Management*. New York: Mary Ann Liebert, 1991.

53. Johnston, C., Pelham, W. E., & Hoza, J. Psychostimulant Rebound in Attention Deficit Disordered Boys. *Journal of the American Academy of Child and Adolescent Psychiatry*, 27: 806–810, 1988.

54. Kaplan, S. L., Busner, J., Kupietz, S., *et al.* Effects of Methylphenidate on

Adolescents with Aggressive Conduct Disorder and ADDH: A Preliminary Report. *Journal of the American Academy of Child and Adolescent Psychiatry*, 29: 719–723, 1990.

55. Kelly, K. L., Rapport, M. D., & DuPaul, G. J. Attention Deficit Disorder and Methylphenidate: A Multi-Step Analysis of Dose-Response Effects on Children's Cardiovascular Functioning. *International Clinics in Psychopharmacology*, 3: 167–181, 1988.

56. Klorman, R., Brumaghim, J. T., Salzman, L. F., *et al.* Effects of Methylphenidate on Attention-Deficit Hyperactivity Disorder with and without Aggressive/Noncompliant Features. *Journal of Abnormal Psychology*, 97: 413–422, 1988.

56a. Kupietz, S. S., Winsberg, B. G., Richardson, E., *et al.* Effects of Methylphenidate Dosage in Hyperactive Reading-Disabled Children: I. Behavior and Cognitive Performance Effects. *Journal of the American Academy of Child and Adolescent Psychiatry*, 22: 70–77, 1988.

57. Leckman, J. F., Detlor, J., Harcherik, D. F., *et al.* Short- and Long-Term Treatment of Tourette's Syndrome with Clonidine: A Clinical Perspective. *Neurology*, 35: 343–351, 1985.

58. Loney, J., Whaley-Klahn, M. M., Kosier, T., *et al.* Hyperactive Boys and Their Brothers at 21: Predictors of Aggressive and Antisocial Outcomes. In K. T. Van Dusen & S. A. Mednick (Eds.), *Prospective Studies of Crime and Delinquency*. Boston: Kluwer-Nijhoff, 1983.

59. Medical Letter. Sudden Death in Children Treated with a Tricyclic Antidepressant. *Medical Letter Drugs Therapy*, 32: 53, 1990.

60. Patrick, S. K., Mueller, R. A., Gualtieri, C. T., *et al.* Pharmacokinetics and Actions of Methylphenidate. In H. Y. Meltzer (Ed.), *Psychopharmacology: The Third Generation of Progress*. New York: Raven Press, 1987.

61. Pelham, W. E., Jr., Greenslade, K. E., Vodde-Hamilton, M., *et al.* Relative Efficacy of Long-Acting Stimulants on ADHD Children: A Comparison of Standard Methylphenidate, Ritalin SR-20, Dexedrine Spansule, and Pemoline. *Pediatrics*, 86: 226–237, 1990.

62. Pelham, W. E., Sturges, J., Hoza, J., *et al.* Sustained Release and Standard Methylphenidate Effects on Cognitive and Social Behavior in Children with Attention Deficit Disorder. *Pediatrics*, 80: 491–501, 1987.

63. Perel, J. W., & Dayton, P. G. Methylphenidate. In E. Usdin & I. Forrest (Eds.), *Psychotherapeutic Drugs, Part II*. New York: Marcel Dekker, 1976.

64. *Physicians' Desk Reference* (45th Ed.). Oradell, NJ: Medical Economics, 1991.

65. Pliszka, S. R. Tricyclic Antidepressants in the Treatment of Children with Attention Deficit Disorder. *Journal of the American Academy of Child and Adolescent Psychiatry*, 26: 127–132, 1987.

66. Pliszka, S. R. Effect of Anxiety on Cognition, Behavior and Stimulant Response in ADHD. *Journal of the American Academy of Child and Adolescent Psychiatry*, 28: 882–887, 1989.

67. Porrino, L. J., Rapoport, L. J., Behar, D., *et al.* A Naturalistic Assessment of the Motor Activity of Hyperactive Boys: II. Stimulant Drug Effects. *Archives of General Psychiatry*, 40: 688–697, 1983.

68. Porrino, L. J., Rapoport, L. J., Behar, D., *et al.* A Naturalistic Assessment of the Motor Activity of Hyperactive Boys: I. Comparison with Normal Controls. *Archives of General Psychiatry*, 40: 681–687, 1983.

69. Rapoport, J., Buchsbaum, M., & Weingartner, H. Dextroamphetamine: Its Cognitive and Behavioral Effects in Normal and Hyperactive Boys and Normal Men. *Archives of General Psychiatry*, 37: 933–943, 1980.

70. Rapport, M. D., & DuPaul, G. J. Hyperactivity and Methylphenidate: Rate-Dependent Effects on Attention. *International Clinics in Psychopharmacology*, 1: 45–52, 1986.

71. Rapport, M. D., Quinn, S. O., DuPaul, G. J., *et al.* Attention Deficit Disorder with

Hyperactivity and Methylphenidate: The Effects of Dose and Mastery Level on Children's Learning Performance. *Journal of Abnormal Child Psychology,* 17: 669–689, 1989.

72. Rapport, M. D., Stoner, G., DuPaul, G. J., *et al.* Methylphenidate in Hyperactive Children: Differential Effects of Dose in Academic Learning and Social Behavior. *Journal of Abnormal Child Psychology,* 13(2): 227–244, 1985.

73. Rapport, M. D., Stoner, G., DuPaul, G. J., *et al.* Attention Deficit Disorder and Methylphenidate: A Multilevel Analysis of Dose–Response Effects on Children's Impulsivity Across Settings. *Journal of the American Academy of Child and Adolescent Psychiatry,* 27: 60–69, 1988.

74. Reeve, E., & Garfinkel, B. Neuroendocrine and Growth Regulation: The Role of Sympathomimetic Medication. In L. L. Greenhill & B. Osman (Eds.), *Ritalin: Theory and Patient Management.* New York: Mary Ann Liebert, 1991.

75. Riddle, M. A., King, R. A., Hardin, M. T., *et al.* Behavioral Side Effects of Fluoxetine in Children and Adolescents. *Journal of Child and Adolescent Psychopharmacology,* 1: 193–198, 1990–1991.

76. Roche, A. F., Lipman, R. S., Overall, J. E., *et al.* The Effects of Stimulant Medication on the Growth of Hyperactive Children. *Pediatrics,* 63: 847–849, 1979.

77. Safer, D. J., & Allen, R. P. Stimulant Drug Treatment of Hyperactive Adolescents. *Diseases of the Nervous System,* 36: 454–457, 1975.

78. Safer, D. Allen, R. P., & Barr, E. Depression of Growth in Hyperactive Children on Stimulant Drugs. *New England Journal of Medicine,* 287: 217–220, 1972.

79. Safer, D. J., & Krager, J. M. A Survey of Medication Treatment for Hyperactive/Inattentive Students. *Journal of the American Medical Association,* 260: 2256–2258, 1988.

80. Satterfield, J. H., Cantwell, D. P., Schell, A., *et al.* Growth of Hyperactive Children Treated with Methylphenidate. *Archives of General Psychiatry,* 36: 212–217, 1979.

81. Schachar, R., Taylor, E., Wieselberg, M., *et al.* Changes in Family Function and Relationships in Children Who Respond to Methylphenidate. *Journal of the American Academy of Child and Adolescent Psychiatry,* 26: 728–732, 1987.

82. Schroeder, J. S., Mullin, A. V., Elliott, G. R., *et al.* Cardiovascular Effects of Desipramine in Children. *Journal of the American Academy of Child and Adolescent Psychiatry,* 28: 376–379, 1989.

83. Sebrechts, M. M., Shaywitz, S. E., Shaywitz, B. A., *et al.* Components of Attention, Methylphenidate Dosage, and Blood Levels and Children with Attention Deficit Disorder. *Pediatrics,* 77: 222–228, 1986.

84. Shapiro, S. K., & Garfinkel, H. D. The Prevalence of Behavior Disorders in Children: The Interdependence of Attention deficit Disorder and Conduct Disorder. *Journal of the American Academy of Child and Adolescent Psychiatry,* 25: 809–819, 1986.

85. Simeon, J. G., Ferguson, H. B., & Fleet, J. V. W. Bupropion Effects in Attention Deficit and Conduct Disorder. *Canadian Journal of Psychiatry,* 31: 581–585, 1986.

86. Solanto, M. V., & Wender, E. H. Does Methylphenidate Constrict Cognitive Functioning? *Journal of the American Academy of Child and Adolescent Psychiatry,* 28: 897–902, 1989.

87. Sprague, R. L., & Sleator, E. K. Methylphenidate in Hyperkinetic Children: Differences in Dose Effects on Learning and Social Behavior. *Science,* 198: 1274–1276, 1977.

88. Swanson, J. M., Granger, D., & Kliewer, W. Natural Social Behaviors in Hyperactive Children: Dose Effects of Methylphenidate. *Journal of Consulting and Clinical Psychology,* 55: 187–193, 1987.

89. Tannock, R., Ickowicz, A., & Schachar, R. Effects of Comorbid Anxiety Disorder on Stimulant Response in Children with Attention Deficit Hyperactivity Disorder (Abstract). *American Academy of Child and Adolescent Psychiatry: Scientific Proceedings of the Annual Meeting,* 7: 56–57, 1991.

90. Tannock, R., Schachar, R. J., Carr, R. P., et al. Effects of Methylphenidate on Inhibitory Control in Hyperactive Children. *Journal of Abnormal Child Psychology,* 17: 473–491, 1989.

91. Tannock, R., Schachar, R. J., Carr, R. P., et al. Dose–Response Effects of Methylphenidate on Academic Performance and Overt Behavior in Hyperactive Children. *Pediatrics,* 84: 648–657, 1989.

92. Varley, C. K., & Trupin, E. W. Double-Blind Assessment of Stimulant Medication for Attention Deficit Disorder: A Model for Clinical Application. *American Journal of Orthopsychiatry,* 53: 542–547, 1983.

93. Vincent, J., Varley, C. K., & Leger, P. Effects of Methylphenidate on Early Adolescent Growth. *American Journal of Psychiatry,* 147: 501–502, 1990.

94. Weiss, G., Kruger, E., Danielson, R., et al. Effect of Long Term Treatment of Hyperactive Children with Methylphenidate. *Canadian Medical Association Journal,* 112: 159–165, 1975.

95. Werry, J., Aman, M. G., & Diamond, E. Imipramine and Methylphenidate in Hyperactive Children. *Journal of Child Psychology and Psychiatry,* 21: 27–35, 1980.

96. Whalen, C. K. Does Stimulant Medication Improve the Peer Status of Hyperactive Children? *Journal of Consulting and Clinical Psychology,* 57: 545–549, 1989.

97. Whalen, C. K., Henker, B., Dotemoto, S., et al. Hyperactivity and Methylphenidate: Peer Interaction Styles. In K. D. Gasow & J. Loney (Eds.), *Psychosocial Aspects of Drug Treatment for Hyperactivity.* Boulder, CO: Westview Press, 1981.

98. Whalen, C. K., Henker, B., & Granger, D. A. Social Judgement Processes in Hyperactive Boys: Effects of Methylphenidate and Comparisons with Normal Peers. *Journal of Abnormal Child Psychology,* 18: 297–316, 1990.

99. Wilens, T. E., & Biederman, J. The Stimulants. *Psychiatric Clinics of North America,* 14: 191–222, 1992.

100. Zametkin, A. J., & Rapoport, J. L. Neurobiology of Attention Deficit Disorder with Hyperactivity: Where Have We Come in 50 Years? *Journal of the American Academy of Child and Adolescent Psychiatry,* 26: 676–686, 1987.

101. Zametkin, A. J., Rapoport, J., Murphy, D. L., et al. Treatment of Hyperactive Children with Monoamine Oxidase Inhibitors: I: Clinical Efficacy. *Archives of General Psychiatry,* 42: 962–968, 1985.

CHAPTER 24

1. Abikoff, H. An Evaluation of Cognitive Behavior Therapy for Hyperactive Children. In B. B. Lahey & A. E. Kazdin (Eds.), *Advances in Clinical Child Psychology* (Vol. 10). New York: Plenum Press, 1987.

2. Abikoff, H., Ganeles, D., Reiter, G., et al. Cognitive Training in Academically Deficient ADHD Boys Receiving Stimulant Medication. *Journal of Abnormal Child Psychology,* 12: 33–44, 1985.

3. Barkley, R. A. *Defiant Children: A Clinician's Manual for Parent Training.* New York: Guilford Press, 1987.

4. Brown, R. T., Borden, K. A., Wynne, M. E., et al. Methylphenidate and Cognitive Therapy with ADD Children: A Methodological Reconsideration. *Journal of Abnormal Child Psychology,* 14: 481–498, 1986.

5. Cantwell, D. P., & Satterfield, J. H. The Prevalence of Academic Underachievement in Hyperactive Children. *Journal of Pediatric Psychology,* 3: 168–171, 1981.

6. Carlson, C. L., Pelham, W. E., Milich, R., et al. Single and Combined Effects of Methylphenidate and Behavior Therapy on the Classroom Performance of Children with

Attention Deficit-Hyperactivity Disorder. *Journal of Abnormal Child Psychology*, 20: 213–232, 1992.

7. Conrad, W. G., Dworken, E. S., Shai, A., & Tobisen, J. E. Effects of Amphetamine Therapy and Presciptive Tutoring on the Behavior and Achievement of Lower Class Hyperactive Children. *Journal of Learning Disabilities*, 5: 509–517, 1971.

8. Dodge, K. A. Problems in Social Relationships. In E. J. Mash & R. A. Barkley (Eds.), *Treatment of Childhood Disorders*. New York: Guilford Press, 1989.

9. Forehand, R. L., & McMahon, R. J. *Helping the Noncompliant Child: A Clinician's Guide to Parent Training*. New York: Guilford Press, 1981.

10. Gardner, R. A. Dramatized Story Telling in Child Psychotherapy. *Acta Paedopsychiatrica*, 41: 110, 1975.

11. Gittelman, R., Klein, D., & Feingold, I. Children with Reading Disorders: II. Effects of Methylphenidate in Combination with Reading Remediation. *Journal of Child Psychology and Psychiatry*, 24: 193–212, 1983.

12. Gittelman-Klein, R., Abikoff, H., Pollack, E., *et al.* A Controlled Trial of Behavior Modification and Methylphenidate in Hyperactive Children. In C. K. Whalen & B. Henker (Eds.), *Hyperactive Children: The Social Ecology of Identification and Treatment*. New York: Academic Press, 1980.

13. Greenfield, B., Gottlieb, S., & Weiss, G. Psychosocial Intervention: Individual Therapy with the Child. *Child and Adolescent Psychiatric Clinics of North America*, 2: 481–494, 1992.

14. Hechtman, L. T., Weiss, G., & Perlman, T. Young Adult Outcome of Hyperactive Children Who Received Long-Term Stimulant Treatment. *Journal of the American Academy of Child Psychiatry*, 23(2): 261–269, 1984.

15. Hinshaw, S. P. Stimulant Medication and the Treatment of Aggression in Children with Attentional Deficits. *Journal of Clinical Child Psychology*, 20: 301, 1991.

16. Hinshaw, S. P., & Erhardt, D. Attention-Deficit Hyperactivity Disorder. In P. C. Kendall (Ed.), *Child and Adolescent Therapy: Cognitive–Behavioral Procedures*. New York: Guilford Press, 1991.

17. Hinshaw, S. P., Henker B., & Whalen, C. K. Cognitive–Behavioral and Pharmacologic Intervention for Hyperactive Boys: Comparative and Combined Effects. *Journal of Consulting and Clinical Psychology*, 52: 739–749, 1984.

18. Hinshaw, S. P., Henker, B., & Whalen, C. K. Self-Control in Hyperactive Boys in Anger-Inducing Situations: Effects of Cognitive-Behavioral Training and of Methylphenidate. *Journal of Abnormal Child Psychology*, 12: 55–77, 1984.

19. Hinshaw, S. P., Henker, B., Whalen, C. K., *et al.* Aggressive, Prosocial, and Nonsocial Behavior in Hyperactive Boys: Dose Effects of Methylphenidate in Naturalistic Settings. *Journal of Consulting and Clinical Psychology*, 57: 636–643, 1989.

20. Hinshaw, S. P., & McHale, J. P. Stimulant Medications and the Social Interactions of Hyperactive Children: Effects and Implications. In J. G. Gilbert & J. J. Connolly (Eds.), *Personality, Social Skills, and Psychopathology: An Individual Differences Approach*. New York: Plenum Press, 1991.

21. Hoza, B., Pelham, W. E., Sams, S. E., *et al.* An Examination of the "Dosage" Effects of Both Behavior Therapy and Methylphenidate on the Classroom Performance of ADHD Children. *Behavior Modification*, 16: 164–192, 1992.

22. Kazdin, A. E., Bass, D., Siegel, T., *et al.* Cognitive–Behavioral Therapy and Relationship Therapy in the Treatment of Children Referred for Antisocial Behavior. *Journal of Consulting and Clinical Psychology*, 57: 522, 1989.

23. Kernberg, P. F., & Chazan, S. E. *Children with Conduct Disorders: A Psychotherapy Manual*. New York: Basic Books, 1991.

24. Lochman, J. E., White, K. J., & Wayland, K. J. Cognitive–Behavioral Assessment

and Treatment with Aggressive Children. In P. C. Kendall (Ed.), *Child and Adolescent Therapy: Cognitive–Behavioral Procedures.* New York: Guilford Press, 1991.

25. Meichenbaum, D., & Goodman, J. Training Impulsive Children to Talk to Themselves: A Means of Developing Self-Control. *Journal of Abnormal Psychology,* 77: 115–126, 1971.

26. Milich, R., & Dodge, K. A. Social Information Processing in Child Psychiatry Populations. *Journal of Abnormal Child Psychology,* 12: 471, 1984.

27. Minde, K., Lewin, D., Weiss, G., *et al.* The Hyperactive Child in Elementary School: A 5-Year Controlled Follow-up. *Exceptional Children,* 33: 215–221, 1971.

28. Murphy, D. A., Pelham, W. E., & Lang, A. R. Aggression in Boys with Attention Deficit Hyperactivity Disorder: Methylphenidate Effects on Naturalistically Observed Aggression, Response to Provocation, and Social Information Processing. *Journal of Abnormal Child Psychology,* in press.

29. Newby, R. F., Fisher, M, & Romans, M. A. Parent Training for Families of Children with ADHD. *School Psychology Review,* 20: 252–265, 1991.

30. Parker, J. G., & Asher, S. R. Peer Relations and Later Personal Adjustment: Are Low-Accepted Children at Risk? *Psychological Bulletin,* 102: 357, 1987.

31. Patterson, G. R. *Living with Children: New Methods for Parents and Teachers.* Champaign, IL: Research Press, 1976.

32. Pelham, W. E. Behavior Therapy, Behavioral Assessment and Psychostimulant Medication in the Treatment of Attention Deficit Disorders: An Integrative Approach. In L. M. Bloomingdale & J. Swanson (Eds.), *Attention Deficit Disorders* (Vol. 4). Oxford: Pergamon Press, 1989.

33. Pelham, W. E., Bender, M. E., Caddell, J., *et al.* Methylphenidate and Children with Attention Deficit Disorder: Dose Effects on Classroom, Academic and Social Behavior. *Archives of General Psychiatry,* 42: 948–952, 1985.

34. Pelham, W. E., Carlson, C. L., Sams, S. E., *et al.* Separate and Combined Effects of Methylphenidate and Behavior Modification on the Classroom Behavior and Academic Performance of ADHD Boys: Group Effects and Individual Differences. *Journal of Consulting and Clinical Psychology,* 60: 259–283, 1992.

35. Pelham, W. E., & Murphy, H. A. Behavioral and Pharmacological Treatment of Attention Deficit and Conduct Disorders. In M. Hersen (Ed.), *Pharmacological and Behavioral Treatment: An Integrative Approach.* New York: Wiley, 1986.

36. Pelham, W. E., Schnedler, R. W., Bender, M. E., *et al.* The Combination of Behavior Therapy and Methylphenidate in the Treatment of Hyperactivity: A Therapy Outcome Study. In L. M. Bloomingdale (Ed.), *Attention Deficit Disorders: Vol. 3. New Research in Attention, Treatment and Psychopharmacology.* Oxford: Pergamon Press, 1988.

37. Price, J. M., & Dodge, K. A. Reactive and Proactive Aggression in Childhood: Relations to Peer Status and Social Context Dimensions. *Journal of Abnormal Child Psychology,* 17: 455, 1989.

38. Rapport, M. D., Murphy, H. A., & Bailey, J. S. Ritalin vs. Response-Cost in the Control of Hyperactive Children: A Within-Subject Comparison. *Journal of Applied Behavior Analysis,* 15: 205–216, 1982.

39. Rapport, M., Stoner, G., DuPaul, G., *et al.* Methylphenidate in Hyperactive Children: Differential Effects of Dose in Academic Learning and Social Behavior. *Journal of Abnormal Child Psychology,* 13(2): 227–244, 1985.

40. Rosen, L. A., O'Leary, S. G., Joyce, S. A., *et al.* The Importance of Prudent Negative Consequences for Maintaining the Appropriate Behavior of Hyperactive Students. *Journal of Abnormal Child Psychology,* 12: 81, 1984.

41. Satterfield, J. H., Hoppe, C., & Schell, A. E. A Prospective Study of Delinquency

in 110 Adolescent Boys with Attention Deficit Disorder and 88 Normal Adolescent Boys. *American Journal of Psychiatry*, 139: 795–798, 1982.

42. Satterfield, J. H., Satterfield, B. T., & Cantwell, D. P. Three-Year Multimodality Treatment Study of 100 Hyperactive Boys. *Journal of Pediatrics*, 98: 650–655, 1981.

43. Satterfield, J. H., Satterfield, B. T., & Schell, A. E. Therapeutic Interventions to Prevent Delinquency in Hyperactive Boys. *Journal of the American Academy of Child and Adolescent Psychiatry*, 26: 56–64, 1987.

44. Smith, H. F. The Elephant on the Fence: Approaches to Psychotherapy of Attention Deficit Disorder. *American Journal of Psychotherapy*, 40: 252–264, 1986.

45. Stephens, R. S., Pelham, W. E., & Skinner, R. State-Dependent and Main Effects of Methylphenidate and Pemoline on Paired-Associate Learning and Spelling in Hyperactive Children. *Journal of Consulting and Clinical Psychology*, 52(1): 104–113, 1984.

46. Sullivan, M. A., & O'Leary, S. G. Differential Maintenance Following Reward and Cost Token Programs with Children. *Behavior Therapy*, 21: 139–151, 1989.

47. The Ungame (A Self-Expression Game). Tattco.

48. Wender, P. H. The Minimal Brain Dysfunction Syndrome. *Annual Review of Medicine*, 26: 45, 1975.

49. Whalen, C. K., & Henker, B. The Social Worlds of Hyperactive Children. *Clinical Psychology Review*, 5: 1, 1985.

50. Whalen, C. K., & Henker, B. Therapies for Hyperactive Children: Comparisons, Combinations, and Compromises. *Journal of Consulting and Clinical Psychology*, 59: 126, 1991.

51. Whalen, C. K., Henker, B., Buhrmester, D., *et al.* Does Stimulant Medication Improve the Peer Status of Hyperactive Children? *Journal of Consulting and Clinical Psychology*, 57: 545, 1989.

52. Winnicott, D. W. *Paediatric Consultations in Child Psychiatry.* London: Hogarth Press, 1971.

CHAPTER 25

1. American Psychiatric Association. *Diagnostic and Statistical Manual of Mental Disorders* (3rd ed.). Washington, DC: Author, 1980.

2. American Psychiatric Association. *Diagnostic and Statistical Manual of Mental Disorders* (3rd ed., rev.). Washington, DC: Author, 1987.

3. Barkley, R. A. *Attention-Deficit Hyperactivity Disorder: A Handbook for Diagnosis and Treatment.* New York: Guilford Press, 1990.

4. Biederman, J., Faraone, S. V., & Keenan, K. Evidence of Familial Association between Attention Deficit Disorder and Major Affective Disorders. *Archives of General Psychiatry*, 48: 633–642, 1991.

5. Denckla, M. B. Attention Deficit Hyperactivity Disorder—Residual Type. *Journal of Child Neurology*, 6(Supplement): S44–S50, 1991.

6. Derogatis, L. *Manual for the Symptom Checklist 90—Revised (SCL-90R).* Baltimore: Author, 1986.

7. Gittelman, R. *Relationship between Childhood Hyperactivity and Adult Affective Antisocial and Substance Use Disorders.* Paper presented at the 3rd Annual Research Conference of the New York State Office of Mental Health, Albany, December 7, 1990.

8. Gittelman, R., Mannuzza, S., Shenker, R., & Bonagura, N. Hyperactive Boys Almost Grown Up: I. Psychiatric Status. *Archives of General Psychiatry*, 42: 937–947, 1985.

9. Gualtieri, T. C., Ondrusek, M. G., & Finley, C. Attention Deficit Disorders in Adults. *Clinical Neuropsychopharmacology*, 8: 343–356, 1985.

10. Heaton, R. K. *A Manual for the Wisconsin Card Sorting Test.* Odessa, FL: Psychological Assessment Resources, 1981.

11. Klee, S. H., & Garfinkel, B. D. The Computerized CPI: A New Measure of Inattention. *Journal of Abnormal Child Psychology,* 11: 487–496, 1983.

12. Laufer, M. W. Long Term Management and Some Follow-Up Findings on the Use of Drugs with Minimal Cerebral Syndromes. *Journal of Learning Disability,* 4: 55–58, 1971.

13. Laufer, M. W., Denhoff, E. Hyperkinetic Behavior Syndrome in Children. *Journal of Pediatrics,* 50: 463–474, 1957.

14. Mattes, J., Boswell, L., & Oliver, H. Methylphenidate Effects on Symptoms of Attention Deficit Disorder in Adults. *Archives of General Psychiatry,* 41: 1059–1067, 1984.

15. Mirsky, A. F. The Neuropsychology of Attention: Elements of a Complex Behavior. In E. Perecman (Ed.), *Integrating Theory and Practice in Clinical Neuropsychology.* Hillsdale, NJ: Erlbaum, 1989.

16. Ratey, J. J. *Paying Attention to Attention in Adult Psychiatry.* Paper presented at the annual meeting of the American Psychiatric Association. New York, 1990.

17. Ratey, J. J., Greenberg, M. S., Bemporad, J. R., & Lindem, K. J. Unrecognized Attention Deficit Hyperactivity Disorder in Adults Presenting for Outpatient Psychotherapy. *Child and Adolescent Psychopharmacology,* 4: 267–275, 1992.

18. Reimherr, F. W., Wender, P. H., Wood, D. R., & Ward, M. An Open Trial of L-Tyrosine in the Treatment of Attention Deficit Disorder—Residual Type. *American Journal of Psychiatry,* 144: 1071–1073, 1987.

19. Reitan, R. M. Validity of the Trail Making Test as an Indication of Organic Brain Damage. *Perceptual and Motor Skills,* 8: 271–276, 1958.

20. Wechsler, D. *Manual for the Wechsler Adult Intelligence Scale—Revised.* New York: Psychological Corporation, 1981.

21. Weiss, G., Hechtman, L., Milroy, T., & Perlman, T. Psychiatric Status of Hyperactives as Adults: A Controlled 15-Year Follow-Up of 63 Hyperactive Children. *Journal of the American Academy of Child Psychiatry,* 24: 211–220, 1985.

22. Weiss, G., Minde, K., Werry, J. S., Douglas, V. I., Nemeth, E. Studies on the Hyperactive Child: VIII. Five Year Follow Up. *Archives of General Psychiatry,* 24: 409–414, 1971.

23. Wender, P. H. *The Hyperactive Child, Adolescent and Adult: Attention Deficit Disorder through the Life Span.* New York: Oxford University Press, 1987.

24. Wender, P. H., & Reimherr, F. W. Bupropion Treatment of Attention Deficit Hyperactivity Disorder in Adults. *American Journal of Psychiatry,* 147: 1018–1020, 1990.

25. Wender, P. H., Reimherr, F. W., & Wood, D. R. Attention Deficit Disorder (Minimal Brian Dysfunction) in Adults: A Replication Study of Diagnosis and Drug Treatment. *Archives of General Psychiatry,* 38: 449–456, 1980.

26. Wender, P. H., Reimherr, F. W., Wood, D., & Ward, M. A Controlled Study of Methylphenidate in the Treatment of Attention Deficit Disorder, Residual Type in Adults. *American Journal of Psychiatry,* 142: 547–552, 1985.

27. Wood, D. R., Reimherr, F. W., Wender, P. H., & Johnson, G. E. Diagnosis and Treatment of Minimal Brain Dysfunction in Adults. *Archives of General Psychiatry,* 33: 1453–1460, 1976.

AUTHOR INDEX

Aarskog, D., 168 (433, *n*.60)

Abate, F., 163, 164 (431, *n*.15)

Abelson, H., 127, 181, 228, 232 (428, *n*.28; 434, *n*.4; 437, *n*.10, 21)

Abikoff, H., 48, 351, 355 (420, *n*.57; 446, *n*.1, 2)

Abrams, N., 125 (428, *n*.23)

Achenbach, T., 14 (416, *n*.64)

Ackerman, P. T., 6, 56, 82, 85, 152, 163, 202, 222, 226, 227, 239, 241 (414, *n*.23; 422, *n*.26; 423, *n*.27; 424, *n*.85; 429, *n*.8; 430, *n*.5; 436, *n*.4, 39; 439, *n*.4)

Adams, D., 45 (419, *n*.28)

Adams, P., 224 (436, *n*.10)

Adney, K., 167 (433, *n*.58)

Albert, J., 242 (440, *n*.19)

Alkus, S. R., 45 (419, *n*.28)

Allen, K., 48 (420, *n*.54)

Allen, N., 125 (428, *n*.23)

Allen, R. P., 3, 47, 48, 166, 168, 282, 283, 355 (413, *n*.1; 420, *n*.49, 55; 432, *n*.44, 45; 433, *n*.46; 441, *n*.5; 451, *n*.78)

Allen, T. W., 39 (418, *n*.12)

Aman, M. G., 364 (447, *n*.3, 4)

American Psychiatric Association, 7, 71, 108, 387 (414, *n*.25; 423, *n*.25; 427, *n*.2; 455, *n*.1, 2)

Amsel, R., 105, 221, 257 (426, *n*.53; 436, *n*.2; 440 *n*.1)

Andersen, G. M., 168 (433, *n*.59)

Anderson, C. M., 52 (431, *n*.14)

Anderson, G., 342 (444, *n*.41)

Arnold, L. E., 284 (441, *n*.11)

Asher, S. R., 374 (454, *n*.30)

Ayllon, T., 48 (420, *n*.51)

Backman, J. F., 48, (420, *n*.52)

Baer, D., 48 (420, *n*.54)

Bailey, J. S., 367 (454, *n*.38)

Bakwin, H., 6, 52 (414, *n*.21; 421, *n*.9)

Bakwin, R. M., 6, 52 (414, *n*.21; 421, *n*.9)

Baldessarini, R. J., 346 (442, *n*.9)

Ballard, J. E., 164 (431, *n*.22)

Baonpane, N., 123, 128 (428, *n*.15)

Barcai, A., 46, 349 (419, *n*.33; 448, *n*.23)

Barker, C., 121, 141, 256 (427, *n*.11; 440, *n*.29)

Barkley, R. A., 3, 12, 16, 48, 163, 164, 184, 185, 232, 332, 333, 345, 346, 349, 351, 353, 369, 370, 389–391, 404 (413, *n*.3; 415, *n*.46, 47, 60; 420, *n*.59; 431, *n*.17; 434, *n*.14, 16; 435, *n*.18; 438, *n*.15; 442, *n*.4–6; 447, *n*.5, 8, 9; 452, *n*.3; 455, *n*.3)

Barnard, K., 24 (417, *n*.11)

Barnes, K. R., 46 (419, *n*.38)

Barr, E., 47, 166, 168, 355 (420, *n*.49; 432, *n*.44; 433, *n*.46; 451, *n*.78)

Barr, R. G., 349 (448, *n*.25)

Barratt, E., 224 (436, *n*.10)

Barrickman, L., 363 (447, *n*.10)

Battle, E. S., 26, 183, 185, 232, (417, *n*.15; 434, *n*.8; 438, *n*.11)

Bechtoldt, H. P., 14, 58, 203, (416, *n*.65; 422, *n*.29; 436, *n*.41)

Beck, L., 38, 120, 121, 128, 167, 170, 282, 283 (418, *n*.10; 427 *n*.6; 433, *n*.57; 441, *n*.4)

Behar, D., 37, 350 (418, *n*.4; 450, *n*.67, 68)

Bell, R. Q., 24, 183, (417, *n*.13, 434, *n*.11)

Bemporad, J. R., 402–403 (456, *n*.17)

Ben Yun, Y., 345 (444, *n*.29)

Benn, R., 189, 190, 203 (435, *n*.34)

Bender, L., 6 (414, *n*.20)

Bender, M. E., 27 (417, *n*.17)

Bennett, A., 108 (433, *n*.59)

Benson, F., 340 (442, *n*.7)

Bergman, A., 358 (447, *n*.11)

Bernfeld, G., 29, 37, 43, 44 (417, *n*.2, 22)

Bettelheim, B., 183 (434, *n*.9)

Bialer, I., 46 (419, *n*.31)

Biederman, J., 284, 333, 334, 346, 348, 349, 356, 357, 377, 385 (441, *n*.10; 442, *n*.9–12, 14; 443, *n*.28; 452, *n*.99; 455, *n*.4)

Birch, H. G., 6, 330 (418, *n*.18; 446, *n*.66)
Birmaher, B. B., 358 (447, *n*.15)
Blair, C. L., 285 (441, *n*.13)
Blair-Broeker, C. T., 233–236 (438, *n*.17)
Blaschke, T., 167, 168 (433, *n*.55)
Bloom, N., 156 (430, *n*.19)
Blouin, A. G. A., 8, 46, 54, 82, 87, 119–121, 241, 255 (414, *n*.30; 420, *n*.46; 421, *n*.17; 423, *n*.28; 424, *n*.15; 427, *n*.3; 434, *n*.13)
Boileau, R. A., 164, 167 (431, *n*.22; 433, *n*.51)
Boles Ponto, L., 167 (433, *n*.58)
Bonagura, N., 80, 93, 127, 128, 386, 387 (424, *n*.30; 426, *n*.39; 428, *n*.30; 455, *n*.8)
Bond, E., 4, (413, *n*.8)
Borcherding, B. G., 351 (447, *n*.16)
Borgstedt, A. D., 283 (441, *n*.9)
Borland, B. L., 8, 63, 70, 82, 90, 92, 104, 105, 125, 126, 128, 140, 142, 148, 154, 180, 181 (414, *n*.34; 422, *n*.4; 425, *n*.33; 428, *n*.25; 429, *n*.3; 430, *n*.14; 434, *n*.1)
Borstein, R., 8, 46, 54, 82, 87, 119, 120, 121, 241, 255 (414, *n*.30; 420, *n*.46; 421, *n*.17; 423, *n*.28; 424, *n*.15; 427, *n*.3; 439, *n*.13)
Boswell, L., 89, 123, 124, 287, 401 (425, *n*.30; 428, *n*.17; 442, *n*.21; 456, *n*.14)
Bower, M. B., 342 (446, *n*.69)
Bradley, C., 4, 46, 52, 348 (413, *n*.9; 419, *n*.30; 421, *n*.10; 447, *n*.17)
Bransome, E. D., 38 (418, *n*.10)
Breaux, A. M., 22, 30 (416, *n*.8, 9)
Brown, R. T., 363 (447, *n*.18; 452, *n*.4)
Brown, T. E., 363 (448, *n*.34)
Bruhn, P., 339, 342 (445, *n*.50)
Brumaghim, J. T., 351 (450, *n*.56)
Brumback, R. A., 43 (419 *n*.23)
Bryne, T., 338 (446, *n*.70)
Buchsbaum, M. S., 4, 10, 11, 165, 282, 354 (413, *n*.10; 414, *n*.39; 432, *n*.34; 441, *n*.3; 450, *n*.69)
Buckley, R. E., 163 (430, *n*.3)
Bugental, D. B., 121, 141, 256 (427, *n*.11; 440, *n*.29)
Bunney, W. E., 37 (418, *n*.4)
Busner, J., 351 (449, *n*.54)

Cadoret, R. J., 332, 333 (443, *n*.17)
Campbell, S. B., 22, 29, 30, 31, 37, 40, 43, 44, 46, 183–185, 232 (416, *n*.8, 9; 417,

n.2, 22, 23; 418, *n*.14; 419, *n*.24, 25; 434, *n*.11, 12; 438, *n*.12, 13)
Cantwell, D. P., 10, 42, 49, 88, 117, 153, 161, 163–168, 173, 179, 186, 187, 189, 202, 230, 242, 332, 356, 381–382 (415, *n*.50; 418, *n*.21; 420, *n*.60; 425, *n*.18; 427, *n*.6; 430, *n*.13; 431, *n*.12; 432, *n*.28, 30; 433, *n*.55; 435, *n*.21, 22; 437, *n*.1; 439, *n*.16; 433, *n*.18; 451, *n*.80; 455, *n*.42)
Capper, L., 364, 365 (449, *n*.51)
Capute, A. J., 164, 165 (431, *n*.23)
Carlson, C. L., 368, 369 (452, *n*.6; 454, *n*.34)
Carlström, G., 11, 12 (415, *n*.54)
Carr, R., 167, 340, 350 (433, *n*.56; 446, *n*.74; 452, *n*.90, 91)
Chadwick, O. F., 50 (421, *n*.6)
Chambers, C., 86, 87, 121, (424, *n*.14; 427, *n*.10)
Chambers, W., 356 (449, *n*.42)
Chapel, J. L., 11, 33 (415, *n*.53; 417, *n*.25)
Charles, L., 8, 46, 241 (414, *n*.31; 420, *n*.48; 439, *n*.14)
Chelune, G. J., 340 (443, *n*.20)
Chen, T.-C., 10 (415, *n*.41)
Chen, W. J., 334 (443, *n*.28)
Chess, S., 237 (438, *n*.29)
Cheuns, M. N., 164 (431, *n*.21)
Clark, K. W., 155, 156, 159 (430, *n*.18; 440, *n*.27)
Clemens, R., 12 (415, *n*.58)
Clemens, S. D., 6, 163 (413, *n*.17; 414, *n*.23; 430, *n*.5)
Clemmens, R. L., 5 (413, *n*.14)
Clopton, P. L., 65, 82, 89 (423, *n*.10; 425, *n*.28)
Cluss, R., 44 (419, *n*.44)
Cohen, A. H., 52 (421, *n*.8)
Cohen, D. J., 10, 11, 168, 342 (415, *n*.48, 52; 431, *n*.59; 444, *n*.41; 446, *n*.69)
Cohen, J., 237, 259 (438, *n*.29; 440, *n*.2)
Cohen, L., 4 (413, *n*.7)
Cohen, M., 163, 167, 286 (431, *n*.11; 433, *n*.51; 442, *n*.20)
Cohen, N. J., 27, 31, 41, 56, 151, 156, 159, 160, 202, 243 (417, *n*.19; 418, *n*.16; 422, *n*.23, 25; 429, *n*.2; 426, *n*.40; 440, *n*.26)
Cohen, P., 259 (440, *n*.2)
Cohen, S. M., 285 (441, *n*.3)

Collar, B. S., 24 (417, *n*.11)

Collins, B. E., 45, (419, *n*.28)

Comings, B. G., 335 (443, *n*.21)

Comings, D. E., 335 (443, *n*.21)

Comly, H. H., 45 (438, *n*.27)

Conboy, J., 63, 79, 80, 91, 101, 102, 104, 127, 140, 141, 181, 225–229, 231, 233, 235–237, 242 (422, *n*.6; 425, *n*.34; 428, *n*.27; 434, *n*.3; 437, *n*.7, 15; 440, *n*.18)

Conners, C. K., 33, 46, 275, 349 (417, *n*.24; 419, *n*.32, 33, 36, 37; 441, *n*.1; 448, *n*.22, 23)

Conrad, W. G., 237, 241 (438, *n*.26; 439, *n*.9)

Coons, H. W., 283 (441, *n*.9)

Cooper, M. A., 358 (447, *n*.15)

Copeland, A. P., 48 (420, *n*.59)

Cornblatt, B., 358 (447, *n*.11)

Costello, A., 331 (443, *n*.24)

Cote, F., 340 (443, *n*.27)

Covi, L., 70, 71, 99, 243 (423, *n*.22; 426, *n*.50; 440, *n*.23)

Cox, A., 57, 67, 79, 102 (422, *n*.28; 423, *n*.18; 426, *n*.51)

Cruikshank, W. M., 5 (413, *n*.13)

Crumrine, P., 355 (448, *n*.29)

Cummings, C., 14, 88, 187, 189 (416, *n*.68; 425, *n*.20; 435, *n*.28)

Cunningham, C. E., 10, 184, 185, 232 (415, *n*.47; 434, *n*.14, 16; 438, *n*.15)

Cvejic, H., 11, 27, 31 (417, *n*.19)

Danielson, R., 352 (452, *n*.94)

Danielson, U., 8, 46, 166, 171, 236, 237, 240 (414, *n*.28; 420, *n*.43; 433, *n*.47; 438, *n*.25; 439, *n*.7)

Davidson, H., 151, 156, 159, 243 (429, *n*.4; 440, *n*.24)

Davis, A., 46 (419, *n*.35)

Dawson, M. E., 163, 164 (431 *n*.7)

Day, D., 242 (440, *n*.19)

de Blois, C. S., 14, 88, 124, 187–189, 231, 232 (416, *n*.68; 425, *n*.20; 428, *n*.21; 435, *n*.28, 30; 437, *n*.3)

DeFries, J. C., 330 (444, *n*.31, 32)

Dekirmenjian, H., 11 (415, *n*.53)

Delameter, A. M., 202 (435, *n*.38)

Denckla, M. B., 354, 386 (448, *n*.23a; 455, *n*.5)

Denhoff, E., 6, 46, 52, 54, 57, 63, 70, 81, 87, 92, 104, 105, 120, 121, 125, 126, 128, 140–142, 152, 153, 161, 163, 181, 242, 384 (414, *n*.22; 419, *n*.35; 421, *n*.12, 18; 422, *n*.5; 425, *n*.16; 427, *n*.5; 429, *n*.2; 430, *n*.1, 10; 434, *n*.2; 440, *n*.17; 456, *n*.13)

Denhoff, J., 54, 57, 63, 70, 81, 87, 91, 104, 105, 120, 121, 125, 126, 128, 140–142, 152, 153, 161, 181, 242 (421, *n*.18; 422, *n*.5; 425, *n*.16; 427, *n*.5; 429, *n*.2; 430, *n*.10; 434, *n*.2; 440, *n*.17)

Derogatis, L., 70, 71, 99, 243 (423, *n*.22; 426, *n*.50; 440, *n*.23)

Detlor, J., 365 (450, *n*.57)

Deutsch, C. K., 334 (443, *n*.22)

DeVeaugh-Geiss, J., 285 (442, *n*.16)

Dickey, T. O., 340 (443, *n*.20)

Dixon, J. R., 164 (431, *n*.25)

Dodge, K. A., 374, 375 (454, *n*.26, 37)

Dogan, K., 10, 164 (415, *n*.42; 432, *n*.26)

Dolemoto, S., 44, 352 (419, *n*.27; 452, *n*.97)

Douglas, V. I., 6, 9, 22, 23, 37–43, 46, 48, 55–57, 61, 66, 85, 118, 150, 163, 224–229, 349, 386 (414, *n*.24, 37; 416, *n*.7; 418, *n*.5–9, 14, 18–20; 419, *n*.22, 34; 420, *n*.58; 421, *n*.19, 21, 22; 422, *n*.1, 24; 423, *n*.16, 17; 424, *n*.3, 4; 427, *n*.1; 429, *n*.1; 430, *n*.2; 431, *n*.11, 19; 436, *n*.8; 437, *n*.13; 448, *n*.25; 456, *n*. 22)

Drake, L., 202 (435, *n*.38)

Drasgow, F., 164 (431, *n*.21)

Drorbaugh, J. E., 24 (417, *n*.12)

Dulcan, M., 358 (448, *n*.26)

DuPaul, G. J., 345, 349–351 (442, *n*.4, 5; 450, *n*.70, 71; 451, *n*.72, 73)

Dyk, R. B., 243 (440, *n*.20)

Dykman, R. A., 6, 56, 82, 85, 152, 163, 202, 222, 226, 227, 239, 241 (414, *n*.23; 422, *n*.26; 423, *n*.27; 424, *n*.6; 429, *n*.8; 430, *n*.5; 436, *n*.4, 39; 439, *n*.4)

Ebaugh, F. G., 4 (413, *n*.6)

Edelbrock, C., 331–333, 353 (442, *n*.6; 443, *n*.24; 447, *n*.8, 9)

Eeg-Olofsson, O., 164 (432, *n*.27)

Eisenberg, L., 46, 52, 167, 275, 348 (419, *n*.32, 33, 37; 421, *n*.11; 433, *n*.52; 441, *n*.1; 448, *n*.23, 26a)

Elardo, P. T., 202 (436, *n*.39)

Elders, J., 167 (433, *n*.56)

Elia, J., 349 (448, n.27)

Elman, M., 8, 27, 31, 46, 166, 171, 236, 237, 240 (414, n.28; 417, n.19; 420, n.43; 433, n.47; 438, n.25; 439, n.7)

Emerich, W., 28 (417, n.21)

Endicott, I., 71, 72, 91, 97, 99, 108, 127, 225, 228, 232, 243, 286 (423, n.26; 425, n.35; 426, n.1; 428, n.29; 437, n.8, 16; 440, n.22; 442, n.19)

Endman, M. W., 29, 37, 43, 44 (417, n.2, 22)

Erikson, E., 51 (421, n.7)

Everett, J., 340 (443, n.27)

Ewing, L. J., 22, 30, 31,(416, n.8, 9)

Famularo, R., 349 (448, n.28)

Faraone, S. V., 333, 334, 346, 349, 385 (442, n.10–12; 448, n.28; 455, n.4)

Farkas, L. G., 334 (443, n.22)

Feingold I., 46 (420, n.41)

Feldman, H., 355 (448, n.29)

Feldman, S., 54, 57, 63 70, 81, 87, 91, 92, 104, 105, 120, 121, 125, 126, 128, 140–142, 152, 153, 161, 181, 242 (421, n.18; 422, n.5; 425, n.16; 427, n.5; 429, n.2; 430, n.10; 434, n.2; 440, n.17)

Fenton, T., 349 (448, n.28)

Ferguson, H. B., 10, 48, 163, 164 (415, n.45; 420, n.52,; 431, n.10, 16)

Ferguson, W., 340 (443, n.20)

Fevang, F. O., 168 (433, n.60)

Fiedler, M. F., 24, 41 (417, n.12; 418, n.15)

Finkelstein, J., 189, 190, 203 (435, n.34)

Finley, C., 401, 402 (455, n.9)

Firestone, P., 41 (418, n.15)

Fishburne, P., 127, 181, 228, 232 (428, n.28; 434, n.4; 437, n.10, 21)

Fischer, M., 332, 333 (442, n.6)

Forehand, R. L., 369 (453, n.9)

Frank, G., 345 (444, n.29)

Franks, G. J., 164 (431, n.21)

Freibergs, V., 41, 163 (418, n.18; 430, n.2)

Freud, A., 50, 117 (421, n.3; 427, n.5)

Fried, J., 354 (448, n.30)

Friedman, N., 167 (433, n.56)

Fuller, P. W., 165 (432, n.37)

Gadow, K., 46, 348, 349, 351 (419, n.40; 448, n.31–33)

Gammon, G. D., 363 (448, n.34)

Garfinkle, B. D., 240 (439, n.8)

Gastfriend, D. R., 284 (441, n.10)

Gauthier, M., 285 (354, n.14)

Gilger, J. W., 330 (444, n.32)

Gillberg, C., 11, 12 (415, n.54)

Gillis, J. J., 330 (444, n.32)

Gittelman(-Klein), R., 39, 46, 48, 80, 93, 127, 128, 166, 168, 281, 283, 349–351, 355, 356, 386, 387, 390 (418, n.13; 420, n.41, 57; 424, n.30; 426, n.39; 428, n.30; 433, n.50; 441, n.1; 446, n.2; 448, n.35; 449, n.36–38; 455, n.7, 8)

Gluck, D. S., 22, 30 (416, n.8)

Glueck, E., 86 (424, n.9)

Glueck, S., 86 (424, n.9)

Gohrer, R. E., 164 (431, n.21)

Gomez, R. L., 65, 82, 89 (423, n.10; 425, n.28)

Goodenough, D. R., 243 (440, n.20)

Goodman, R., 329, 368 (444, n.34; 454, n.25)

Goodwin, D. W., 65, 122, 123, 128, 187 (423, n.9; 427, n.12; 435, n.26)

Gorenstein, E. E., 340 (444, n.35)

Gorham, D. R., 69, 259 (423, n.2; 440, n.3)

Gottlieb, S., 378 (453, n.13)

Gouch, R. 166, 170 (432, n.42)

Gough, H., 69, 71 (423, n.21)

Graham, P., 13, 50 (416, n.61; 421, n.6)

Granger, D., 352 (452, n.88, 98)

Green, W. H., 361, 365 (449, n.40)

Greenberg, L., 163, 164 (431, n.13)

Greenberg, M. S., 402–403 (456, n.17)

Greenfield, B., 378 (453, n.13)

Greenhill, L. L., 9, 166, 169, 354–356, 358, 359 (414, n.38; 432, n.40; 433, n.49; 447, n.15; 448, n.30; 449, n.41–43)

Greenslade, K. E., 358 (450, n.61)

Greenspan, S. I., 89, 285 (425, n.29; 441, n.15)

Griffin, R. B., 165 (432, n.35)

Gross, M. B., 283 (441, n.7)

Gross, M. D., 167, 339, 355 (433, n.53; 446, n.80; 449, n.44)

Grünewald, G., 165 (432, n.31)

Grünewaid-Zuberbier, E., 165 (432, n.31)

Gualtieri, C. T., 401, 402 (455, n.9)

Guze, S. B., 65, 122, 123, 128, 187 (423, n.9; 427, n.12; 435, n.26)

Guzman, A., 10, 164 (415, n.42; 432, n.26)

Hacker, M., 233–236 (438, *n*.17)
Hagen, J., 151, 159, 243 (429, *n*.5; 440, *n*.25)
Hall, G. S., 50 (421, *n*.1)
Hall, R. A., 165 (432, *n*.35)
Hallahan, D. P., 5 (413, *n*.13)
Halverson, C. F., 10, 14 (415, *n*.44; 417, *n*.13)
Handen, B. L., 355 (448, *n*.29)
Harcherik, D. F., 365 (450, *n*.57)
Hardin, M. T., 363 (451, *n*.75)
Harper, L. V., 183 (434, *n*.10)
Harris, F., 48 (420, *n*.54)
Hastings, J. E., 10 (415, *n*.46)
Hauser, P., 335 (444, *n*.36)
Hawkins, R., 46 (419, *n*.35)
Hay, D., 330 (445, *n*.47)
Hays, M., 86, 121, (424, *n*.13; 427, *n*.9)
Hechtman, L., 8, 22, 66, 70, 79, 82, 93, 94, 97, 102, 104, 105, 129, 136, 140, 142, 144, 154, 155, 158, 169, 171, 172, 184, 189, 190, 203, 205, 221, 224, 257, 341, 352, 356, 386, 387 (414, *n*.32, 33; 416, *n*.5; 423, *n*.11–15, 23, 24; 426, *n*.40–45, 48, 49, 52, 53; 428, *n*.32, 34; 429, *n*.5–7; 430, *n*.16, 17, 20, 21; 433, *n*.61–63; 435, *n*.33, 34; 436, *n*.1, 2, 11; 440, *n*.1; 444, *n*.37; 449, *n*.47, 48; 456, *n*.21)
Heckman, H. K., 8, 63, 70, 82, 90, 92, 104, 105, 125, 126, 128, 140, 142, 148, 154, 180, 181 (414, *n*.34; 422, *n*.4; 425, *n*.33; 428, *n*.25; 429, *n*.3; 430, *n*.14; 434, *n*.1)
Heffron, W. A., 335 (444, *n*.38)
Heilman, K. M., 340 (444, *n*.39)
Helper, M. M., 239 (439, *n*.5)
Henke, L., 48 (420, *n*.54)
Henker, B., 44, 45, 121, 141, 256, 351, 352, 374, 375 (419, *n*.27, 28; 427, *n*.11; 440, *n*.29; 449, *n*.50; 452, *n*.97, 98; 453, *n*.17–19; 455, *n*.49)
Henriksen, L., 339, 342 (445, *n*.50)
Hermansen, L., 65, 122, 123, 128, 187 (423, *n*.9; 427, *n*.12; 435, *n*.26)
Hinshaw, S. P., 351, 374, 375 (449, *n*. 49, 50; 453, *n*.15, 17–20)
Hinton, G. G., 46, 165, 167 (419, *n*.39; 432, *n*.29)
Hogarty, G. E., 191 (435, *n*.36)
Hohman, L. B., 4 (413, *n*.5)
Hollingshead, A. B., 94, 151 (426, *n*.46; 429, *n*.3)

Hopkins, J., 8, 22, 66, 93, 154, 155 (414, *n*.32; 416, *n*.5; 423, *n*.11, 15; 426, *n*.41; 430, *n*.16)
Hopkins, K. H., 165 (432, *n*.35)
Hoppe, C. M., 57, 80, 85, 104, 105, 118, 236, 242, 381–382 (422, *n*.27; 424, *n*.7; 427, *n*.2; 438, *n*.24; 439, *n*.15; 454, *n*.41)
Hopwood, J., 163, 164 (431, *n*.43)
Hoy, E., 10, 41, 56, 151, 156, 159, 160, 164, 243 (415, *n*.42; 418, *n*.16; 422, *n*.23; 429, *n*.2; 432, *n*.26; 440, *n*.26)
Hoza, J. 358 (450, *n*.62)
Hudson, B., 12 (415, *n*.58)
Huessy, H. R., 52, 92, 104, 105, 118, 235, 285 (421, *n*.8; 426, *n*.37; 438, *n*.21; 441, *n*.12, 13)
Huey, L., 65, 82, 89 (423, *n*.10; 425, *n*.28)
Hughes, J. R., 170 (434, *n*.65)
Hughes, T., 325
Humphries, T., 183, 185, 232 (434, *n*.13; 438, *n*.14)
Hung, W., 166, 168 (432, *n*.43)
Hunt, R. D., 168, 342, 364, 365 (433, *n*.59; 444, *n*.41; 449, *n*.51, 52)

Ickowitz, A., 357 (451, *n*.89)
Insel, J., 237, 241 (436, *n*.26; 439, *n*.9)
Ismond, D. R., 37 (418, *n*.4)

Jackson, T. L., Jr., 163, 164 (431, *n*.17)
Janowsky, D, 65, 82, 89 (423, *n*.10; 425, *n*.28)
Jatlow, P., 168 (433, *n*.59)
Jellineck, M. S., 284 (441, *n*.10)
Johnson, G. E., 64, 65, 89, 123, 388, 401 (422, *n*.7; 425, *n*.25; 428, *n*.16; 456, *n*.27)
Johnson, N. E., 53, 57, 61, 84, 85, 120, 124, 142, 152, 225, 228, 231, 232, 237, 238 (421, *n*.15, 16; 422, *n*.2; 424, *n*.1, 2; 427, *n*.4; 429, *n*.4, 6, 7; 436, *n*.12; 437, *n*.4; 439, *n*.1)
Johnston, C., 26, 184, 185, 354 (417, *n*.16; 434, *n*.15, 17; 435, *n*.19; 449, *n*.53)
Joseph, A., 285 (442, *n*.16)
Joyce, S. A., 368 (454, *n*.40)

Kagan, J., 242 (440, *n*.19)
Kahn, E., 4 (413, *n*.7)
Kandel, H. I., 48 (420, *n*.51)

Kaplan, S. L., 351 (449, n.54)
Karp, S. A., 243 (440, n.20)
Katz, F., 48 (420, n.57)
Katz, M. M., 191 (435, n.36)
Keenan, K., 333, 334, 385 (442, n.10, 11; 455, n.4)
Kelman, H. R., 202 (435, n.37)
Kenny, T. J., 5, 12 (413, n.14; 415, n.58)
Kephart, N. C., 5 (413, n.12)
Keren, 164 (431, n.21)
Kessler, M. D., 331 (443, n.24)
Kilby, 27 (413, n.18)
King, R. A., 363 (451, n.75)
Kinsbourne, M., 183, 185, 232 (434, n.13; 438, n.14)
Klein, A. R., 37 (418, n.3)
Klein, D. F., 46, 48 (420 n.41, 57)
Kliewer, W., 352 (451, n.88)
Klinderfuss, G. H., 164 (431, n.24)
Klopper, J. H., 342 (446, n.71)
Klorman, R., 351 (450, n.56)
Klove, H., 168 (433, n.60)
Klovman, R., 283 (441, n.3)
Knights, R. M., 46, 165, 167 (419, n.39; 432, n.29)
Knobloch, H., 5, 10 (413, n.15)
Kohlberg, L., 94, 96, 97 (426, n.47)
Koon, R., 340 (443, n.20)
Korb, R. J., 163, 164 (431, n.18)
Korn, S., 237, 330 (438, n.29; 446, n.66)
Kosier, T., 63, 79, 80, 91, 101, 102, 104, 127, 140, 141, 181, 225–229, 233, 235–237, 242 (422, n.6; 425, n.34; 428, n.27; 434, n.3; 437, n.7, 15; 439, n.8)
Kovelowsky, C. J., 342 (446, n.68)
Krager, J. M., 348 (451, n.79)
Kramer, J., 86, 91, 105, 120, 121, 128, 221–223, 226–229, 232, 233, 235–237, 242 (424, n.10, 11; 425, n.36; 427, n.7, 8; 436, 1; 437, n.9, 18, 20; 438, n.16; 439, n.11; 440, n.5)
Krause, M., 86 (424, n.12)
Kringlen, E., 330 (446, n.75)
Kruger, E., 8, 27, 31, 46, 166, 171, 236, 237, 240, 352 (414, n.28; 417, n.19; 420, n.43; 433, n.47; 438, n.25; 439, n.7; 452, n.94)
Krynicki, V., 166 (432, n.41)
Kuperman, S., 363 (447, n.10)
Kupietz, S., 46, 350, 351 (419, n.31; 449, n.54; 450, n.56a)

Lacey, B. A., 26, 183, 185, 232 (417, n.15; 434, n.8; 438, n.11)
Lachman, R. 348 (448, n.26a)
Lahey, B. B., 202, 332 (435, n.38; 444, n.44)
Lambert, N. M., 12, 13, 21, 128 (415, n.50; 416, n.1; 428, n.31)
Lampl-de-Groot, J., 116 (427, n.3)
Landa, B., 355, 356 (449, n.37)
Landau, S., 27 (417, n.18)
Lang, G., 151, 156, 159, 243 (429, n.4; 440, n.24)
Lange, P. H., 164 (431, n.24)
Langford, W. S., 120, 121, 128 (427, n.6; 433, n.57)
Langhorne, J. E., 14, 58, 152, 153, 203, 233–236 (416, n.65; 422, n.29, 30; 430, n.11, 12; 436, n.41; 438, n.17, 19)
Laprade, K., 14 (416, n.67)
Lapey, 346 (443, n.12)
Lau, S., 364 (449, n.52)
Laufer, M. W., 6, 52, 90, 92, 104, 125, 126, 128, 140, 141, 163, 384 (414, n.22; 421, n.12, 13; 425, n.32; 428, n.24; 430, n.1; 456, n.13)
Lavigueur, H., 42, 43, 56, 85, 225, 226, 229 (419, n.22; 422, n.24; 424, n.4; 437, n.13)
Layman, D., 48 (420, n.51)
Leckman, J. F., 365 (450, n.57)
Leger, P., 355 (452, n.93)
Lehtinen L. E., 39 (418, n.11)
Lenneberg, E. H., 24 (417, n.12)
Leone, L., 188, 189 (435, n.29)
Levy, F., 330 (445, n.47)
Lesser, L. I., 163–166 (431, n.12)
Lewin, D., 42, 43, 56, 85 (419, n.22; 422, n.24; 424, n.4)
Lilienfeld, A., 5 (413, n.16)
Limbeck, G. A., 166, 170 (432, n.42)
Lindem, K. J., 402–403 (456, n.17)
Lipman, R. S., 47, 70, 71, 99, 166, 168, 243, 356 (420, n.50; 423, n.22; 426, n.50; 432 n.43; 440, n.23; 451, n.76)
Little, B. C., 163, 164 (431, n.15)
Lochman, J. E., 375 (453, n.24)
Loiselle, D. L., 224 (436, n.9)
Loney, J., 8, 14, 58, 63, 79, 80, 86, 91, 101, 102, 104, 105, 120, 121, 127, 128, 140, 141, 152, 153, 167, 181, 203, 221–223, 225–229, 231–237, 241, 242, 269, 339

(414, *n*.35; 416, *n*.65, 66; 422, *n*.6, 29, 30; 424, *n*.10, 11; 425, *n*.34, 36; 427, *n*.7, 8; 428, *n*.27; 430, *n*.11, 12; 433, *n*.58; 434, *n*.3; 436, *n*.1, 41; 437, *n*.7, 9, 15, 17, 18, 20; 438, *n*.16, 19, 27; 439, *n*.10, 11; 440, *n*.5, 18; 445, *n*.59)

Long, B., 243 (440, *n*.25)

Lopez, R. E., 10, 182, 329 (415, *n*.51; 434, *n*.6; 445, *n*.48)

Lord, I. M., 243 (440, *n*.28)

Lou, H. C., 339, 342 (445, *n*.50)

Ludlow, C., 4, 10, 11, 282 (413, *n*.10; 414, *n*.39; 441, *n*.3)

Mackay, M. C., 120, 121, 128, 167, 170, 282, 283 (427, *n*.6; 433, *n*.57; 441, *n*.4)

Mackeith, R., 6 (413, *n*.19)

Maitinsky, S., 224 (436, *n*.9)

Majovski, L. V., 166, 170 (432, *n*.42)

Mammato, C. A., 340 (444, *n*.35)

Mann, H. B., 89, 285 (425, *n*.29; 441, *n*.15)

Mannuzza, S., 80, 93, 127, 128, 356, 386, 387, (424, *n*.30; 426, *n*.39; 428, *n*.30; 449, *n*.38; 455, *n*.8)

Marks, R. E., 364 (447, *n*.3, 4)

Martin, C. A., 335 (444, *n*.38)

Martin, J. E., 41, 55, 66 (418, *n*.15; 421, *n*.21; 423, *n*.16)

Mash, E. J., 26, 184, 185 (417, *n*.16; 434, *n*.15, 17; 435, *n*.19)

Massey, B. H., 164 (431, *n*.22)

Mattes, J. M., 48, 89, 123, 124, 166, 168, 287, 289, 355, 356, 401 (420, *n*.57; 425, *n*.30; 428, *n*.17; 433, *n*.50; 442, *n*.21, 22; 449, *n*.37; 456, *n*.14)

Matthysse, S., 334 (443, *n*.22)

McBride, N., 123, 128 (428, *n*.15)

McBurnett, M., 332 (444, *n*.44)

McCraken, J. A., 342 (445, *n*.52)

McGee, R. O., 11, 14, 33 (414, *n*.25; 415, *n*.56; 416, *n*.69)

McHale, J. P., 375 (453, *n*.20)

McLaughlin, B., 24 (413, *n*.13)

McMahon, R. F., 189 (435, *n*.32)

McMahon, R. J., 369 (453, *n*.9)

McMurray, M. B., 345, 351, 353 (442, *n*.4, 5; 447, *n*.8, 9)

McNutt, B. A., 167 (433, *n*.51)

Mead, M., 50 (421, *n*.2)

Meichenbaum, D., 368 (454, *n*.25)

Mellsop, G. W., 235 (438, *n*.22)

Mendelson, N., 55–57, 85, 225, 227, 231, 234–240 (421, *n*.20; 424, *n*.5; 437, *n*.6, 14; 439, *n*.2)

Mendelson, W. B., 53, 57, 61, 84, 85, 120, 121, 142, 152, 225, 228, 231, 232, 237, 238 (421, *n*.15, 16; 422, *n*.2; 424, *n*.1, 2; 427, *n*.4; 429, *n*.4, 6, 7; 436, *n*.12; 437, *n*.4; 439, *n*.1)

Menkes, J. H., 62, 63, 81, 82, 90, 104, 142, 189, 223, 224, 226, 237, 239 (422, *n*.3; 425, *n*.31; 429, *n*.1; 435, *n*.35; 436, *n*.6; 438, *n*.28; 439, *n*.6)

Metrakos, K., 93, 172, 224 (426, *n*.44; 433, *n*.63; 436, *n*.11)

Mikkelsen, E. J., 4, 10, 11, 282 (413, *n*.10; 414, *n*.39; 441, *n*.3)

Milich, R. S., 8, 27, 86, 105, 120, 221–223, 226–229, 233, 235–237, 241, 269, 369, 374 (414, *n*.35; 417, *n*.18; 424, *n*.11; 427, *n*.8; 436, *n*.1; 438, *n*.16; 439, *n*.11; 440, *n*.5; 452, *n*.6; 454, *n*.26)

Miller, R. G., 13 (416, *n*.62)

Millichap, J. G., 167 (433, *n*.54)

Millichap, M., 167 (433, *n*.54)

Milman, D. H., 93, 104, 105, 126, 128, 140, 141, 154, 158, 223, 225, 226, 235–237, 269 (426, *n*.38; 428, *n*.26; 430, *n*.15; 436, *n*.5; 438, *n*.20; 440, *n*.4)

Milman, M., 8 (414, *n*.26)

Milroy, T., 70, 82, 97, 102, 158, 386, 387 (423, *n*.24; 426, *n*.48; 430, *n*.20; 456, *n*.21)

Milstein, V., 165, 173 (432, *n*.36; 434, *n*.64)

Minde, K. K., 10, 38, 41–43, 46, 55–57, 61, 66, 85, 118, 150, 151, 156, 159, 160, 164, 202, 224–229, 231, 233–240, 243, 386 (415, *n*.42; 418, *n*.6, 9, 16; 419, *n*.22, 34; 421, *n*.19, 20, 22; 422, *n*.1, 24, 25; 423, *n*.17; 424, *n*.3, 4, 5; 427, *n*.1; 429, *n*.1, 2; 432, *n*.6; 436, *n*.8, 40; 437, *n*. 5, 6, 13, 14; 439, *n*.2; 440, *n*.26; 456, *n*.22)

Minkoff, K., 89 (425, *n*.27)

Mirsky, A. F., 38, 336, 391 (418, *n*.10; 445, *n*.53; 456, *n*.15)

Mitleman, D., 335 (443, *n*.21)

Mittelman, M., 237 (438, *n*.29)

Molling, P., 348 (448, *n*.26a)

Montagu, J. D., 163, 164 (431, *n*.14)

Morgenstern, G., 28, 38, 40, 46 (417, *n*.20; 418, *n*.8, 14)

Morrison, J. L, 331, 332, 334 (445, *n*.54–57)

Morrison, J. R., 10, 87–89, 117, 122, 124, 125, 186–189 (415, *n*.49; 425, *n*.17, 19, 21–23, 27; 427, *n*.7; 428, *n*.14, 18, 22; 435, *n*.20, 23–25, 27, 31; 437, *n*.1)

Morton, P., 48 (420, *n*.58)

Moyer, D. L., 165 (432, *n*.35)

Murphy, D. L., 360, 362 (452, *n*.101)

Murphy, H. A., 367, 369 (454, *n*. 35, 38)

Murray, J. M., 116 (427, *n*.4)

Nadeau, S. E., 340 (444, *n*.39)

Nahas, A. D., 166 (432, *n*.41)

Nasrallah, H. A., 339 (445, *n*.59)

Nemeth, E., 38, 55–57, 61, 85, 118, 150, 224, 226–229, 386 (418, *n*.6; 421, *n*.19; 422, *n*.1; 424, *n*.3; 427, *n*.1; 429, *n*.1; 436, *n*.8; 456, *n*.22)

Neumann, A., 46 (420, *n*.45)

Newcorn, J., 357 (447, *n*.14)

Nichamin, S. J., 22, 23 (416, *n*.6)

Nichols, P., 10 (415, *n*.41)

Niedermeyer, E. F., 164, 165 (431, *n*.23)

Nolan, E. E., 351 (448, *n*.33)

Nordahl, T. E., 339 (446, *n*.80)

Novacenko, H., 356, 359 (449, *n*.43)

Noyes, R., 363 (447, *n*.10)

O'Connell, P., 364, 365 (449, *n*.51)

Oettinger, L., 166, 170, 283 (432, *n*.42; 441, *n*.6)

Offer, D., 50 (421, *n*.4, 5)

Offord, D. R., 125 (428, *n*.23)

O'Leary, J., 164 (431, *n*.24)

O'Leary, K., 48 (420, *n*.56)

O'Leary, S. G., 368 (454, *n*.40; 455, *n*.46)

Oliver, H., 89, 123, 124, 287, 401 (425, *n*.30; 428, *n*.17; 442, *n*.21; 456, *n*.14)

Omenn, G. S., 334 (445, *n*.61)

Ondrusek, M. G., 401, 402 (455, *n*.9)

O'Neill, I., 240 (439, *n*.8)

O'Neill, M. E., 349 (448, *n*.25)

Olsen, S. C., 339 (445, *n*.59)

Overall, J. E., 69, 166, 168, 259, 356 (423, *n*.20; 432, *n*.43; 440, *n*.3; 451, *n*.76)

Overall, P. E., 47 (420, *n*.50)

Palkes, H. S., 13, 182 (416, *n*.62; 434, *n*.5)

Pappas, B. A., 10 (415, *n*.45)

Parker, J. B., Jr., 164 (431, *n*.25)

Parker, J. G., 374 (454, *n*.30)

Parry, P., 42, 48 (418, *n*.20; 420, *n*.58)

Pasamanick, B., 5, 10 (413, *n*.15, 16)

Paternite, C. E., 14, 58, 152, 153, 203, 233–236 (416, *n*.65; 422, *n*.29; 422, *n*.30; 430, *n*.12; 436, *n*.41; 438, *n*.17, 19)

Patterson, G. R., 369 (454, *n*.31)

Paulauskas, S. L., 44 (419, *n*.25)

Pauls, D. L., 334 (445, *n*.62)

Pelham, W. E., 27, 45, 48, 358, 368, 369 (417, *n*.17; 419, *n*.29; 420, *n*.56; 450, *n*.61, 62; 452, *n*.6; 454, *n*.34, 35)

Pennington, B. F., 330 (444, *n*.31, 32)

Perlman, T., 8, 22, 66, 70, 79, 82, 93, 102, 105, 129, 140, 142, 144, 154, 155, 158, 169, 171, 172, 205, 221, 257, 352, 356, 386, 387 (414, *n*.32, 33; 416, *n*.5; 423, *n*.11, 13–15, 23, 24; 426, *n*.40–43, 48, 52, 53; 428, *n*.32; 429, *n*.5–7; 430, *n*.16, 17, 20; 433, *n*.61, 62; 436, *n*. 1, 2; 440, *n*.1; 449, *n*.47, 48; 456, *n*.21)

Peters, J. E., 6, 56, 85, 152, 163, 222, 226, 227, 239, 241 (413, *n*.17; 419, *n*.23; 422, *n*.26; 424, *n*.6; 429, *n*.8; 430, *n*.5; 436, *n*.4; 399, *n*.4)

Peters, K. G., 42 (418, *n*.19)

Peterson, D. R., 238 (439, *n*.3)

Phillips, W., 242 (440, *n*.19)

Piacentini, J., 332 (444, *n*.44)

Pierce, R., 168 (433, *n*.59)

Pihl, R. F., 48 (419, *n*.53)

Platt, J. J., 156 (430, *n*.19)

Pliszka, S. R., 357 (445, *n*.63; 450, *n*.65, 66)

Plymate, H. B., 52 (421, *n*.14)

Pollack, E., 48 (420, *n*.57)

Porges, S. W., 163, 164 (431, *n*.18, 21)

Porrino, C. J., 37 (418, *n*.4)

Porrino, L. J., 350 (450, *n*.67, 68)

Pososim, R. L., 163–166 (431, *n*.12)

Price, G., 48 (420, *n*.56)

Price, J. M., 375 (454, *n*.37)

Puig-Antich, J., 166, 169, 356 (432, *n*.40; 433, *n*.49; 449, *n*.42, 43)

Quay, H. C., 14, 238 (416, *n*.63; 439, *n*.3)

Quinlan, B., 57, 67, 79, 102 (422, *n*.28; 423, *n*.18; 426, *n*.51)

Quinn, P. O., 10, 165, 166 (415, *n*.43; 432, *n*.38; 433, *n*.48)

Quinn, S. O., 349, 350 (450, *n*.71)

Radosh, A., 39 (418, *n.*13)

Rafferty, F., 86 (424, *n.*12)

Rapoport, J. L., 4, 8, 10, 11, 37, 46, 163, 165, 166, 222, 226, 228, 241, 282, 336, 341, 343, 349, 350, 354, 360, 362 (413, *n.*10; 414, *n.*29, 39; 415, *n.*43; 418, *n.*4; 420, *n.*44; 431, *n.*10; 432, *n.*35, 38; 433, *n.*48; 436, *n.*3; 439, *n.*12; 441, *n.*3; 446, *n.*81, 82; 448, *n.*27; 450, *n.*67–69; 452, *n.*101)

Rapport, M. D., 349–351, 367 (450, *n.*70, 71; 451, *n.*72, 73; 454, *n.*38)

Rasche, A., 165 (432, *n.*31)

Rasmussen, P., 11, 12 (415, *n.*54)

Ratey, J. J., 393–394, 402–403 (456, *n.*16, 17)

Redlich, F. C., 94, 151 (426, *n.*46; 429, *n.*3)

Reimherr, F. W., 64, 65, 89, 122, 123, 128, 285, 388, 401 (422, *n.*7; 425, *n.*25; 428, *n.*13, 16; 442, *n.*17, 18; 456, *n.*18, 24–27)

Reynard, C. L., 46 (420, *n.*47)

Reynolds, N., 48 (420, *n.*54)

Richardson, E., 350 (450, *n.*56a)

Richardson, F., 164, 165 (431, *n.*23)

Riddle, K. D., 8, 22, 46, 226, 228, 241 (414, *n.*29; 420, *n.*44; 436, *n.*3; 439, *n.*12)

Riddle, M. A., 363 (451, *n.*75)

Riester, A., 64, 65, 89 (422, *n.*8; 425, *n.*26)

Ringdahl, I., 167 (433, *n.*56)

Rivera, R., 86 (424, *n.*12)

Robins, A. J., 33 (417, *n.*25)

Robins, E., 286 (442, *n.*19)

Robins, L. N., 44, 86, 136, 228, 236 (419, *n.*26; 424, *n.*8; 427, *n.*33; 437, *n.*19; 438, *n.*23)

Roche, A. F., 47, 166–168, 356 (420, *n.*50; 432, *n.*43; 433, *n.*56; 451, *n.*76)

Roeltgen, D., 342 (445, *n.*64)

Rogers, M. E., 5 (413, *n.*16)

Rolfe, U. T., 24 (417, *n.*12)

Rood, P., 285 (441, *n.*13)

Rosen, L. A., 368 (454, *n.*64)

Rosenbaum, A., 48 (420, *n.*56)

Rosenthal, R. H., 39 (418, *n.*12)

Rosman, B. L., 242 (440, *n.*19)

Ross, D. M., 3, 7, 8 (413, *n.*3)

Ross, S. A., 3, 7, 8 (413, *n.*3)

Rosvold, H. E., 38 (418, *n.*10)

Rothchild, G., 46 (419, *n.*36)

Rowe, J. S., 62, 63, 81, 82, 90, 104, 142, 189, 223, 224, 226, 237, 239 (422, *n.*3; 425,

*n.*31; 429, *n.*1; 435, *n.*35; 436, *n.*6; 438, *n.*28; 439, *n.*6)

Rutter, M., 11–14, 21, 36, 50, 57, 67, 79, 102, 330 (415, *n.*55, 57; 416, *n.*2, 61; 417, *n.*36; 421, *n.*50; 422, *n.*28; 423, *n.*18, 19; 426, *n.*51; 446, *n.*66)

Ryu, J., 364 (449, *n.*52)

Sachar, E. J., 166, 169 (432, *n.*40; 433, *n.*49)

Sachdev, K., 165, 173 (432, *n.*36; 434, *n.*64)

Safer, D. J., 3, 47, 48, 166, 168, 182, 282, 283, 331, 348, 355 (413, *n.*1; 420, *n.*49, 55; 432, *n.*44, 45; 433, *n.*46; 434, *n.*7; 441, *n.*5; 446, *n.*67; 451, *n.*78, 79)

Salzman, L. F., 351 (450, *n.*56)

Sams, S. E., 368 (454, *n.*34)

Sandoval, J., 12, 13, 21 (415, *n.*59; 321, *n.*1)

Sandy, J. M., 340 (444, *n.*35)

Sarason, I., 38 (321, *n.*10)

Sassin, J., 166, 169 (432, *n.*40; 433, *n.*49)

Sassone, D., 12, 13, 21 (415, *n.*59; 416, *n.*1)

Satterfield, B. T., 49, 153, 161, 242, 381–382 (420, *n.*60; 430, *n.*13; 439, *n.*16; 455, *n.*42, 43)

Satterfield, J. H., 42, 49, 57, 80, 85, 104, 105, 118, 153, 161, 163–168, 173, 178, 179, 224, 236, 242, 356, 381–382 (418, *n.*21; 420, *n.*60; 422, *n.*27; 424, *n.*7, 29; 427, *n.*2; 430, *n.*13; 431, *n.*7, 12; 432, *n.*30, 33; 433, *n.*55; 436, *n.*7; 438, *n.*24; 439, *n.*15, 16; 451, *n.*80; 454, *n.*41; 455, *n.*42, 43)

Saul, R. E., 165, 173, 179 (432, *n.*30)

Sceery, W., 37 (418, *n.*4)

Schachar, R., 11–14, 21, 67, 79, 340, 350, 357 (415, *n.*55; 416, *n.*2; 423, *n.* 19; 446, *n.*74; 452, *n.*90, 91)

Schain, R., 8, 46 (414, *n.*31; 420, *n.*48)

Schell, A. M., 57, 80, 85, 104, 105, 167, 168, 236, 242, 356, 381–382 (422, *n.*27; 424, *n.*55; 438, *n.*24; 439, *n.*15; 451, *n.*80; 454, *n.*41, 43)

Schleifer, M., 27, 31 (417, *n.*19)

Schneider, D. U., 123, 128 (428, *n.*15)

Schneider, J. S., 342 (445, *n.*64; 446, *n.*68)

Schulsinger, F., 65, 122, 123, 128, 187 (423, *n.*9; 427, *n.*12; 435, *n.*16)

Scoot, J., 163, 164 (431, *n.*13)

Shaffer, D., 9 (414, *n.*38)

Sharpe, L., 46, 275 (419, *n.*37; 441, *n.*1)

Shaywitz, B. A., 10, 11, 168, 338, 342 (415, n.48, 52; 433, n.59; 446, n.69–71)

Shaywitz, S. E., 10, 11, 168, 338, 342 (415, n.48, 52; 433, n.59; 446, n.70)

Shekim, W. O., 11 (415, n.53)

Shelley, E. M., 64, 65, 89 (422, n.8; 425, n.26)

* Shenker, R., 80, 93, 127, 128, 386, 387 (424, n.30; 426, n.39; 428, n.30; 455, n.8)

Shetty, T., 165 (432, n.32, 39)

Silva, P. A., 11, 14, 33 (415, n.56; 416, n.9; 417, n.25)

Simon, B., 237 (438, n.27)

Simpson, S., 163, 164 (431, n.16)

Singer, S., 14, 124, 188, 189, 231, 232 (416, n.68; 428, n.21; 435, n.30; 437, n.3)

Sivage, A. C., 48 (420, n.59)

Sleator, E. K., 8, 46, 164, 349 (414, n.27; 420, n.42, 45; 431, n.22; 451, n.87)

Sloman, L., 240 (439, n.8)

Smith, A., 11–14, 21, 67, 79 (415, n.55; 416, n.2; 423, n.19)

Smith, H. L., 378 (455, n.44)

Smith, L. H., 4 (418, n.8)

Smith, M. D., 151, 159, 243 (429, n.5; 440, n.25)

Smith, R. S., 10, 11, 21, 152, 234 (414, n.40; 416, n.3; 430, n.9; 438, n.18)

Solanto, M. V., 350 (451, n.86)

Solomons, S., 163 (430, n.1)

Sonies, B. C., 164 (431, n.20)

Spitzer, R. L., 71, 72, 91, 97, 99, 108, 127, 225, 228, 232, 243, 286 (423, n.26; 425, n.35; 426, n.1; 428, n.29; 437, n.8, 16; 440, n.22; 442, n.19)

Spivack, G., 156 (430, n.19)

Sprague, R. L., 8, 46, 163, 164, 286, 349 (414, n.27, 36; 419, n.38; 420, n.42, 45; 431, n.18, 22; 442, n.20; 451, n.87)

Sprich, S., 357 (447, n.14)

Spring, C., 163, 164 (431, n.13)

Sroufe, L. A., 164 (431, n.20)

Stamm, J. S., 224 (436, n.9)

Stapp, J., 45 (419, n.28)

Stein, R. M., 46, 241 (420, n.47; 439, n.14)

Stevens, J. R., 165, 173 (432, n.36; 434, n.64)

Stevenson, J., 329, 330 (444, n.34; 446, n.72)

Stewart, M. A., 10, 13, 14, 53, 57, 61, 84, 85, 88, 117, 120, 121, 124, 125, 128, 142, 152, 182, 186–189, 225, 228, 230–232, 237, 238, 331–334 (415, n.49; 416, n.62, 68; 421, n.15, 16; 422, n.2; 424, n.1, 2; 425, n.17, 19, 20; 427, n. 4, 7; 428, n.18, 20, 21; 429, n.4, 6, 7; 434, n.5; 435, n.20, 23–25, 27–30; 436, n.12; 437, n.1, 3, 4; 439, n.1; 443, n.17; 445, n.55–57; 446, n.78)

Still, G. G., 4 (413, n.4)

Stoa, K. F., 168 (433, n.60)

Stoner, G., 349 (451, n.72, 73)

Strauss, A. A., 5, 39 (413, n.12; 418, n.11)

Strobl, D., 284 (441, n.11)

Stroop, J. R., 243 (440, n.21)

Sturges, J., 358 (450, n.62)

Sullivan, M. A., 368 (455, n.46)

Sullivan, N., 125 (428, n.23)

Sum, G., 120, 121, 128, 167, 170 (427, n.6; 433, n.57)

Sverd, J., 351 (448, n.33)

Swanson, J., 183, 185, 232, 334, 352 (434, n.13; 438, n.14; 443, n.22; 451, n.88)

Sykes, D. H., 38, 42, 43, 46, 55, 66 (418, n.8, 9; 419, n.22, 34; 421, n.22; 423, n.17)

Sykes, E., 56, 85, 225, 226, 229 (422, n.24; 424, n.4; 437, n.13)

Szumowski, E. K., 22, 30 (416, n.8, 9)

Tallmadge, J., 185 (435, n.18)

Tannock, R., 340, 350, 351, 357 (446, n.74; 451, n. 89; 452, n.90, 91)

Tarter, R. E., 123, 128 (428, n.15)

Taylor, R., 282, 283 (441, n.4)

Thomas, A., 237 (438, n.29)

Thomas, J., 167, 340 (433, n.56; 443, n.27)

Thorsen, T., 168 (433, n.60)

Tobias, J., 46 (419, n.31)

Torgerson, A. M., 330 (446, n.75)

Torres, D., 354 (448, n.30)

Townsend, M., 92, 104, 105, 235 (426, n.37; 438, n.21)

Trites, R. L., 8, 14, 46, 48, 54, 82, 87, 119–121, 163, 164, 241, 255 (414, n.30; 416, n.67; 420, n.46, 52; 421, n.17; 423, n.28; 424, n.15; 427, n.3; 431, n.16; 439, n.13)

Tuck, D., 8, 70, 105, 144, 205 (414, n.33; 423, n.23; 426, n.52; 429, n.6, 7; 436, n.1)

Turbott, S. H., 364 (447, n.3, 4)

Varley, C., 283, 355 (441, *n*.8; 452, *n*.93)
Vincent, J., 355 (452, *n*.93)
Vitiello, B., 335 (444, *n*.39)
Vodde-Hamilton, M., 358 (450, *n*.61)
Voeller, K. S., 340 (444, *n*.39)
Von Neumann, A., 8 (414, *n*.27)

Waldrop, M. F., 10, 24 (415, *n*.44; 417, *n*.13)
Walter, G. F., 163, 164 (431, *n*.18)
Ward, M. A., 388, 401 (456, *n*.26)
Weinberg, W. A., 43, 164 (419, *n*.23; 431, *n*.24)
Weingartner, H., 4, 10, 11, 282, 354 (413, *n*.10; 414, *n*.39; 441, *n*.3; 450, *n*.69)
Weisenberg, A., 284 (441, *n*.11)
Weiss, G., 8, 10, 22, 23, 27, 31, 38, 41, 46, 55–57, 61, 66, 70, 79, 82, 85, 93, 97, 102, 104, 105, 118, 129, 136, 140, 142, 144, 150, 151, 154–156, 158–160, 164, 166, 169, 171, 172, 189, 190, 203, 205, 221, 224–229, 231, 233–240, 243, 257, 282, 322, 323, 325, 352, 356, 378, 386, 387 (414, *n*.28, 32, 33; 415, *n*.42; 416, *n*.4, 5, 7; 417, *n*.19; 418, *n*.6, 9, 16; 419, *n*.34; 420, *n*.43; 421, n19–22; 422, *n*.1, 23–25; 423, *n*.11–15, 17, 23, 24; 424, *n*.3–5; 426, *n*.40–44, 48, 49, 52, 53; 427, *n*.1; 428, *n*.32, 34; 429, *n*.1, 2, 5–7; 430, *n*.16, 17, 20, 21; 432, *n*.26; 433, *n*.47, 61–63; 435, *n*.34; 436, *n*.2, 8, 11; 437, *n*.5, 6, 13, 14; 438, *n*.25; 439, *n*.2, 7; 440, *n*.1, 26; 441, *n*.2; 449, *n*.47, 48; 452, *n*.94; 453, *n*.13; 456, *n*.21, 22)
Welner, A., 182 (434, *n*.5)
Welner, H., 331 (446, *n*.78)
Welner, Z., 182, 331 (434, *n*.5; 446, *n*.78)
Welsh, R. J., 335 (444, *n*.38)
Wender, P. H., 4, 41, 64, 65, 88, 89, 122, 123, 128, 163–165, 240, 285, 350, 378, 388–390, 392 (413, *n*.11; 418, *n*.17; 422, *n*.7; 425, *n*.24, 25; 428, *n*.13, 16; 430, *n*.4; 431, *n*.8, 15; 432, *n*.34; 439, *n*.8; 442, *n*.17, 18; 451, *n*.86; 455, *n*.48; 456, *n*.18, 23–27)
Wener, A., 8, 22, 66, 154, 155, 189, 190, 203 (414, *n*.32; 416, *n*.5; 423, *n*.11; 430, *n*.16; 435 *n*.34)
Werner, E. E., 10, 11, 21, 152, 234 (414, *n*.40; 416, *n*.3; 430, *n*.9; 437, *n*.18)

Werry, J. S., 10, 22, 23, 38, 46, 55–57, 61, 66, 85, 118, 150, 163, 164, 224, 226–229, 231, 233–236, 286, 386 (415, *n*.42; 416, *n*.7; 418, *n*.6; 419, *n*.34, 38; 421, *n*.19, 21, 22; 422, *n*.1; 423, *n*.16, 17; 424, *n*.3; 427, *n*.1; 429, *n*.1; 431, *n*.6; 432, *n*.26; 436, *n*.8; 437, *n*.5; 442, *n*.20; 456, *n*.22)
West, W. D., 164 (431, *n*.20)
Whalen, C. K., 44, 45, 121, 141, 256, 351, 352, 374 (419, *n*.27, 28; 427, *n*.11; 440, *n*.29; 449, *n*.50; 452, *n*.96–98; 453, *n*.17–19; 455, *n*.49)
Whaley-Klahn, M. A., 63, 79, 80, 91, 101, 102, 104, 127, 140, 141, 167, 181, 225–229, 231–237, 242 (422, *n*.6; 425, *n*.34; 425, *n*.36; 428, *n*.27; 433, *n*.58; 434, *n*.3; 437, *n*.7, 9, 15, 20; 438, *n*.17; 440, *n*.18)
Whillen, P., 27 (417, *n*.18)
White, J., 224 (436, *n*.10)
Wikler, A., 164 (431, *n*.25)
Wilens, T. E., 348, 349, 356 (452, *n*.99)
Wilkin, H. A., 243 (440, *n*.20)
Willerman, L., 330 (446, *n*.79)
Williams, S. M., 11, 14, 33 (415, *n*.56; 416, *n*.69; 417, *n*.25)
Wilson, W. C., 283 (441, *n*.7)
Winnicott, D. W., 25, 276 (417, *n*.14; 441, *n*.2)
Winokur, G., 65, 122, 123, 128, 187 (423, *n*.9; 427, *n*.12; 435, *n*.26)
Winsberg, B., 46, 350 (419, *n*.31; 450, *n*.56a)
Winters, L., 358 (447, *n*.11)
Wish, E., 182 (434, *n*.5)
Wolff, P. H., 23 (417, *n*.10)
Wood, D. R., 64, 65, 89, 122, 123, 128, 285, 388, 401 (422, *n*.7; 425, *n*.25; 428, *n*.13, 16; 442, *n*.17, 18; 456, *n*.18, 25–27)
Wright, F. S., 164 (431, *n*.20)
Wright, V., 346 (442, *n*.9)

Yager, R. D., 342 (446, *n*.71)
Yule, B., 57, 67, 79, 102 (422, *n*.28; 423, *n*.18; 426, *n*.51)
Yule, W., 13, 50 (416, *n*.61; 421, *n*.6)
Yusin, A., 165, 173, 179 (432, *n*.30)
Young, J. G., 168 (433, *n*.59)
Young, R. D., 37 (418, *n*.3)

Zahn, T. P., 4, 10, 11, 163, 164, 282 (413, *n*.10; 414, *n*.39; 431, *n*.15; 441, *n*.3)

Zambelli, A. J., 224 (431, *n*.9)

Zametkin, A. J., 335, 336, 339–341, 343, 360, 362 (444, *n*.36; 446, *n*.80–82; 452; *n*.100, 101)

Zeitin, M., 65, 82, 89 (423, *n*.10; 425, *n*.28)

Zentall, S. S., 163 (431, *n*.9)

Ziller, R. C., 151, 159, 243 (429, *n*.5; 440, *n*.25)

SUBJECT INDEX

Academic performance, 68, 246, 318, 349, 376–377
  initial, 228–229
Actometer readings, 13, 30, 37
ADD(H), *see* Attention Deficit Disorder with Hyperactivity
Adolescence, 38, 50–58, 321, 384, 385, 386
  stimulant therapy, 281–284
Adolescent outcome studies, 84–87, 352
Adoptees, 64–65, 88, 122, 186–187, 331–332
Adult Brain Dysfunction (ABD), 285
Adulthood, 59–218
  ADHD in, 301–325, 384–406, 411
  stimulant therapy, 284–289
Affection, craving for, 320
Aggression, 29, 95, 99, 111, 188, 210, 227, 248, 269, 351, 375
Alcohol offenses, 87
Alcohol usage, 54, 118–141, 248–253, 265–266
Alcoholism, 54, 65, 88, 186–189, 225–226, 232
Amitriptyline, 285, 286
Antipsychotic agents, 363–364
Antisocial behavior, 56–58, 80, 84–106, 214–218, 407
Antisocial Personality Disorder, 74, 77, 82, 88–90, 332, 333–334, 386
  criteria, 91
  diagnosis, 100–101
Anxiety, 32, 329, 334
  generalized, 399–400
  stimulant treatment, 346, 357
Appearance, 24–25
Area Test, 156, 157, 160
Arrests, 57–58, 85–86, 89, 236
Assessment 15–17
  referrals for, 27, 35
Association Deficit Pathology, 52
Attention, 336, 388, 391–392
  brain areas, 336–337
  difficulties, 37–39
  selective, 38

Attention Deficit Disorder (ADD), 324, 345–346
Attention Deficit Disorder with Hyperactivity (ADD[H]), 7, 37
  adult, 286
  operational criteria for diagnosis, 16, 286
  Residual Type, 387
  Utah Criteria, 286, 287
Attention-Deficit Hyperactivity Disorder (ADHD)
  in adults, 301–325, 384–406, 411
  comorbidity in, 329, 332, 345–347, 357, 358, 364, 365, 386, 400
  with Conduct Disorder, 332–334
  hypotheses, 338–345
  neuroanatomical studies, 338–341
  treatment, *see* Behavior modification; Stimulants
Autonomic measures, 163–164

Babbling, 24
Barbiturates, 134–135, 251
Behavior modification, 48, 49, 366–369
Behavioral rebound, 354
Beliefs, 107–117
Benzedrine, 4, 46
Bipolar Affective Disorder, 187
Borderline Personality Disorder, 399
BPRS, *see* Brief Psychiatric Rating Scale
Brain damage, 4, 5
Brief Psychiatric Rating Scale (BPRS), 259, 260
Briquet's Syndrome (hysteria), 188
Bupropion hydrochloride, 363, 400, 402, 404

California Psychological Inventory (CPI), 69, 70, 77, 80
Car accidents, 68, 206, 211, 215, 246, 264, 265, 269

Cardiovascular effects, 356–357, 362
Catecholamine hypothesis, 343
Central nervous system (CNS)
  abnormality, 222–224
  underarousal, 163
Cerebral dysfunction, 11
Character disorder, 65
Child-rearing practices, 193, 194
Chlorpromazine, 46, 294, 297
Classroom behavior, 351
Clonidine, 364–365
CNS, see Central nervous system
Cocaine, 134, 251, 267, 268
Cognitive–behavioral strategies, 368–
  370, 375
Colic, 23
Concurrent validity, 9–12
Conduct Disorder, 329, 332–334, 346, 364,
  365
Contingency management, 367–368
Continuous Performance Test (CPT), 29,
  38, 39, 41, 393
Counseling, 238–240
Court records, 79, 86, 87, 94, 95, 98, 101,
  102, 269
CPI, see California Psychological Inven-
  tory
CPT, see Continuous Performance Test
Crime and Punishment Survey (CAPS),
  91, 92
Crying, 23
Cuddling, 25
Cylert, see Pemoline

DALST, see Draw a Line Slowly Test
Davidson and Lang Checklist, 156, 157,
  160, 161
Debts, 244
Depression, 36, 43, 44, 215, 320, 324, 329,
  399
Desipramine, 284, 346–347, 362, 403, 411
Developmental Hyperactivity, 6
Developmental Lag, 93
Dexedrine, see Dextroamphetamine
Dextroamphetamine, 45, 47, 167, 168,
  285, 358–361, 365, 404
Diagnosis, 22
  clinical aspects, 15–17
  differential, 398–400
  DSM-III, see DSM-III diagnosis

Diagnostic criteria scales, 103, 104
Difficult infant, 25, 26
Disruptive behavior, 37
Distractibility, 39
Dopamine D_2 receptor gene, 335
Dopamine hypothesis, 342
Draw a Line Slowly Test (DALST), 28–30
Drug holidays, 356
Drug offenses, 86
Drug selling, 139
Drug treatment 240–242, 400–404, 411
Drug use, 129–135, 137–139, 181, 288, 357
DSM-III diagnosis, 7, 12, 55, 74–79, 387,
  408
  Attention Deficit Disorder with Hyper-
    activity (ADD[H]), 7, 16, 37, 387
  impulsivity, 40

Early Childhood Matching Familiar Fig-
  ures Test (ECMFFT), 28–30
ECMFFT, see Early Childhood Matching
  Familiar Figures Test
EEG, see Electroencephalogram
EFT, see Embedded Figures Test
Ego ideal, 107, 116–117
Ego identity, 51
Electroencephalogram (EEG), 5, 164–166,
  172–179, 224
Elementary school, 35–49
Embarrassment 297–299
Embedded Figures Test (EFT), 28–30, 40
Employers' Rating Scale, 144, 145
Encephalitis lethargica, 4
Epigenetic stage theory, 51
External values, 111–113

Failed socialization, 117, 318–319
Families of hyperactives, 87, 88, 124–125,
  180–204, 214
  assessment of, 199–203
  child-rearing practices, 232–234
  emotional climate, 194, 320
  health of, 193, 194
  long-term follow-up, 189–204
  mental health, 230–233, 269
  overall functioning, 236–237
  parental control, 233, 234
  parental psychopathology, 231, 232,
    332–334
  parental short temper, 231, 232

retrospective ratings, 195, 200, 201
socioeconomic status, 234–236, 269
substance abuse, 333
Feeding difficulties, 24
Feeling different, 297–299, 410
Field independence, 28–30, 40
Fluoxetine hydrochloride, 363, 404
Follow-back studies, 62, 64–66
Free-play period, 28
Friends, 68, 206, 210, 214
Frontal lobe dysfunction, 340

Generalized Anxiety Disorder, 399–400
Generalized resistance to thyroid
    hormone (GRTH), 335
Genetic studies, 329–336, 385, 411
Global Assessment Scale (GAS), 99, 100
Glucose metabolism tests, 339–340
Good-enough mother, 25, 26
Growth suppression, 47, 166–169, 283,
    355–356

Hallucinogens, 133, 267, 268
Hashish, 133, 250, 267, 268
Height, 166–169
Heroin, 134, 251
Home token economy system, 372
Hyperactive–aggressive children, 13
Hyperactivity
    core features, 407
    developmental aspects, 21–58
    initial measures, 226, 227
    measures, 13, 30
    operational criteria, 16
    overview, 3–17
    pervasive, 12–15, 21
    referrals for, 27, 35
    situational, 12–15, 28–30
    symptoms, 9–15
    treatment issues, 273–289
    true, 28–30
Hyperkinetic Impulse Disorder, 6
Hypomania, 399
Hysteria, 88, 187–189

Ideal fantasy person, 111
Imipramine, 167, 285, 286
Impaired Interpersonal Relationships, 91
Impulsivity, 16, 40, 41, 56, 351, 388,
    392–393
Inattention, 16

Industry, 51
Infancy, 21–26
Institutionalization for delinquency, 57,
    86
Intelligence, 72, 223–226, 269
IQ, see Intelligence
Isolated cubicles, 5, 7, 39

Job changes, 143, 148, 209, 210

Katz Scale of Psychopathology, 191, 195,
    198

L-Dopa, 168
L-Tyrosine, 400, 402
Life-styles, 205–218
Living arrangements, 244
Loss of subjects, 66, 67, 79, 102

Major Depression, 334
Mandrax, 134, 135
Marijuana, 133, 250, 267, 268
Matching Familiar Figures Test (MFFT), 41
Maternal behavior, 183–186
Maturation, 296
Maturational lag, 6
MBD, see Minimal Brain Dysfunction
Methylphenidate, 28, 45–49, 54, 282, 283,
    285–289, 345, 348, 349–361, 365, 411;
    see also Ritalin; Stimulants
    adolescent outcome, 240
    in adult ADHD, 400–402
    and cerebral blood flow, 339
    and growth, 167–169
    for preschoolers, 31–33, 47
    side effects, 32, 47, 167, 353–358
MFFT, Matching Familiar Figures Test
Minimal Brain Damage Syndrome, 5
Minimal Brain Dysfunction (MBD), 4, 6,
    285; see also Attention-Deficit Hyper-
    activity Disorder
Monoamine oxidase inhibitors (MAOIs),
    360, 362
Mood, 206
Moral behavior, 108–111
Moral development, 94, 96
Mothers' groups, 32, 33
Motor impulsivity, 28–30, 350–351, 388, 392
Moves, 244
Multimodal treatment, 153, 242, 300,
    381–383, 411

Neuroticism, 238
Neurotransmitters, 341–345
Nomenclature, *see* Terminology
Nonmedical drug use, 129–135, 137–139, 181, 248–250, 265–268
Noradrenergic hypothesis, 342–343
Norepinephrine, 364
Normative crisis, 51

Occupational performance, 91, 142–149
Off-task behavior, 29, 30, 37
Oppositional Defiant Disorder, 329, 346, 364, 365
Organic Brain Syndrome, 93
Organizational skills training, 376–377
Out-of-seat behavior, 29, 30, 37
Outcome groups, 205–218

Paradoxical quietening effect, 4, 282, 283
Parent support groups, 373–374
Parental control, 233, 234
Parental studies, genetic aspects, 186–189, 329–336, 385, 411
Parental training, 369–373, 405, 406
Parenting skills, 48, 185, 232–234, 370–373
Part-time jobs, 143
Peer relationships, 27, 44, 45, 54, 352
Pemoline, 286, 288, 358–360, 400, 401
Perception of childhood, 69
Perinatal distress, 22
Personal qualities, 111–113
Personality development, 51
Personality-trait disorders, 68–70
Pervasive hyperactivity, 12–15, 21
Physical anomalies, 24, 25
Physiological measures, 162–179
  in adulthood, 169–179
Play therapy, 275, 276, 377
Police involvement, 263, 264, 269
Postdictive validity, 9, 10
Predictive factors, 219–289
  academic performance, 246, 260, 261
  car accidents, 264, 265
  child, 221–229
  drug treatment, 240–242
  family, 230–237
  interrelationship of, 257–272
  nonmedical drug use, 265–268
  police involvement, 263, 264, 269

  treatment, 238–256
  work record, 261–263
Predictive validity, 10
Prenatal variables, 10
Preschooler, 27–31
  treatment of, 31–34
Prognostic factors, *see* Predictive factors
Prolactin, 168, 169
Prospective studies, 8, 53, 55–61
  adolescent outcome studies, 84–87, 352
  adult outcome studies, 92, 93, 125–128, 386, 387
  fifteen-year follow-up, 70–81, 97–102, 136–141, 158–161
  ten-year follow-up, 66–70, 93–97, 129–136, 154–158
Psychiatric assessment, 68–72, 74, 75
Psychiatric illness, 64–66, 88–90, 122–124, 214–218
Psychoeducation, 404, 405
Psychosis, 354–355
Psychotherapy, 238, 240, 275–280, 377–381, 394, 403
  therapeutic alliance in, 378, 379
Punishment, 233

Real admired person, 113–115
Rebelliousness, 53
Referral for assessment, 27, 35
  age at, 222
  symptoms at, 226–229
Reflectivity–impulsivity, 28–30
Reinforcement, 41–42, 371, 372
Remedial education, 238–240, 377
Restlessness, 68, 73, 74, 80, 199
Retrospective studies, 8, 52–55, 62–64
  adolescent outcome studies, 84–87
  adult outcome studies, 90–92, 125–128
  types of, 62
Ritalin, 283, 320–323, 348, 357, 400, 405
  dosage, 358
  side effects, 323

SADS-L, *see* Schedule for Affective Disorders and Schizophrenia, Lifetime Version
Schedule for Affective Disorders and Schizophrenia, Lifetime Version (SADS-L), 91, 139, 140
School achievement, *see* Academic performance; Underachievement

SCL-*90*, 70, 77
Secobarbital, 285
Seizure disorders, 355
Self-control, 368
Self-esteem, 29, 30, 36, 52, 56, 206, 211, 215, 254, 379
  and aggression, 153
  and depression, 43, 44, 320
  maternal, 25, 26
  and social skills, 150–161, 386
  tests, 156
Self-paced tasks, 39
Self-rating scales, 69, 70
Self-report, 53, 54, 108–111
Serotonin hypothesis, 343
Siblings, 180–183
Side effects, 297–299, 410
Situational Social Skills Inventory (SSSI), 155–157
Sleep difficulties, 23, 24
Smiling, 25
Social isolation, 151, 255
Social skills, 150–161, 251, 254, 321, 353, 374–376, 386, 393
Sociocultural factors, 191–194
Socioeconomic status, 234–236
Sociopathy, 88
Soft neurological signs, 10
Special education classes, 5
Speeding, 98
Stealing, 95, 96, 206, 248
Stimulants, 8, 45–48, 250, 251, 411
  and aggression, 375
  and alcohol use, 119–121, 126, 136, 141
  amphetamines, 133, 134, 348
  combined with behavior modification, 369
  efficacy of, 349–353
  growth effects, 355–356
  interactions, 360–361
  limits, 366
  long-acting, 358–359
  mechanisms of action, 359
  metabolism, 359–360
  side effects, 47, 353–358

slow-release, 358, 360
speed, 133, 134
therapy of adolescents, 281–284
therapy of hyperactive adults, 284–289
treatment, 240–256, 348–365
Stress intolerance, 389
Subjective view of treatment, 293–300, 409–410
  autobiography, 302–325
  effect of medication, 296–299
  maturation, 296
  parents, 295
  teachers, 295, 296
Substance Use Disorder, 93
Superego, 113, 116, 117

Teachers, 44, 45, 295, 296
Terminology, 3–7, 37
Tics, 354, 365
Toddlers, 27–31
Toxic substances, 10
Tranylcypromine, 360, 362
Treatment issues, 273–289
Tricyclic antidepressants, 285, 286, 347, 361–363, 365; *see also* Desipramine
Twin studies, 329–331

Underachievement, 36, 42, 43
Unipolar Affective Disorder, 187
University of Massachusetts Medical Center (UMMC) protocol, 388–391
Utah Criteria, 286, 287

Values and beliefs, 107–117
Vigilance task, 38
Vocalization, 24

Weapons, 58, 79, 104
Weight gain, 33, 47, 166–169
Work record, 142–149, 214, 244, 247, 261–263
Worldly success, 111–113

Ziller Self–Other Test, 156, 157, 160